S0-BCP-505

Basic & Applied

Concepts of Immunohematology

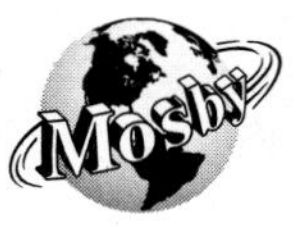
Mosby

BASIC & APPLIED

Concepts of Immunohematology

KATHY D. BLANEY, MS, BB(ASCP) SBB
University of Central Florida
Medical Laboratory Sciences
Department of Molecular Biology & Microbiology
Orlando, Florida

PAULA R. HOWARD, MS, MT(ASCP) SBB
Micro Typing Systems, Inc.
Pompano Beach, Florida

with **128** *illustrations*

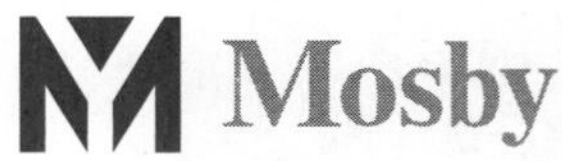

St. Louis Baltimore Boston Carlsbad Chicago Minneapolis New York Philadelphia Portland
London Milan Sydney Tokyo Toronto

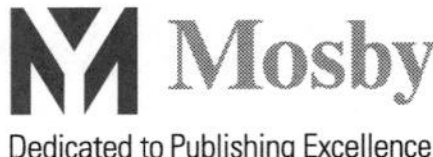
Dedicated to Publishing Excellence

Editor-in-Chief: Andrew Allen
Acquisitions Editor: Janet Russell
Developmental Editor: Sarahlynn Lester
Project Manager: Patricia Tannian
Production Editor: Richard Hund
Design Manager: Gail Morey Hudson
Cover Design: Teresa Breckwoldt

NOTICE
Pharmacology is an ever-changing field. Standard safety precautions must be followed, but as new research and clinical experience broaden our knowledge, changes in treatment and drug therapy may become necessary or appropriate. Readers are advised to check the most current product information provided by the manufacturer of each drug to be administered to verify the recommended dose, the method and duration of administration, and contraindications. It is the responsibility of the treating physician, relying on experience and knowledge of the patient, to determine dosages and the best treatment for each individual patient. Neither the publisher nor the editor assumes any liability for any injury and/or damage to persons or property arising from this publication.

Mosby, Inc.
A Harcourt Health Sciences Company
11830 Westline Industrial Drive
St. Louis, Missouri 63146

Printed in the United States of America

International Standard Book Number 0-323-00165-3

99 00 01 02 03 GW/KPT 9 8 7 6 5 4 3 2 1

CONTRIBUTORS

BARBARA V. ANDERSON, MS, MT(ASCP) SBB
Assistant Professor/Director
Undergraduate Program in Medical Laboratory Technology
Florida International University
Miami, Florida

SARAH L. DOPP, MA, MT(ASCP) SBB, CLS(IH)
Blood Bank Computer Specialist, Fletcher Allen Healthcare
Burlington, Vermont
Clinical Instructor, Department of Biomedical Technology
University of Vermont
Burlington, Vermont

CAROL J. GRANT, MS, MT(ASCP) SBB
Education Officer, American Red Cross
National Testing Laboratory
Philadelphia, Pennsylvania

DORILYN HITCHCOCK, MS, MT(ASCP)
Program Director, Medical Laboratory Sciences
University of Central Florida
Orlando, Florida

ANNE E. HUOT, PhD
Associate Professor/Chairperson
Department of Biomedical Technologies, University of Vermont
Burlington, Vermont

AWILDA ORTA, MT(ASCP) SBB
Quality Control Manager
Micro Typing Systems, Inc.
Pompano Beach, Florida

WILLIAM W. SAFRANEK, PhD
Manager Molecular Science
Wuestoff Reference Laboratory
Melborne, Florida

JO ANN WILSON, PhD
Associate Professor/Chairperson
Department of Clinical Laboratory Science
Florida Gulf Coast University
Fort Myers, Florida

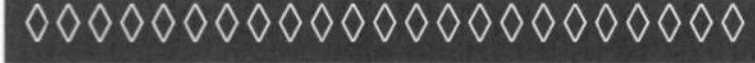

REVIEWERS

AWILDA ORTA, MT(ASCP) SBB
Quality Control Manager
Micro Typing Systems, Inc.
Pompano Beach, Florida

DONNA C. PFEIFFER, BS, MT(ASCP) SBB
Program Director, Clinical Laboratory Science
Lakeland Community College
Mentor, Ohio

ANNE T. ROGERS, PhD, MT(ASCP), CLS(NCA)
Associate Professor, Medical Technology Program
Armstrong Atlantic State University
Savannah, Georgia

This book is dedicated to my husband

Tommy

and my son

Sean

who always support and encourage my dreams and ambitions,

and to my parents

Alice and Edward Donahue

who taught me the value of education and hard work.

KDB

To all of my

former CLS students

who energized my personal joy of learning and

inspired my desire for excellence in teaching.

PRH

PREFACE

Basic and Applied Concepts of Immunohematology was developed for students in 2- or 4-year clinical laboratory science programs, laboratory professionals undergoing retraining, and other healthcare professionals who desire knowledge in routine blood banking practices. Basic didactic concepts are introduced, and an emphasis on the practical application of these theories to modern transfusion and blood bank settings is described.

This textbook provides important features to assist both the student and the instructor. Each chapter features:

- Chapter outlines listing the important elements in each chapter
- Educational objectives for use by both the student and the instructor
- Study questions for self-assessment
- Key words with definitions on the same page
- Chapter summaries, in varying formats, to provide a succinct overview of the chapter's important points
- Critical thinking exercises to illustrate the practical applications to the clinical environment
- Illustrations, boxes, and tables designed to reinforce and summarize the most important information found in the chapter

The text is divided into six sections and begins with a "foundations" section, which includes an overview of immunology and genetics designed for the immunohematologist. A unique chapter on reagents is included in this section, which defines the specific immunologic principles of common laboratory reagents used in the blood bank laboratory. Students performing laboratory exercises concurrently with the didactic lectures will especially benefit from this chapter, because it reinforces applied concepts. An appreciation of the uses and limitations of reagents is important for laboratory workers who are being cross trained in the blood bank and for those reentering the field.

Following the introduction, an overview of the major blood groups is presented. The essentials of pretransfusion testing follow with chapters on antibody detection and identification and compatibility testing. A section on blood collection, processing, and component production and therapy is included with updated information on viral marker testing. The clinical applications associated with immunohematology are presented in chapters covering adverse complications of blood transfusions, hemolytic disease of the newborn, and transfusion therapy for selected patient populations. The final section of the text outlines quality issues relevant to current laboratory practices. Quality assurance and regulations are presented in addition to an overview of safety.

The accompanying Instructor's Guide outlines laboratory exercises to incorporate and reinforce the immunohematologic theories presented in each chapter. It also provides a bank of additional study questions as well as answers to the critical thinking exercises that follow each chapter in the text.

We are grateful to all our contributors, who wrote comprehensive chapters and contributed their collective wisdom, based on professional experiences, to this text. We are also very appreciative of the editors at Mosby for their patience and professionalism in the manuscript review and publication process. We hope that, after reading this text, our readers have the same enthusiasm that we do for the exciting field of immunohematology.

Kathy D. Blaney
Paula R. Howard

CONTENTS

PART V
CLINICAL CONSIDERATIONS IN IMMUNOHEMATOLOGY

PART VI
QUALITY AND SAFETY ISSUES

DETAILED CONTENTS

Basic & Applied Concepts of Immunohematology

FOUNDATIONS: BASIC SCIENCES AND REAGENTS

IMMUNOLOGY
Basic Principles and Applications in the Blood Bank

1

Anne E. Huot
Paula R. Howard
Kathy D. Blaney

CHAPTER OUTLINE

Overview of the Immune System
Innate and Acquired Immunity
Cells and Mediators of the Immune System
Characteristics of Antigens
General Properties
Red Blood Cell Antigens
Human Leukocyte Antigens
Platelet Antigens
Characteristics of Antibodies
General Properties
Comparison of IgM and IgG Antibodies
Primary and Secondary Immune Response
Antigen-Antibody Interactions
Properties That Influence Binding
Immunohematology: Antigen-Antibody Reactions in Vivo
Transfusion, Pregnancy, and the Immune Response
Clearance of Antigen-Antibody Complexes
Immunohematology: Antigen-Antibody Reactions in Vitro
Overview of Agglutination
Hemolysis as an Indicator of Antigen-Antibody Reactions
Principles of the Antiglobulin Test
Direct Antiglobulin Test
Indirect Antiglobulin Test
Sources of Error in Antiglobulin Testing
Principles of Antibody Potentiators
Low–Ionic Strength Solution
Bovine Serum Albumin
Polyethylene Glycol Additive
Proteolytic Enzymes

LEARNING OBJECTIVES

Upon completion of this chapter, the reader should be able to:

1. Describe the role of innate and acquired immunity in the overall process of immunity.
2. Describe the role of phagocytes, T cells, B cells, cytokines, and complement proteins in the immune system.
3. Define the following key terms: *antigen, immunogen, epitopes, antigenic determinants,* and *specificity.*
4. Discuss the general properties of antigens and relate these characteristics to the antigens considered important in immunohematology that are located on red blood cells, white blood cells, and platelets.
5. Identify the components of the molecular structure of the basic immunoglobulin molecule, including the fragment, antigen-binding (Fab) and fragment, crystallizable (Fc) fragments.
6. Compare and contrast immunoglobulin M and immunoglobulin G antibodies.
7. Describe the major events in the primary and secondary immune response and identify the major differences between these two responses.
8. Identify the major forces that influence the binding of an antigen and antibody.
9. Discuss the potential immunologic consequences of transfusion and pregnancy.
10. Define the two stages of the agglutination reaction and describe the factors that influence these stages in vitro.
11. Describe the different gradings associated with the interpretation of agglutination reactions.
12. Discuss the significance of hemolysis in immunohematologic testing.
13. Describe the basic principles of antiglobulin testing.
14. Distinguish between direct and indirect antiglobulin tests.
15. Identify the indications for implementing the direct and indirect antiglobulin tests.
16. Discuss the different sources of possible errors in the performance of antiglobulin testing.
17. Discuss the role of potentiators in immunohematologic testing.
18. Describe the function of the following potentiators in immunohematologic testing: low–ionic strength solution, bovine serum albumin, polyethylene glycol, and proteolytic enzymes.

Immunohematology: study of blood group antigens and antibodies.

The science of **immunohematology** embodies the study of blood group antigens and antibodies. Immunohematology, in part, depends on the field of immunology because it involves the immune response to the transfusion of cellular elements. To enable the reader's appreciation of the physiology involved in this immune response, this text begins with an overview of the cells and soluble mediators that constitute the immune system. Emphasis is placed on the clinical and serologic nature of antibodies and antigens because these fundamentals are essential to the immunohematologist.

OVERVIEW OF THE IMMUNE SYSTEM

Innate and Acquired Immunity

The immune system is a compilation of an integrated network of cells, tissues, organs, mechanical barriers, and secreted molecules. The immune system serves the following purposes:

- Prevents the entry of infectious agents
- Eliminates these infectious agents, should they gain entry, to prevent systemic disease

The immune defense is often classified into two categories of responses: innate and acquired immunity.

Innate immunity: nonspecific host defense that exists before exposure to an antigen; involves the anatomic and inflammatory response.
Phagocytic cells: cells that engulf microorganisms, other cells, and foreign particles; include neutrophils, macrophages, and monocytes.
Chemical mediators: factors secreted by certain cells that when activated promote or inhibit a response from another cell or tissue.
Vasodilatation: increase in the diameter of blood vessels.
Edema: tissue swelling caused by an increase in fluid from the vasculature.
Neutrophil: circulating granulocyte involved in the early immune response.

Innate (or natural) **immunity** is nonspecific and provides the first line of defense against invading pathogens. The skin, mucosal linings, normal flora, and chemical secretions (tears, saliva, etc.) provide an unfriendly environment for most pathogens (Fig. 1-1). Thus the pathogens' first challenge is to gain entry into host tissues. The second line of natural defense includes the **phagocytic cells** and **chemical mediators** working in concert to promote an inflammatory response. Inflammation is marked by the following:

- **Vasodilatation:** increased blood flow in the area, increased tissue temperature
- **Edema:** increased capillary permeability with an increase of fluid
- Phagocyte migration into tissue: **neutrophil** accumulation in the area of injury

As the cells of the immune system are widely distributed throughout the body, the inflammation process helps to concentrate the cells of the immune system in the area they are needed.[1]

Innate immunity is also distinguished for its consistency of response. Regardless of the number of times an individual encounters a particular pathogen, the innate response is of the same magnitude and is governed by the same regulatory mechanisms. In other words, the innate response has no memory.

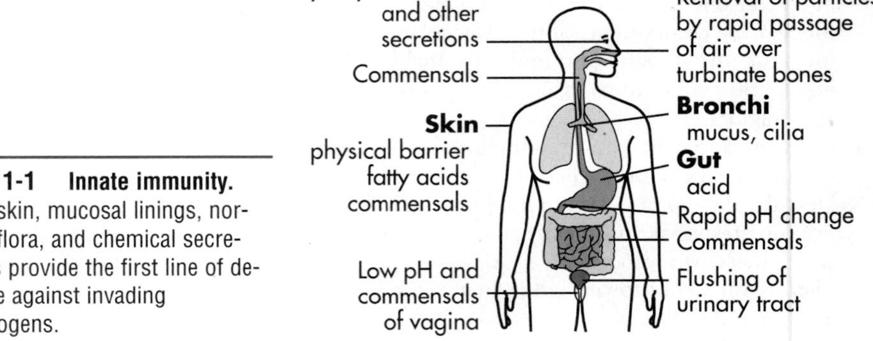

Fig. 1-1 Innate immunity. The skin, mucosal linings, normal flora, and chemical secretions provide the first line of defense against invading pathogens.

When an invading pathogen or foreign substance eludes the innate defense mechanisms, a specific immune response is enlisted.[1] In **acquired** (or adaptive) **immunity**, the cells involved have the ability to recognize the specific infectious agent and, on subsequent exposure, are capable of mounting a more powerful response. The acquired immune response involves **lymphocytes** that have recognition receptors capable of discriminating many molecular configurations. Antibodies are products of the adaptive immune system and are highly specific for invading foreign substances. The acquired immune response supplements the innate defense mechanism to produce a more effective total response.[1] Table 1-1 compares innate and acquired immunity. The cells and molecules involved in the immune response are described in the following sections.

Acquired immunity: host defenses mediated by lymphocytes following exposure to an antigen that exhibits specificity, memory, and self/nonself recognition.
Lymphocytes: mononuclear leukocyte that mediates humoral or cell-mediated immunity.

Cells and Mediators of the Immune System

Phagocytes

Phagocytic cells are capable of binding to microorganisms, internalizing them and killing them. Since they are nonspecific, these cells are part of the innate response and act as a first line of defense against infection. **Mononuclear phagocytes** include monocytes that are found in the blood and macrophages that are found in the tissue. Macrophages are also **antigen-presenting cells** (APCs), since they present the foreign material to lymphocytes that will initiate the adaptive immune response. Other phagocytic cells, the **polymorphonuclear neutrophils,** are found in the peripheral blood and migrate into tissues when signaled by the inflammatory mediators. In response to infection the bone marrow releases more neutrophils into the circulation. Neutrophils contain lytic enzymes and bactericidal substances within their granules, which makes them effective in killing ingested microorganisms. These lytic enzymes are also released outside of the cell and can cause damage to nearby healthy cells and tissue.

Mononuclear phagocytes: leukocytes that circulate (monocytes) or are fixed (macrophages) that are involved in phagocytosis and antigen presenting.
Antigen-presenting cells: cells that process and present antigenic peptides in association with class II MHC molecules and activate T cells.
Polymorphonuclear neutrophils: another name for neutrophils.

Lymphocytes

The adaptive immune response depends on the lymphocytes, particularly the **T lymphocytes** (T cells) and **B lymphocytes** (B cells). T cells generally combat intracellular pathogens, whereas B cells recognize and clear extracellular material.[2] T-cell activity is often referred to as **cellular immunity,** whereas B cells are part of **humoral immunity.** These cells do not function independently; T cells, B cells, and phagocytic cells interact (Fig. 1-2).

Cells of the immune system are products of the same **stem cell** or precursor cells originating in the bone marrow. B cells remain in the bone marrow to mature, whereas T cells migrate to and mature in the thymus. During the maturation, these cells develop their **specificity** and memory that allow for adaptive

T lymphocytes: lymphocytes that mature in the thymus and express specific receptors; involved in cellular immunity.
B lymphocytes: lymphocytes that mature in the bone marrow, differentiate into plasma cells, and produce antibodies.
Cellular immunity: adaptive immunity in which T lymphocytes recognize and react with the antigen through direct cell-to-cell interaction.
Humoral immunity: adaptive immunity in which B lymphocytes and plasma cells produce specific antibodies that recognize and react with an antigen.
Stem cell: cell from which differentiated cells divide.
Specificity: ability of an antibody to distinguish between two antigens.

Table 1-1 Characteristics of Innate and Acquired Immunity

INNATE	ACQUIRED
Nonspecific	Specific
No memory	Memory response
First line of host defense	Lag period in response
Clears most invading microorganisms	Diverse; recognizes many different antigens
Mediated by many cells, cell products, cytokines, and systems	Mediated by lymphocytes

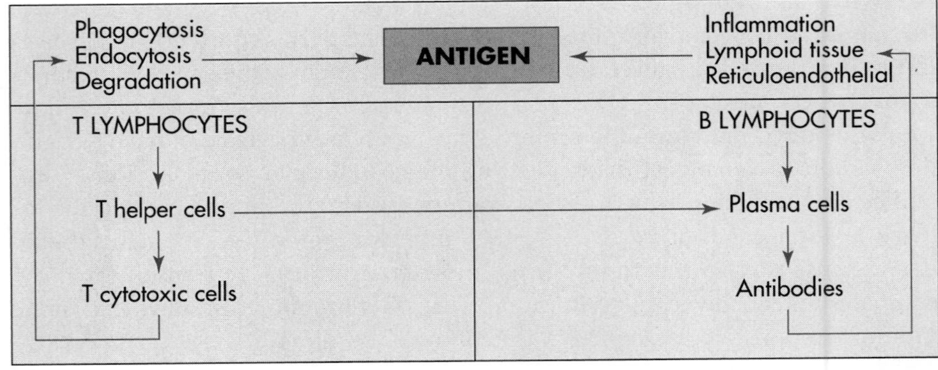

Fig. 1-2 Cellular interaction in the immune response.

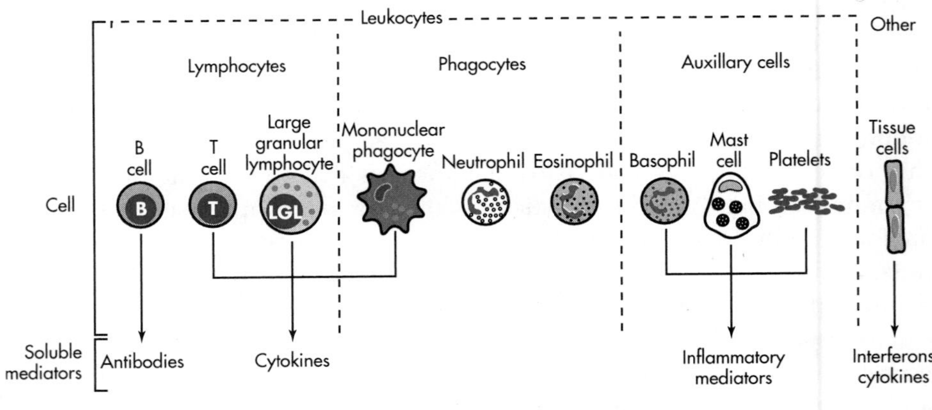

Fig. 1-3 Principal cells of the immune system.

Antibody: protein (immunoglobulin) that recognizes a particular epitope on an antigen and facilitates clearance of that antigen.
Antigen: substance (usually foreign) that binds specifically to an antibody or a T-cell receptor.
Antigenic determinants: site on an antigen that is recognized and bound by a particular antibody or T-cell receptor (also called the *epitope*).
Epitopes: single antigenic determinants; functionally, they are the parts of the antigen that combine with the antibody.
Plasma cell: antibody-producing B cell that has reached the end of its differentiating pathway.
Clone: family of cells or organisms having genetically identical constitution.

or acquired immune responses. The functions of these cells are illustrated in Fig. 1-3 and described in more detail in the section that follows.

B CELLS. The B cells manufacture **antibody** molecules that specifically recognize and bind to a particular target molecule called an **antigen.** An antigen can be a molecule on the surface of a pathogen, a foreign cell (such as transfused red blood cells), or a toxin produced by a microorganism. Antibodies do not bind to the entire infectious agent. Many antibodies to a foreign substance can be produced, each binding to a different antigen on the surface. For example, red blood cells have many different antigens on their surface. When red blood cells from one donor are transfused to a patient, several different antibodies to the red blood cell may be produced. The different **antigenic determinants** or **epitopes** on a red blood cell can elicit the production of a different antibody. The activated B cell, known as the **plasma cell,** produces antibodies. Each plasma cell produces one specific antibody **clone** and predetermines antibody specificity.

Because antibodies are contained in body fluids, the term *humoral immunity* is associated with the B cell response to antigen. *Humoral* is derived from the Latin *humor,* meaning body fluid.[1] The properties of antigens and antibodies as they relate to transfusion are described in greater detail later in this chapter.

CLONAL SELECTION OF B CELLS. Each B cell is genetically programmed to be capable of recognizing only one particular antigen. Once an antigen stimu-

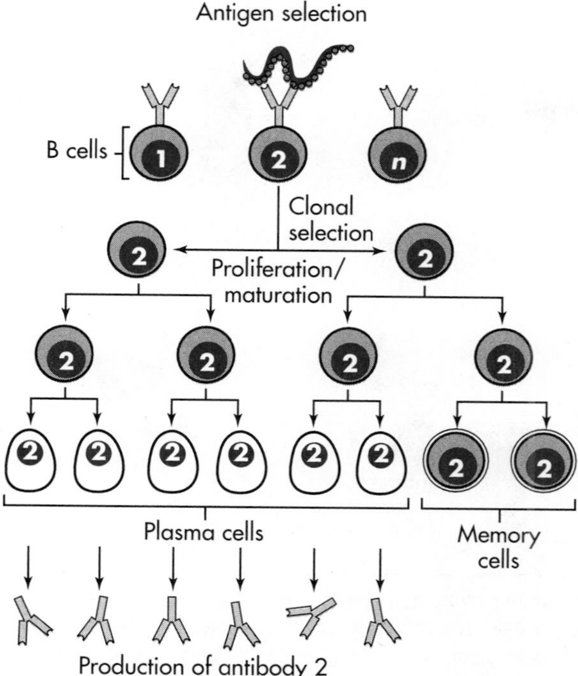

Fig. 1-4 B-cell clonal selection. Each B cell is programmed to produce one antibody. Groups of B cells or plasma cells that produce antibodies with the same specificity are members of the same B-cell clone.

lates a B lymphocyte, the cells divide and proliferate into plasma cells that produce antibody and into memory B cells. **Memory B cells** confer a lasting immunity to a particular antigenic determinant. When the antigen specific to the B cell is encountered again, the response to the foreign substance is therefore quicker and more intense. Groups of B cells or plasma cells that produce antibodies with the same specificity are members of the same **B-cell clone.** The antigen selects a specific clone in a process called clonal selection.[2] Fig. 1-4 illustrates B-cell clonal selection.

Memory B cells: antigen-specific lymphocytes formed after a humoral response; capable of responding to the antigen more quickly and with greater affinity.

B-cell clone: B cells producing antibodies with the same specificity.

T CELLS. There are two types of T-cell populations, and each has unique surface receptors and functions. **T helper** (T_H) **cells** recognize and interact with antigen and produce **cytokines** that activate other cells in the immune response, such as B cells, **T cytotoxic** (T_C) **cells,** and macrophages. T_C cells do not secrete many cytokines and instead are involved in the clearance of viral-infected cells, tumor cells, and cells of foreign tissue graft (Fig. 1-5).

Unlike B cells, T cells recognize antigens only when they are enclosed within the peptide-binding groove of the **major histocompatibility complex** (MHC). The MHC is encoded by a set of genes that will be discussed further in the human leukocyte antigen (HLA) section of this chapter. This concept is illustrated in Fig. 1-6.

To differentiate lymphocytes, reagents that react with unique membrane molecules are used to group cells into a common **cluster of differentiation** (CD).[3] Thus a lymphocyte with a CD4 has a specific membrane molecule that differentiates it from a CD8 lymphocyte. CD4 T cells generally function as T_H cells, and CD8 T cells function as T_C cells. The ratio of T_H to T_C cells can be determined by assaying the number of CD4 and CD8 T cells. This ratio is 2:1 in normal peripheral blood but may be significantly altered in acquired immunodeficiency disease or autoimmune disease.[4]

T cells also have a memory response signaled by a secondary infection in a mechanism similar to that of a B cell.

T helper cells: lymphocytes that interact with mononuclear phagocytes to destroy intracellular pathogens and with B cells to signal cell division and antibody production.

Cytokines: secreted proteins that regulate the intensity and duration of the immune response by mediating interactions between cells.

T cytotoxic cells: lymphocytes responsible for the destruction of host cells that have become infected by virus or other intracellular pathogen.

Major histocompatibility complex: group of genes located on chromosome 6 that determine the expression of the human leukocyte antigen and complement proteins.

Cluster of differentiation: cell membrane molecule used to differentiate human leukocyte subpopulations; determined by specific monoclonal antibodies.

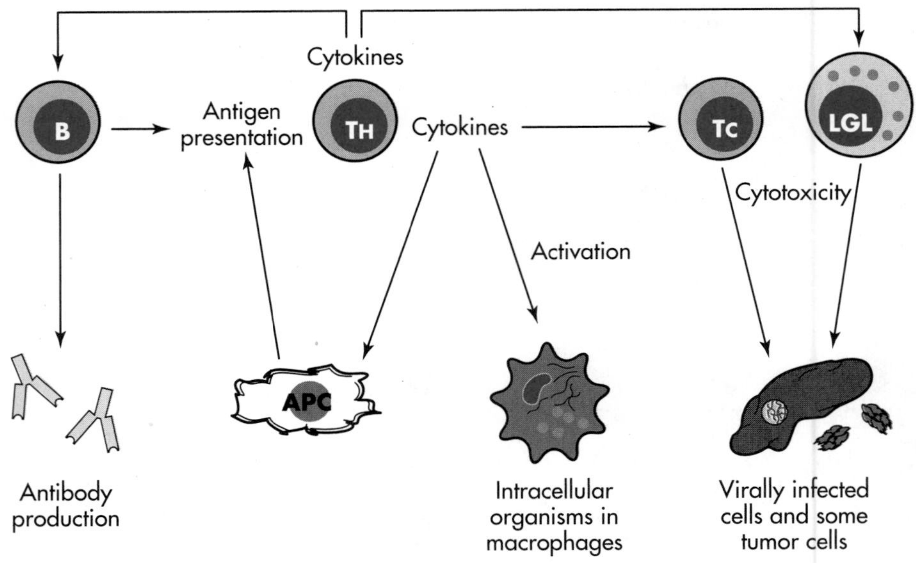

Fig. 1-5 The role of T cells in the immune system. T helper cells are stimulated by antigen-presenting cells and B cells to produce cytokines. T cytotoxic cells are involved in the clearance of virally infected cells and some tumor cells along with large granular lymphocytes. T_H, T helper cells; T_C, T cytotoxic cells; *LGL*, large granular lymphocytes; *APC*, antigen-presenting cells.

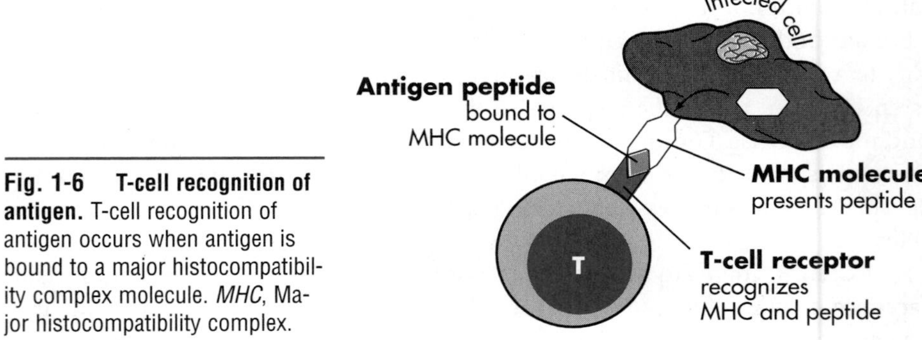

Fig. 1-6 T-cell recognition of antigen. T-cell recognition of antigen occurs when antigen is bound to a major histocompatibility complex molecule. *MHC*, Major histocompatibility complex.

Cytokines

Immune responses are mediated by partisanship with a variety of cells that interact to recognize, process, present, and ultimately clear potentially infectious material. These cells also secrete molecules called cytokines, which have various roles in the signaling between cells during an immune response. They regulate the intensity and duration of an immune response by stimulating or inhibiting the activation and proliferation of various cells. They also regulate inflammation and other cytokines. Examples of cytokines are listed on Table 1-2. It is important to remember that immune response varies with the pathogen or foreign material and whether the individual has previously encountered the material.

Complement Proteins

Complement system: group of serum proteins that participate in an enzymatic cascade, ultimately generating the membrane attack complex that causes lysis of cellular elements.

The **complement system** is a group of serum proteins that have a number of biologic roles related to antigen clearance, cell lysis, and vasodilatation (Box 1-1). These proteins normally circulate in an inactive or proenzyme state. On activation, they are converted into active enzymes that enhance the immunologic processes.

At least nine components of the complement family are designated C1

Table 1-2 Selected Cytokines and Their Functions

CYTOKINE	FUNCTION
Interleukin 1 (IL-1)	Activates T helper cells; promotes inflammatory response and fever
Interferon alpha (IFN-α)	Inhibits viral replication
Tumor necrosis factor (TNF-α)	Kills tumor cells
Interleukin 6 (IL-6) and colony stimulating factors (CSF)	Promote hematopoiesis (cell formation and differentiation)

BOX 1-1

Biologic Effects Mediated by Complement Proteins

- Stimulate increased vascular permeability
- Enhance antibody responses
- Clear immune complexes
- Enhance phagocytosis
- Kill microorganisms by membrane lysis
- Aid in viral neutralization
- Promote platelet aggregation
- Promote release of enzymes from neutrophils

through C9. When activation occurs, each protein is converted into protein fragments and given the distinction of *a* or *b* (e.g., C3 is converted to C3a and C3b). The smaller fragment is designated as *a* and the larger one as *b*.[1] The larger *b* fragment binds to the cell and the smaller *a* fragment enhances the inflammatory response. The fragments also interact with each other to form complexes with enzymatic activity. They are designated by a bar over the number or symbol (e.g., $\overline{C4b2a}$). The final formation of a **membrane attack complex** causes lysis of various cells (**hemolysis** of red blood cells), bacteria, and viruses by disrupting the cell membrane. The direct attachment of the membrane attack complex, consisting of the complement proteins C5 to C9, to the cell surface results in the formation of holes in the cell membrane; this leads to osmotic lysis. If the membrane attack complex becomes attached to transfused red blood cells, hemolysis occurs with a subsequent release of free hemoglobin into the circulation.

Membrane attack complex: C5 to C9 proteins of the complement system that mediate cell lysis in the target cell.
Hemolysis: lysis or rupture of erythrocytes.

The early steps in the activation of the complement proteins can occur in either of two pathways:

- The **classical pathway** is activated by the presence of an antibody bound to an antigen. Red blood cell destruction that may result from antibody-coated red blood cells is caused by the activation of this pathway.
- The **alternative pathway** does not require a specific antibody for activation. Foreign cell–surface constituents, such as bacteria, viruses, and foreign proteins or carbohydrates, initiate it.

Classical pathway: activation of complement that is initiated by antigen-antibody complexes.

Alternative pathway: activation of complement that is initiated by foreign cell–surface constituents.

Regardless of the activation mode, the final steps involved in cell lysis are common to both pathways. In addition, the consequences of complement activation, which serves as an important amplifier of the immune system, are common to both pathways. The peptides generated during the formation of the membrane attack unit have the following additional functions (Fig. 1-7):

- **Anaphylatoxins** C3a, C4a, and C5a assist in the recruitment of phagocytic cells and the promotion of inflammation. These complement proteins attach to mast cells and promote the release of **vasoactive amines** that in turn help make blood vessels permeable for fluid and cells to enter the area.
- Furthermore, the C5a protein is **chemotactic** for neutrophils and attracts these cells to the site of injury.
- Complement also functions as an **opsonin,** which is a substance that binds to an antigen to promote phagocytosis. Phagocytic cells are generally inefficient. However, if the substance they are phagocytosing is coated with an opsonin, the process becomes extremely efficient. **Receptors** on the surface of the phagocytic cell have a higher affinity for opsonins. C3b and antibodies are opsonins, which promote the clearance of bacteria and other cells to which the opsonins are attached. A test to determine if the red blood cell is coated with C3b complement components is a useful serologic tool when red blood cell destruction is being investigated (Fig. 1-8).

Anaphylatoxins: complement split products, C3a, C4a, and C5a, that mediate degranulation of mast cells and basophils, which results in smooth muscle contraction and increased vascular permeability.
Vasoactive amines: products such as histamines released by basophils, mast cells, and platelets that act on the endothelium and smooth muscle of the local vasculature.
Chemotactic: movement of cells in the direction of the antigenic stimulus.
Opsonins: substance (antibody or complement protein) that binds to an antigen and enhances its phagocytosis.
Receptors: molecule on the cell surface that has a high affinity for a particular ligand.

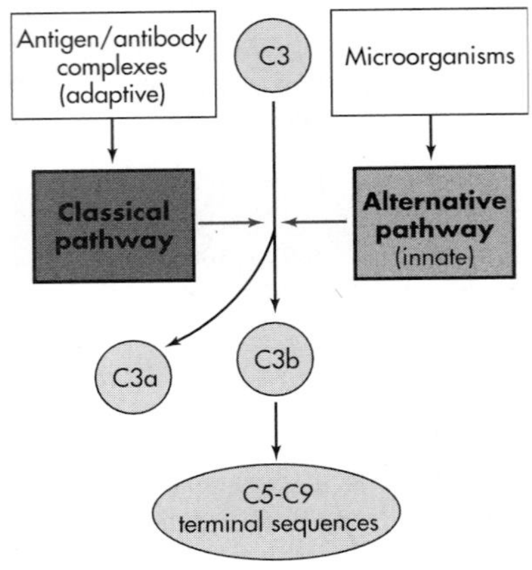

Fig. 1-7 Comparison of the classical and alternative complement systems.

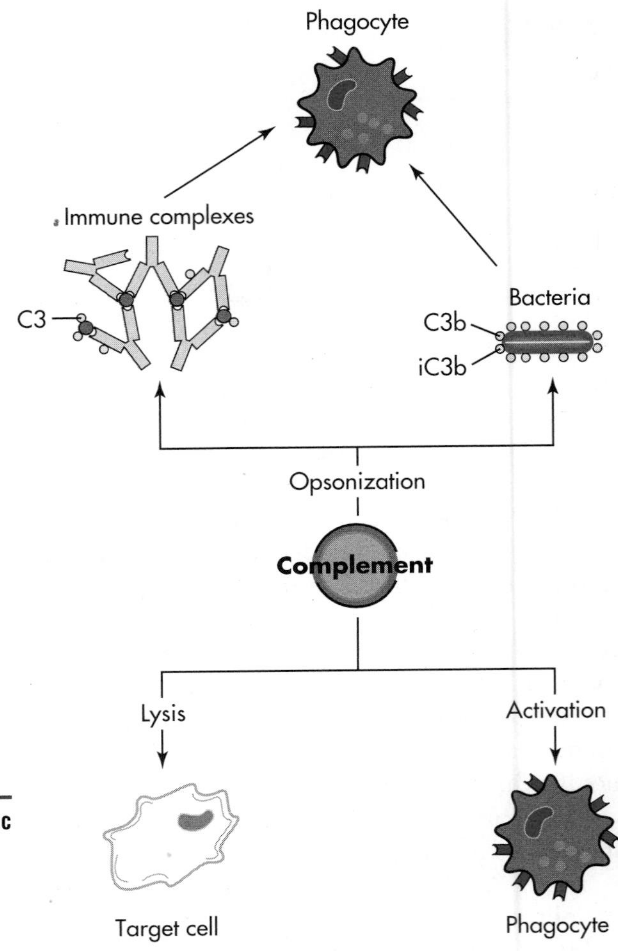

Fig. 1-8 Three major biologic activities of the complement system: opsonization, lysis of target cells, and activation of phagocytes.

CHARACTERISTICS OF ANTIGENS

General Properties

Any substance (usually foreign) that combines with an antibody (in vivo or in vitro) or binds to a T cell is called an antigen. An antigen can be a molecule on the surface of a pathogen, a foreign cell (such as transfused red blood cells), or a toxin produced by a microorganism. This term is often inappropriately used as a synonym for an immunogen. An **immunogen** is an antigen in its role of eliciting an immune response in the body, whether humoral, cellular, or both.[5] Several important characteristics of a molecule contribute to its degree of immunogenicity (Box 1-2). For example, different biologic materials have varying degrees of immunogenicity. Protein is the most immunogenic, followed by **carbohydrates,** and then **lipids,** which tend to be immunologically inert. In addition, complex compounds, such as a protein-carbohydrate combination, are more immunogenic than simpler molecules.[6] Exposure to nonself immunogens through transfusion may elicit antibody production to antigens present on human red blood cells, white blood cells, and platelets. Antigens on these cells vary in their ability to elicit an immune response.

Immunogen: antigen in its role of eliciting an immune response, whether humoral, cellular, or both.

Carbohydrates: simple sugars, such as monosaccharides and starches (polysaccharides).
Lipids: fatty acids and glycerol compounds.

BOX 1-2 Factors Contributing to Immunogenicity: Properties of the Antigen

CHEMICAL COMPOSITION AND COMPLEXITY OF THE ANTIGEN
Proteins are the best immunogens, followed by complex carbohydrates

DEGREE OF FOREIGNNESS
Immunogen must be identified as nonself; the greater the difference from self, the greater likelihood of eliciting an immune response

SIZE
Molecules with a molecular weight greater than 10,000 daltons are better immunogens

DOSAGE AND ANTIGEN DENSITY
Number of red blood cells introduced and the amount of antigen that they carry contribute to the likelihood of an immune response

ROUTE OF ADMINISTRATION
Manner in which the antigenic stimulus is introduced; intramuscular or intravenous injections are generally better routes for eliciting an immune response

Within the immunogen, small regions of the molecule are called epitopes or antigenic determinants. The antigenic determinant is responsible for specificity. The unique configuration of the antigenic determinant allows recognition by a corresponding antibody molecule. The antibody is considered specific for the immunogen, in that the antibody is produced by the immune system to combine with a certain molecular configuration. An immunogen may have multiple epitopes and produce multiple antibodies of varying specificity.

Red Blood Cell Antigens

Twenty-three blood group systems with more than 200 unique red blood cell antigens are recognized. The presence of the red blood cell antigens is determined by the inheritance of many blood group genes. Every individual possesses a unique set of red blood cell antigens determined through genetic inheritance. Because of a diversity of blood group gene inheritance patterns, certain racial populations may possess a greater prevalence of specific red blood cell antigens. Scientific research has determined the biochemical characteristics of many red blood cell antigens and their relationship to the red blood cell membrane. Generally, the red blood cell antigens protrude from the surface of the red blood cell membrane in three-dimensional configurations. Because of this orientation on the surface of the red blood cell, the antigens are accessible to antibody molecules for agglutination reactions. In biochemical terms these antigens may take the form of proteins, proteins coupled with carbohydrate molecules **(glycoproteins)**, or carbohydrates coupled with lipids **(glycolipids)**. Some red blood cell antigens are more immunogenic than others and must be matched to the patient receiving a transfusion. For example, the D antigen within the Rh blood group system is highly immunogenic compared with other antigens. The stimulation of anti-D antibody production is high in an individual who lacks D antigens on red blood cells when that individual is transfused with red blood cells possessing D antigens. Therefore all patients receiving transfusions are matched with the donor's D antigen to prevent anti-D antibody production.

Glycoproteins: compounds containing carbohydrate and protein molecules.
Glycolipids: compounds containing carbohydrate and lipid molecules.

Human Leukocyte Antigens

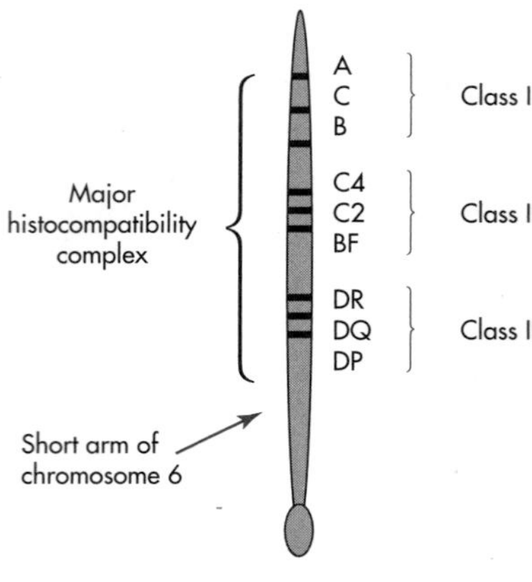

Fig. 1-9 Major histocompatibility complex.

Nucleated cells such as leukocytes and tissues possess many antigens on the cell surface called human leukocyte antigens (HLAs). These antigens readily provoke an immune response if transferred into a genetically different (allogeneic) individual. The genes encoding the expression of these antigens are parts of the MHC gene system. The MHC system is important in the recognition of nonself, the coordination of cellular and humoral immunity, and graft rejection.

The MHC region is located on chromosome 6 and is divided into three categories or classes (Fig. 1-9). Class I includes the A, B, and C locus, Class II includes the DR, DP, and DQ, and Class III includes the complement proteins. The MHC region is called polymorphic because there are so many possible alleles at each location. For example, at least 49 different alleles or possible genetic expressions have been identified at the A locus.[3] At the B locus 97 alleles have been identified. Box 1-3 lists alleles currently recognized for the A and B locus. The probability that any two individuals will express the same HLA antigen is very low.

HLA antigens and the antibodies they elicit are involved in several aspects of transfusion medicine (Box 1-4). Antibodies produced by patients following repeated transfusion of platelets are often directed against HLA antigens. These antibodies can cause poor platelet response, or **refractoriness.** HLA antibodies are

Refractoriness: unresponsiveness to platelet transfusions due to HLA- or platelet-specific antibodies or platelet destruction from fever or sepsis.

BOX 1-3 ***Human Leukocyte A and B Antigens***

A Locus	B Locus	
A1	B5	B49(21)
A2	B7	B50(21)
A203	B703	B51(5)
A210	B8	B5102
A3	B12	B5103
A9	B13	B52(5)
A10	B14	B53
A11	B15	B54(22)
A19	B16	B55(22)
A23(9)	B17	B56(22)
A24(9)	B18	B57(17)
A2403	B21	B58(17)
A25(10)	B22	B59
A26(10)	B27	B60(40)
A28	B35	B61(40)
A29(19)	B37	B62(15)
A30(19)	B38(16)	B63(15)
A31(19)	B39(19)	B64(14)
A32(19)	B3901	B65(14)
A33(19)	B3902	B67
A34(10)	B40	B70
A36	B4005	B71(70)
A43	B41	B72(70)
A66(10)	B42	B73
A68(28)	B44(12)	B75(15)
A69(28)	B45(12)	B76(15)
A74(19)	B46	B77(15)
	B47	B7801
	B48	

BOX 1-4

Human Leukocyte Antigen Testing Applications

- Paternity testing
- Organ and tissue transplants
- Bone marrow and progenitor cell transplants
- Platelet matching
- Disease association

also responsible for reactions that cause chills and fever in some patients receiving transfusions.

Close HLA matching between the donor and the recipient of organ, tissue, bone marrow, and stem cell transplant is important to avoid transplant rejection. The risk of graft versus host disease (GVHD) increases if the HLA matching is not close, especially with bone marrow recipients.[7] GVHD occurs when grafted immunocompetent cells from a donor mount an immune response against the host tissue. Since recipients of these transplants are often immunosuppressed, this process is more likely to occur. Clinical symptoms include rash, diarrhea, and jaundice and can be fatal if left untreated. GVHD can also occur in immunocompromised patients receiving blood components from related donors. Irradiation of these blood components is performed to reduce the risk of leukocytes proliferating in the host.

The lymphocytotoxicity test is used for identification of either the HLA system antigens or antibodies (Fig. 1-10). This test uses the principle of dye inclusion when the antibody-antigen recognition causes membrane damage in the presence of complement.

Platelet Antigens

Platelets possess inherited membrane proteins that can also elicit an immune response. Platelet antibodies are less frequently found because there is less antigen variability in the population. Antibodies to platelet antigens are the major cause of neonatal alloimmune thrombocytopenia, in which maternal **alloantibodies** against antigen inherited from the father can cause fetal platelet destruction. Posttransfusion purpura, in which a transfusion recipient's platelets are destroyed following transfusion, is caused by platelet antibodies. Platelet antibodies can also decrease the expected increment of platelets following a platelet transfusion.

Alloantibodies: antibodies with specificities other than self; stimulated by transfusion or pregnancy.

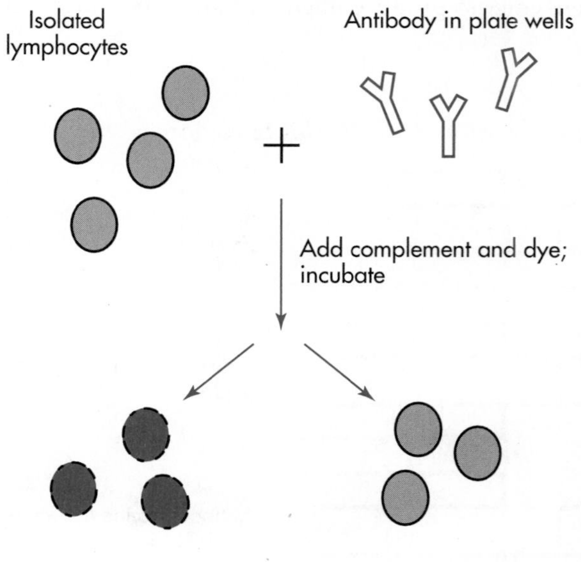

Fig. 1-10 Lymphocytotoxicity test: identification of human leukocyte antigens. Complement-mediated cell membrane damage occurs if the antigen and antibody form a complex. The damaged membrane becomes permeable to the dye, which demonstrates a positive reaction.

Immunoglobulins: antibodies; proteins secreted by plasma cells that bind to specific epitopes on antigenic substances.

Heavy chains: larger polypeptide of an antibody molecule composed of a variable and constant region; five major classes of heavy chains determine the isotype of an antibody.

Light chains: smaller polypeptide of an antibody molecule, composed of a variable and constant region; two major types of light chains exist in humans (kappa and lambda).

Kappa chains: one of the two types of light chains that make up an immunoglobulin.

Lambda chains: one of the two types of light chains that make up an immunoglobulin.

Variable regions: amino-terminal portions of immunoglobulins and T-cell receptor chains that are highly variable and responsible for the antigenic specificity of these molecules.

Constant regions: nonvariable portions of the heavy and light chains of an immunoglobulin and T-cell receptor.

Idiotypes: sets of antigenic determinants characterizing each unique antibody or T-cell receptor.

Hinge region: portion of the immunoglobulin heavy chains between the Fc and Fab region; provides flexibility to the molecule to allow two antigen-binding sites to function independently.

CHARACTERISTICS OF ANTIBODIES

General Properties

Molecular Structure

Antibody molecules are proteins composed of four polypeptide chains joined together by disulfide bonds and classified as **immunoglobulins** (Ig) (Fig. 1-11). Five classifications of antibodies are designated as IgG, IgA, IgM, IgD, and IgE. The five classes are differentiated on the basis of certain physical, chemical, and biologic characteristics. Each antibody molecule has two identical **heavy chains** and two identical **light chains** joined together by disulfide bond (S—S) bridges. These molecular bridges provide flexibility to the molecule to change its three-dimensional shape. Five distinctive heavy chain molecules distinguish antibody classification. Each heavy chain imparts unique features to the five immunoglobulin classes, which permit them to function biologically. For example, the IgA family, which possesses alpha heavy chains, is the only antibody class capable of residing in mucosal linings. There are two types of light chains, **kappa** and **lambda.** Antibodies possess either two kappa or two lambda chains but never one of each. Each heavy chain and light chain molecule also contains **variable** and **constant regions** (or domains). The constant regions of the heavy chain domain impart the unique antibody class functions, such as the activation of complement or the attachment to cells. These constant regions are identical within each immunoglobulin class. The variable regions of both the heavy and light chains are concerned with antigen binding and constitute the area of the antibody that contains **idiotypes** (the idiotypic portion). This area is the binding site or pocket into which the antigen fits (Fig. 1-12). The **hinge region** of the antibody molecule imparts flexibility to the molecule for combination with the antigen.[3,7]

Fab and Fc Regions

In addition to the structural characteristics just described, immunoglobulin molecules may be degraded with enzymes to produce fragments known as fragment,

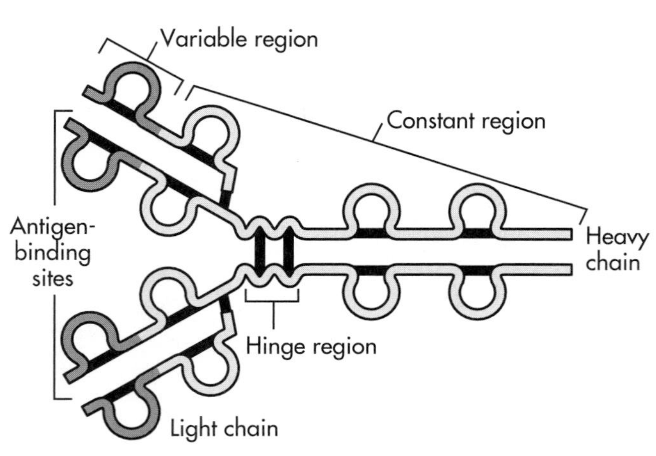

Fig. 1-11 Basic structure of immunoglobulins.

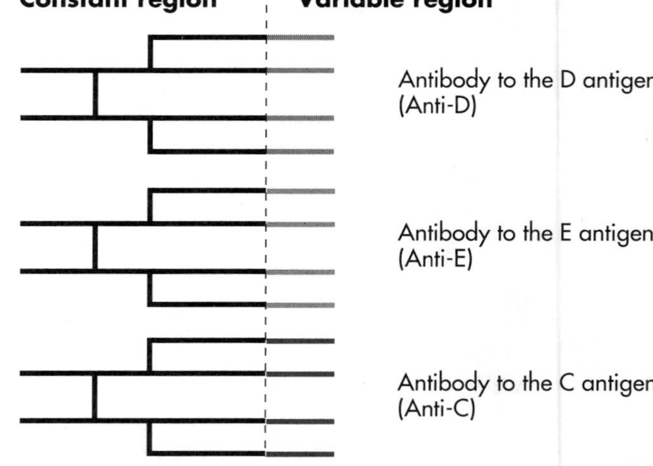

Fig. 1-12 Variable and constant regions of an immunoglobulin.

antigen-binding (Fab) and fragment, crystallizable (Fc) fragments. The study of these fragments has generated information related to immunoglobulin structure and function. Fab contains the portion of the molecule that binds to the antigenic determinant. Fc consists of the remainder of the constant domains of the two heavy chains linked by disulfide bonds (see Fig. 1-11).[7] Certain immune cells, such as macrophages, B cells, and T cells, possess receptors for this portion of the antibody molecule referred to as Fc receptors. These immune cells bind to the Fc portion of antibodies attached to red blood cells and assist in their removal from the systemic circulation.

Comparison of IgM and IgG Antibodies

Since IgM and IgG antibodies have the most significance in immunohematology, the following discussion focuses on these two immunoglobulins (Table 1-3).

IgM Antibodies

When the B cells initially respond immunologically to a foreign antigen, they produce IgM antibodies first. The IgM molecule consists of five basic immunoglobulin units (two mu heavy chains and two light chains) held together by a joining chain, or J chain (Fig. 1-13). Classified as a large pentamer structurally, one IgM molecule contains 10 potential antigen-combining sites or has a

Table 1-3 Comparison of IgM and IgG

CHARACTERISTIC	IgM	IgG
Heavy chain composition	Mu	Gamma
Light chain composition	Kappa or lambda	Kappa or lambda
J chain	Yes	No
Molecular weight (daltons)	900,000	150,000
Valence	10	2
% of total serum concentration	5% to 10%	80%
Serum half-life	5 to 6 days	23 days
Crosses the placenta	No	Yes
Activation of the classical pathway of complement	Yes; very efficient	Yes; not as efficient
Optimal temperature of reaction in immunohematologic tests	Room temperature or below	37° C
Agglutination in antiglobulin tests	No	Yes
Agglutination upon immediate spin	Yes	Usually no

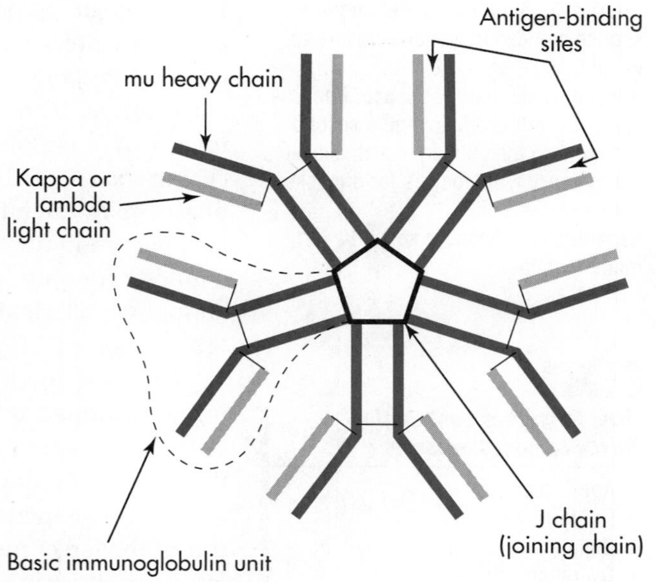

Fig. 1-13 Pentameric structure of the IgM molecule. Five basic immunoglobulin units with 10 antigen-binding sites.

Valency: number of epitopes per molecule of immunogen.
Agglutination: visible clumping of particulate antigens.
Half-life: time required for the concentration of a substance to decrease by half.

valency of 10.[7] Because of their large structure and high valency, these molecules are capable of direct **agglutination** of antigen-positive red blood cells suspended in saline. IgM antibodies constitute about 5% to 10% of the total serum immunoglobulin concentration and possess a short serum **half-life** of 5 to 6 days.[6] A classic functional feature associated with IgM antibodies is the ability to activate the classical pathway of complement with great efficiency. Only one IgM molecule is required for the initiation of the classical pathway in complement activation.

IgG Antibodies

Divalent: combining power of two.

The IgG antibody molecule consists of a four-chain unit with two gamma heavy chains and two light chains, either kappa or lambda in structure. This form of an immunoglobulin molecule is known as a monomer. IgG antibodies constitute about 80% of the total immunoglobulin concentration in serum.[3] These antibodies are also located within the extravascular fluid. The molecule is **divalent;** it possesses two antigen-combining sites. Because of the molecule's relatively small size and divalent structure, most IgG antibodies are not effective in producing a visible agglutinate with antigen-positive red blood cells suspended in saline. The antigen-antibody complexes can be visualized with the antiglobulin test discussed later in this chapter. IgG antibodies possess a serum half-life of 23 days and are capable of crossing the placenta and activating the complement system.[3] However, because of the immunoglobulin structure, two molecules of IgG are necessary to initiate the classical pathway of complement activation.

Four IgG subclasses (IgG1, IgG2, IgG3, and IgG4) exist as a result of minor variations in the gamma heavy chains. The amino acid differences in these heavy chains affect the biologic activity of the molecule.

PRIMARY AND SECONDARY IMMUNE RESPONSE

Primary immune response: immune response induced by initial exposure to the antigen.
Secondary immune response: immune response induced following a second exposure to the antigen, which activates the memory lymphocytes for a quicker response.
Anamnestic response: secondary immune response.

Immunologic response following exposure to an antigen is influenced by the host's previous history with the foreign material. There are two types of immune responses: the primary and the secondary.[6] The **primary immune response** is elicited on the first exposure to the foreign antigen. It is characterized by a lag phase of approximately 5 to 7 days and is influenced by the characteristics of the antigen and immune system of the host (Box 1-5). Lag phases may extend for longer periods. During this period no detectable circulating antibody levels exist within the host. Following this lag period, antibody concentrations rise and sustain a plateau before a decline in detectable antibody levels. IgM antibodies are produced first, followed by the production of IgG antibodies.

BOX 1-5

Host Properties Contributing to the Immune Response

- Age
- Route of inoculation
- Genetic makeup
- Overall health
  - Diet
  - Stress
  - Fatigue

The second contact with the identical antigen initiates a **secondary immune response,** or **anamnestic response,** within 1 or 2 days of exposure. Because of the significant production of memory B cells from the initial exposure, the concentrations of circulating antibody are much higher and are sustained for a much longer period. Antibody levels may be 100 to 1000 times higher as a result of the larger number of plasma cells. In contrast with the primary immune response, the principal antibody produced is of the IgG immunoglobulin class. IgM antibodies are also generated in the secondary immune response (Fig. 1-14). The magnitude of the IgM response is reduced when compared to the IgG response.

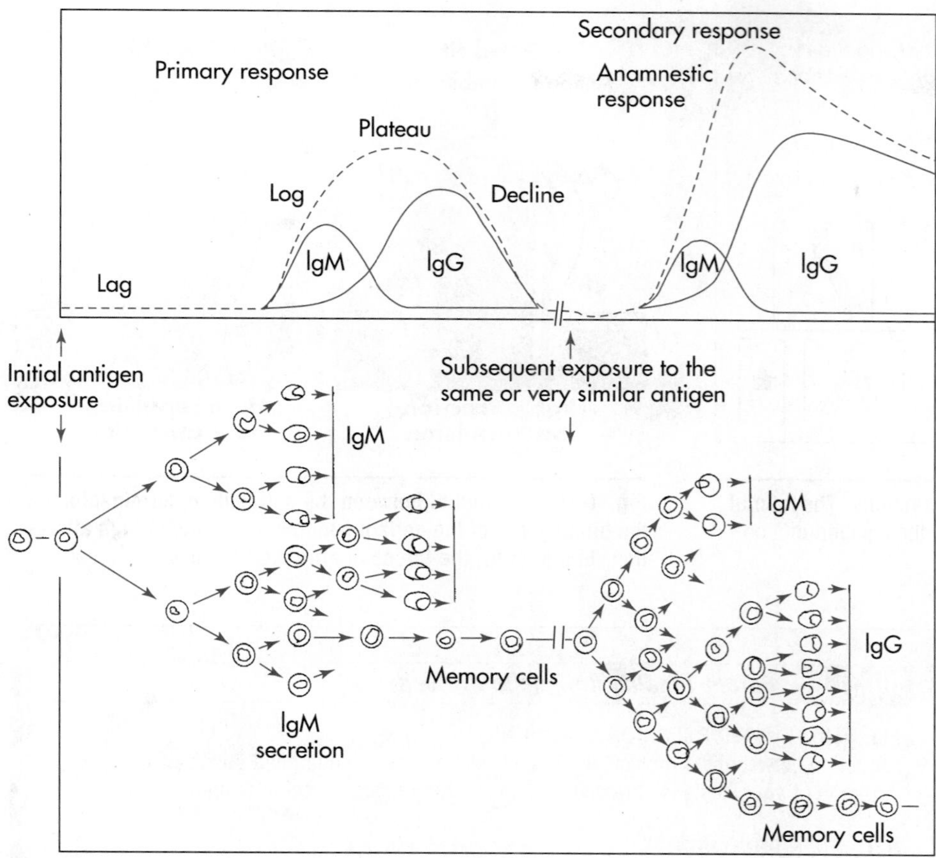

Fig. 1-14 Primary and secondary immune responses.
From Turgeon ML: *Fundamentals of immunohematology*, Baltimore, 1995, Williams & Wilkins.

ANTIGEN-ANTIBODY INTERACTIONS

Properties That Influence Binding

The binding of an antigen and antibody follows the law of mass action and is a reversible process. This union complies with the principles of a chemical reaction that has reached equilibrium. When the antigen and antibody combine, an antigen-antibody complex or immune complex is produced. The amount of antigen-antibody complex formation is determined by the association constant of the reaction. The association constant drives the forward reaction rate, whereas the reverse reaction rate is influenced by the dissociation constant. When the forward reaction rate is faster than the reverse reaction rate, antigen-antibody complex formation is favored. Therefore a higher association constant influences greater immune complex formation at equilibrium (Fig. 1-15).

Several properties influence the binding of antigen and antibody. The goodness of fit and the complementary nature of the antibody for its specific epitope contribute to the strength and rate of the reaction.[2] Factors such as the size, shape, and charge of an antigen determine its binding to the complementary antibody. This concept of goodness of fit is most easily visualized by viewing an antigen-antibody binding as a lock and key fit (Fig. 1-16). If the shape of the antigen is altered, the fit

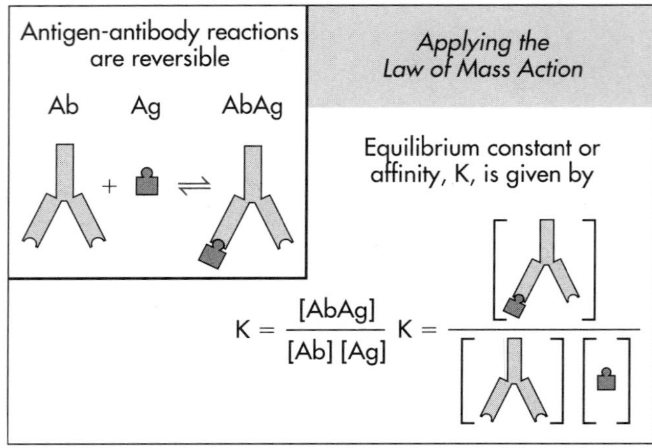

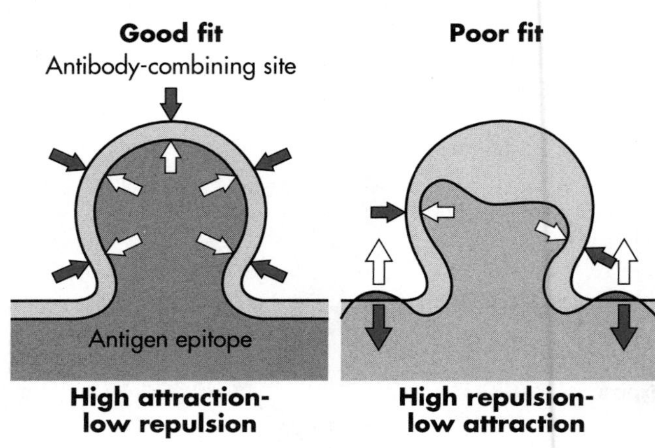

Fig. 1-15 Kinetics of antigen-antibody reactions. The ratio of the forward and reverse reaction rates gives the equilibrium constant. *Ab*, Antibody; *Ag*, antigen.

Fig. 1-16 A good fit between the antigenic determinant and the binding site of the antibody molecule results in high attraction. In a poor fit, the forces of attraction are low.

BOX 1-6 *Forces Binding Antigen to Antibody*

ELECTROSTATIC FORCES (IONIC BONDING)
Attraction between two molecules on the basis of opposite charge; a positively charged region of a molecule is attracted to the negatively charged region of another molecule.

HYDROGEN BONDING
Attraction of two negatively charged groups (X^-) for a H^+ atom

HYDROPHOBIC BONDING
Weak bonds formed as a result of the exclusion of water from the antigen-antibody complex

VAN DER WAALS FORCES
Attraction between the election cloud (−) of one atom and the protons (+) within another atom's nucleus

of the antigen for the antibody is changed. Likewise, if the charge of the antigen is altered, the binding properties of the antigen and antibody are affected.

Once the immune complex has been generated, the complex is held together by noncovalent attractive forces, including electrostatic forces (ionic bonding), hydrogen bonding, hydrophobic bonding, and Van der Waals forces.[6] The influence of these forces on immune complex stability is further described in Box 1-6. The cumulative effect of these forces maintains the union between the antigen and antibody molecules.

IMMUNOHEMATOLOGY: ANTIGEN-ANTIBODY REACTIONS IN VIVO

Transfusion, Pregnancy, and the Immune Response

In vivo: referring to a reaction within the body.

In the transfusion of blood and blood products, the potential for the formation of antigen-antibody complexes **in vivo** (within the patient's body) is a primary concern for blood bank technologists. During transfusion a patient is exposed to many potentially foreign antigens on red blood cells, white blood cells, and platelets that possess varying degrees of immunogenicity. Because of this exposure to foreign antigens in the blood products, a patient's immune system may become activated with the resultant production of circulating antibodies. The antibodies produced in response to transfusion of blood products are classified as alloantibodies. The **antibody screen test** is performed on the patient before transfusion to detect any preformed red blood cell alloantibodies. If a red blood cell alloantibody is detected, a test is performed to identify the specificity of the antibody. Once the specificity is identified, donor units lacking the red blood cell antigen are selected for transfusion.

Antibody screen test: test to determine presence of alloantibodies.

Immunization may also occur during pregnancy as cellular elements from the fetus enter the maternal circulation. Alloantibody production in **multiparous** women may be observed as an immune response to red blood cell, white blood cell, or platelet antigens of fetal origin. Women are also routinely screened during the first trimester of pregnancy for the presence of preformed red blood cell alloantibodies.

Multiparous: having multiple pregnancies.

Clearance of Antigen-Antibody Complexes

Antigen-antibody complexes are removed from the body's circulation through the **reticuloendothelial system.** This system acts as a filter to trap antigens and is present in all secondary lymphoid organs (spleen and lymph nodes), bone marrow, liver, and lungs. The largest lymphoid organ, the spleen, is particularly effective for filtering the blood and clearing the body of antigen-antibody complexes.

Reticuloendothelial system: system of phagocytic cells, associated with the liver, spleen, and lymph nodes, that clear inert particles.

IMMUNOHEMATOLOGY: ANTIGEN-ANTIBODY REACTIONS IN VITRO

Overview of Agglutination

Antigen-antibody reactions occurring **in vitro** (in laboratory testing) are detected by visible agglutination of red blood cells or evidence of hemolysis at the completion of testing. The absence of hemagglutination in immunohematologic testing implies the lack of antigen-antibody complex formation in testing. Hemagglutination occurs in two stages referred to as the **sensitization** step and the **lattice formation** step.[3,6]

In vitro: reaction in an artificial environment, such as in a test tube.

Sensitization: binding of antibody or complement components to a red blood cell.

Lattice formation: combination of antibody and a multivalent antigen to form crosslinks and result in visible agglutination.

Sensitization Stage or Antibody Binding to Red Blood Cells

In the first stage of red blood cell agglutination the antibody binds to an antigen on the red blood cell membrane. This stage requires an immunologic recognition between the antigen and antibody. During this recognition stage antigenic determinants on the red blood cell combine with the antigen-binding site of the antibody molecule. No visible agglutination is observable at this stage.

The physical joining of an antigen and antibody is essentially a random pairing of the two structures determined largely by chance. Whether an antigenic determinant encounters the binding site of an antibody is a matter of chance. Antibody concentration and antigen receptor accessibility and concentration may influence the probability for this collision. An increase in antibody concentration will increase the probability of collision events with the corresponding antigen. This concept is referred to as the overall effect of the **serum to cell ratio** in immunohematologic tests. Increasing the amount of serum placed in the test tube increases the concentration of antibodies available for binding to red blood cell

Serum to cell ratio: ratio of antigen on the red blood cell to antibody in the serum.

antigens. When a patient's serum demonstrates weak reactions in agglutination testing, this simple technique may be used to enhance the first stage of the agglutination reaction.

In addition to the serum to cell ratio, certain environmental factors may influence this first stage of the agglutination reaction. These factors include the following items:

TEMPERATURE OF THE REACTION. Most antibodies of clinical relevance in transfusion are IgG antibodies reacting at approximately 37° C. By combining the sources of antigen and antibody and incubating them at this temperature, the first stage of the agglutination reaction is enhanced. In contrast, IgM antibodies are more reactive at lower temperatures, generally at or below room temperature (22° C).

INCUBATION TIME. Allowing adequate time for the combination of antigen and antibody to attain equilibrium also enhances the first stage of the agglutination reaction. The length of time recommended for optimal antigen-antibody reactivity varies with the test procedure and the reagents used in testing. Some test procedures may indicate a predetermined incubation period performed at variable temperatures such as 37° C, 22° C, or 4° C. Additionally, the test procedures may indicate an **immediate spin** step that indicates a combination of test reagents and sample with no period of incubation.

Immediate spin: interpretation of agglutination reactions immediately following centrifugation and without incubation.

pH. The optimal pH for hemagglutination is around 7.0, which is the physiologic pH range.[3] This pH range is adequate for the majority of important red blood cell antibodies.

IONIC STRENGTH. In an isotonic environment, such as physiologic saline, Na^+ and Cl^- ions are attracted to the oppositely charged groups on antigen and antibody molecules. As a result of this attraction the combination of antigen and antibody is hindered. If the ionic environment is reduced, this shielding effect is reduced and the amount of antibody uptake onto the red blood cell is increased.

Lattice Formation Stage or Cell: Cell Interactions

After the red blood cells have been sensitized with antibody molecules, random collisions between the antibody-coated red blood cells are necessary to develop cross-linkages for the visualization of red blood cell clumping or agglutinates within the test tube. Visible agglutinates form when red blood cells are in close proximity to promote the crosslinkage of antibody-binding sites to antigenic determinants on adjacent red blood cells. This stage of the agglutination reaction is also influenced by the following factors:

DISTANCE BETWEEN RED BLOOD CELLS. The **zeta potential,** or the force of repulsion between red blood cells in a physiologic saline solution, exerts an influence upon the agglutination reaction. Red blood cells possess a net negative charge on the cell surface in a saline suspension. Cations (positively charged ions) from the saline environment are attracted to these negative charges. A stable cationic cloud surrounds each cell and contributes a force of repulsion between molecules of similar charge. As a consequence of this repulsive force, the red blood cells remain a distance from each other.[3] This distance between the cells is proportional to the zeta potential (Fig. 1-17).

Zeta potential: electrostatic potential measured between the red blood cell membrane and the slipping plane of the same cell.

Because of the larger size, pentameric shape, and multivalent properties of IgM molecules, agglutination is facilitated between adjacent red blood cells sensitized with IgM and suspended in a physiologic saline solution. In contrast, IgG antibody molecules are smaller and incapable of spanning the distance between

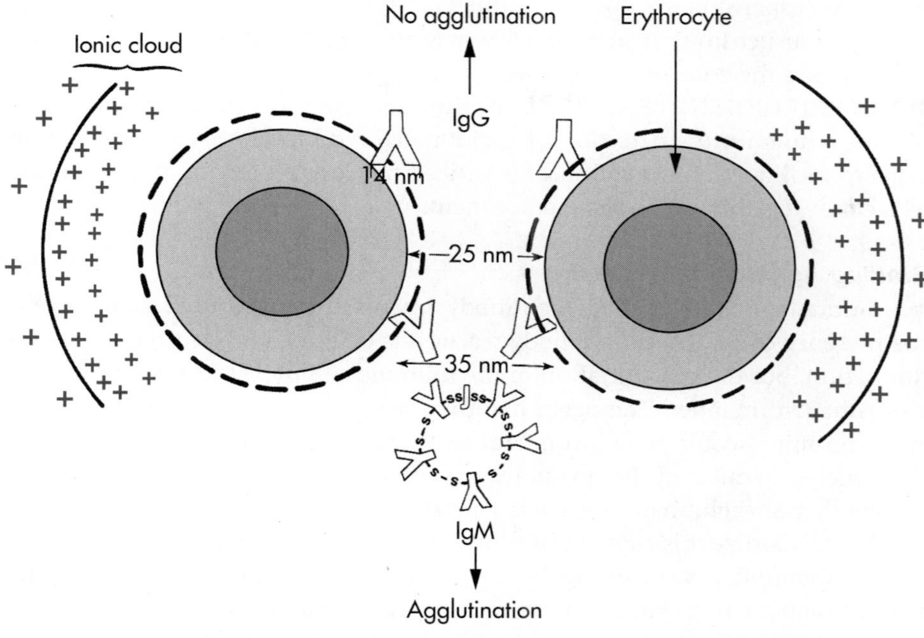

Fig. 1-17 Effect of the zeta potential on the second stage of agglutination.
From Harmening D: *Modern blood banking and transfusion practices*, ed 3, Philadelphia, 1994, FA Davis.

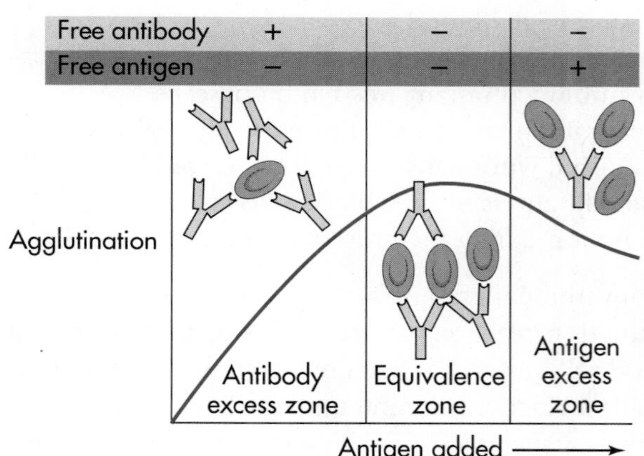

Fig. 1-18 Agglutination reactions. Maximal agglutination is observed when the concentrations of antigens and antibody fall within the zone of equivalence.

adjacent red blood cells generated by the zeta potential. Therefore sensitization without visible agglutination may occur.

OPTIMAL CONCENTRATIONS OF ANTIGEN AND ANTIBODY. Maximum amounts of agglutination are observed when the concentrations of antigens (red blood cells) and antibody (serum) fall within the **zone of equivalence** (Fig. 1-18).[2] When the concentration of antibody exceeds the concentration of antigen, antibody excess, or **prozone,** exists, which decreases the amount of agglutinated red blood cells. In contrast to prozone, antigen excess exists when the concentration of antigen exceeds the number of antibody present. The amount of agglutinates formed under these circumstances is also suboptimal and diminished. Immunohematologic testing is designed to obtain reactions within the zone of equivalence. Commercial antibody preparations are diluted to optimum antibody concentrations for testing. Red blood cell preparations are diluted to a

Zone of equivalence: maximum agglutination or precipitation; equilibrium between antigen and antibody binding.
Prozone: excess antibody causing a false negative reaction.

2% to 5% suspension in saline for optimal antigen concentrations. The use of red blood cell suspensions greater than 5% may affect the ability of the test reaction to fall within the zone of equivalence.

EFFECT OF CENTRIFUGATION. The time and speed of centrifugation are important factors for the detection of agglutinated red blood cells. Centrifugation helps to facilitate the formation of a latticed network by forcing the red blood cells closer together in the test environment.

Grading Agglutination Reactions

Supernatant: fluid above cells or particles following centrifugation.

In immunohematology, antigen-antibody reactions are measured qualitatively. The presence of an antigen-antibody reaction is detected with red blood cell agglutination, but the concentration of the immune complex is not determined in a quantitative manner. The agglutination reactions may be performed in test tubes, on microscopic slides, in microtiter plates, and in microtubes filled with gel particles. Because of the qualitative nature of the measurement, the reading and grading of agglutination reactions are subjective.

To standardize this element of subjectivity among personnel performing the testing, a grading system for agglutination reactions has been established. The conventional grading system for tube testing uses a 0 to 4+ scale[3]:

- 4+ Red blood cell button is a solid agglutinate; clear **supernatant** background
- 3+ Red blood cell button breaks into several large agglutinates; clear supernatant background
- 2+ Red blood cell button breaks into many medium-sized agglutinates; clear supernatant background; no free red blood cells
- 1+ Red blood cell button breaks into numerous medium- and small-sized agglutinates; background is turbid with many free red blood cells
- +^{w} Red blood cell button breaks into many small clumps barely visible macroscopically; background is turbid with many unagglutinated red blood cells
- 0 No agglutinated red blood cells are visible; red blood cells are observed flowing off the red blood cell button during the process of grading (Fig. 1-19)

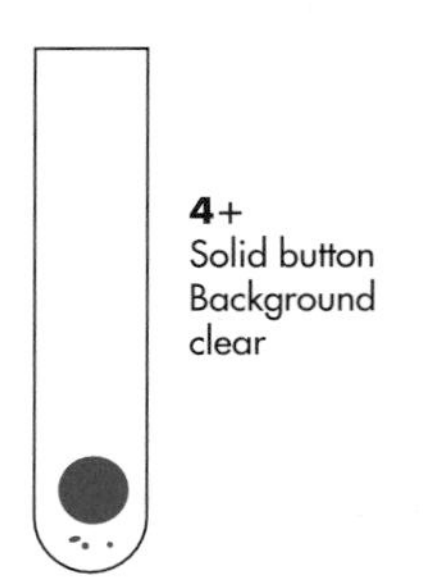

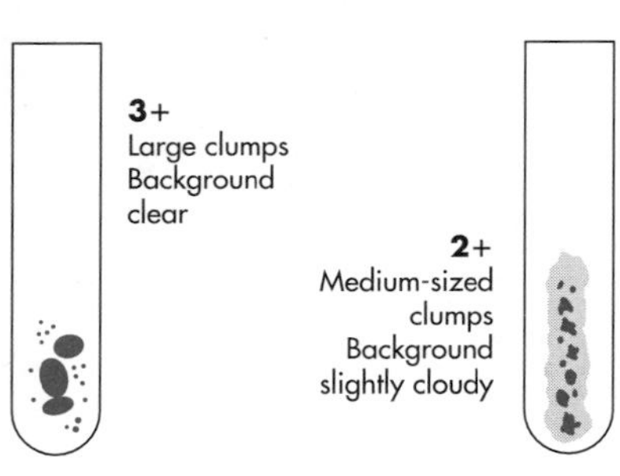

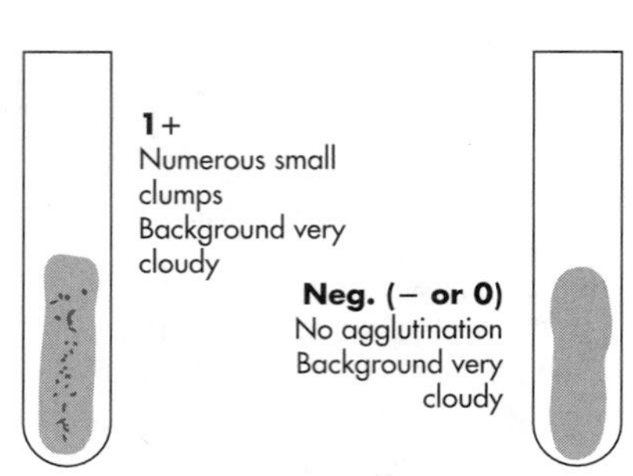

Fig. 1-19 Grading antigen-antibody reactions.

Modified from Gamma Biologicals, Houston, Tex.

Slight variations in this conventional grading system may be established in individual institutions. Agglutination reactions are read by shaking and tilting the test tubes until the red blood cell button has been removed from the bottom of the tube. Negative agglutination reactions are interpreted after the red blood cell button has been completely resuspended. Technologists often use an agglutination viewer lamp with a magnifying mirror to evaluate the agglutination reactions. Laboratories using a microscopic reading in some testing have criteria established for grading these reactions.

Hemolysis as an Indicator of Antigen-Antibody Reactions

In addition to agglutination as an indicator of an antigen-antibody reaction in the immunohematology laboratory, red blood cell hemolysis observed in the tube is an indicator of the reactivity of an antigen and antibody in vitro. The final steps in the process of complement activation initiate the membrane attack complex, thus causing membrane damage. As a consequence of this damage, intracellular fluid is released to the reaction environment. In the case of red blood cell hemolysis, intracellular hemoglobin is released to the reaction environment and imparts a slightly reddish tinge to the supernatant in the tube. Often the red blood cell button is also reduced in size in comparison with the red blood cell button present in other tubes. For grading a tube with hemolysis, an *H* is traditionally used when this phenomenon is observed. Some red blood cell antibodies characteristically display hemolysis in vitro.

PRINCIPLES OF THE ANTIGLOBULIN TEST

Immunohematology can credit the work of Coombs, Mourant, and Race in 1945 for demonstrating that red blood cells may combine with antibodies without producing agglutination.[8] These investigators prepared an antibody that reacted with human globulins (e.g., a family of human proteins) and used this reagent to agglutinate antibody-coated red blood cells. The reagent was called antihuman globulin (AHG); the procedure is referred to as the antiglobulin test. This test is applied to many blood banking testing protocols and provides important information. The antiglobulin test is important because it detects IgG antibodies and complement proteins that have attached to red blood cells either in vitro or in vivo but have not effected visible agglutination in testing.

The principle of the antiglobulin test is not complicated. The test uses a reagent that has been prepared by injecting animals (e.g., rabbits) with human antibody molecules and complement proteins. In these animals the injected proteins are recognized as foreign antigens, stimulating the animal's immune system to produce antibodies to human antibody molecules and complement proteins. The reagent, polyspecific AHG, contains antibodies to IgG molecules (anti-IgG) and complement proteins (anti-C3). This AHG reagent will react with human IgG antibody and complement proteins whether freely present in serum or bound to antigens on the red blood cells. Therefore it is essential that red blood cells first be washed with physiologic saline to remove any unbound molecules before the addition of the AHG reagent. The washing step of an antiglobulin test requires the filling of test tubes with saline to mix with the red blood cells already present in the tube. The saline-suspended red blood cells are centrifuged. The saline wash is decanted from the red blood cell button, and this process is repeated for two additional cycles. On completion of the third wash, the saline is removed, and the tube is blotted dry to remove most traces of the saline. Red blood cell washing is an important technical aspect in the performance of an antiglobulin test. If the test red blood cells are not adequately washed, any unbound antibody or complement present in serum can potentially bind to the AHG reagent and inhibit its reaction with antibody or complement molecules attached to the red blood cells. This effect is known as the **neutralization** of the AHG reagent. Neutralization of the AHG reagent is a source of error in antiglobulin testing since it may mask a positive antiglobulin test.[3]

Neutralization: blocking antibody sites and thus causing a negative reaction.

Following adequate red blood cell washing, the AHG reagent is added to the test. If the red blood cells in the test are sensitized with IgG and/or complement the red blood cells agglutinate on the addition of the AHG reagent. The anti-IgG in the AHG reagent attaches to the Fc portion of the IgG molecule that is bound to the red blood cell; the anti-C3 in the AHG reagent attaches to C3 molecules bound to the red blood cell as the consequence of complement activation. The formation of agglutinated red blood cells is the final step in this process (Fig. 1-20). An antiglobulin test that demonstrates agglutination is interpreted as a positive antiglobulin test. No agglutination at the completion of the antiglobulin test is interpreted as a negative antiglobulin test.

There are two types of antiglobulin tests performed in the immunohematology laboratory: the **direct antiglobulin test** (DAT) and the **indirect antiglobulin test** (IAT). The distinction between these tests is often difficult for individuals

Direct antiglobulin test: test used to detect antibody bound to red blood cells in vivo.

Indirect antiglobulin test: test used to detect antibody bound to red blood cells in vitro.

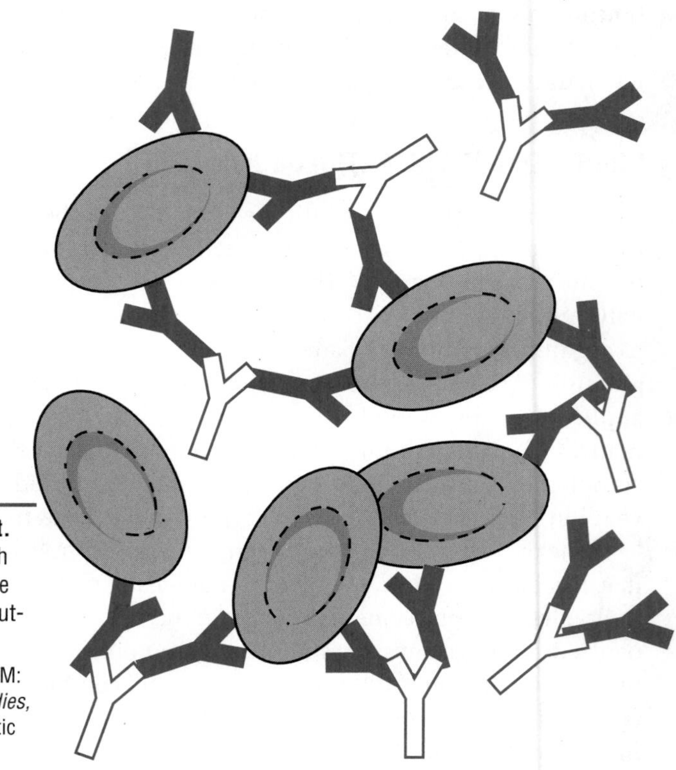

Fig. 1-20 Antiglobulin test. Red blood cells sensitized with IgG molecules (solid color) are agglutinated when anti-IgG (outlined) reagent is added.

Modified from Stroup MT, Treacy M: *Blood group antigens and antibodies,* Raritan, NJ, 1982, Ortho Diagnostic Systems, Inc.

entering this field since both tests use the AHG reagents. The DAT is a test in immunohematology to detect antibody bound to red blood cells in vivo. In contrast the IAT is used in immunohematology testing to detect antibody bound to red blood cells in vitro.

Direct Antiglobulin Test

Autoimmune hemolytic anemia: immune destruction of autologous or self red blood cells.

Hemolytic disease of the newborn: disease caused by destruction of fetal or neonatal red blood cells by maternal antibodies.

Under normal circumstances, red blood cells are not sensitized with either IgG or complement in vivo. The DAT is ordered to detect IgG or complement proteins bound to patient cells, which is a consequence of certain clinical events. These clinical events include **autoimmune hemolytic anemia, hemolytic disease of the newborn,** a drug-related mechanism, or a transfusion reaction. A positive DAT is an important indicator of potential immune-mediated red blood cell destruction in the body. As a consequence of IgG and complement attachment to the patient's red blood cells, the Fc receptors on macrophages and other immune cells bind the antibody-coated red blood cells and clear them using the reticuloendothelial system organs.

In the DAT procedure, patient's red blood cells are first washed several times with physiologic saline to remove unbound proteins. The AHG reagent is added following the washing process. Agglutination with AHG reagent indicates that IgG antibodies, complement molecules, or both are bound to the patient's red blood cells. Agglutination after the addition of the AHG reagent is interpreted as a positive DAT. No agglutination after the addition of the AHG reagent is interpreted as a negative DAT. As noted earlier, a positive DAT recognizes attached antibody or complement as a result of a clinical process or event (Fig. 1-21). The significance of a positive DAT should be assessed in relation to the patient's medical history and clinical condition.

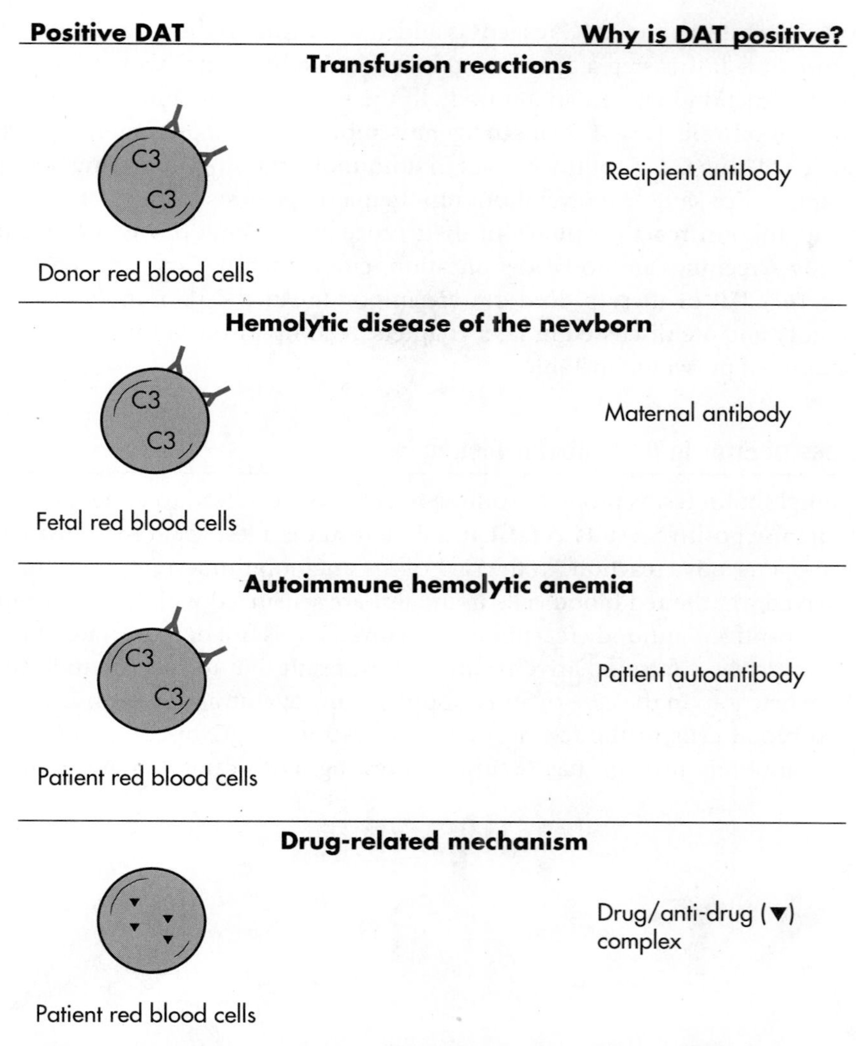

Fig. 1-21 Clinical examples of a positive direct antiglobulin test. The recipient noted above is the patient receiving the transfusion. *DAT*, Direct antiglobulin test.

The sample of choice for a DAT is collected in an ethylenediaminetetraacetic acid (EDTA) tube. Since complement can attach nonspecifically to red blood cells when samples are stored, it is important to use an anticoagulated EDTA sample when performing this test. Because EDTA negates the in vitro activation of the complement pathway, the test will be detecting only complement proteins that have been bound to the red blood cells in vivo.[3]

Indirect Antiglobulin Test

In contrast the IAT is designed to detect in vitro sensitization of red blood cells. This test is performed through a two-stage testing procedure. Antibodies first must combine with red blood cell antigens in vitro through an incubation step. In this first stage a serum source is incubated at body temperature with a red blood cell source to allow the attachment of IgG antibodies to specific red blood cell antigens. The red blood cell suspension is then washed with physiologic saline to remove unbound antibody or complement proteins. Following red blood cell washing, the AHG reagent is added to the test in the second stage. Any agglutination at this step is interpreted as a positive IAT. A positive IAT indicates a specific reaction between an antibody in the serum and an antigen present on the red blood cells (Fig. 1-22). No agglutination at this step is interpreted as a negative IAT. The IAT is routinely used in immunohematology in testing both patient and donor samples. Several immunohematologic tests incorporate an indirect antiglobulin **reaction phase** in their procedures. These procedures include antibody screening, antibody identification, crossmatching, and antigen typing (Table 1-4). All of these procedures are important in the immunohematology laboratory and are discussed in later chapters. A comparison of the DAT and IAT procedures is presented in Table 1-5.

Reaction phase: observation of agglutination at certain temperatures, following incubation, or after the addition of antihuman globulin.

Sources of Error in Antiglobulin Testing

The antiglobulin test is prone to sources of error that can lead to either false negative or false positive results. A **false negative result** is a test result that incorrectly indicates a negative reaction. In the case of the antiglobulin test no agglutination is observed, yet the red blood cells in the test are sensitized with IgG or complement. An antigen-antibody reaction has occurred but is not demonstrated in testing. Conversely, a **false positive result** is a test result that incorrectly indicates a positive reaction. In the case of antiglobulin testing agglutination is observed, yet the red blood cells in the test are not sensitized with IgG or complement. No antigen-antibody reaction has occurred in testing. With careful attention to the

False negative result: test result that incorrectly indicates a negative reaction (the lack of agglutination); an antigen-antibody reaction has occurred but is not demonstrated.

False positive result: test result that incorrectly indicates a positive reaction (the presence of agglutination or hemolysis); no antigen-antibody reaction occurred.

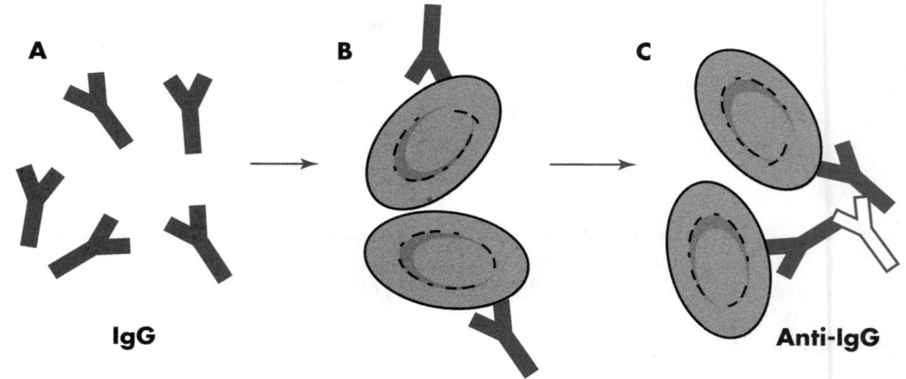

Fig. 1-22 Indirect antiglobulin test. ***A,*** Serum containing blood group antibodies. ***B,*** Red blood cells are added to serum and incubated. Sensitization of the red blood cells occurs during incubation. ***C,*** Sensitized red blood cells are agglutinated by antihuman globulin reagent (anti-IgG).

Modified from Stroup MT, Treacy M: *Blood group antigens and antibodies,* Raritan, NJ, 1982, Ortho Diagnostic Systems, Inc.

Table 1-4 Applications of Indirect Antiglobulin Test in the Immunohematology Laboratory

PROCEDURE	PURPOSE
Antibody screening	Detects antibodies with specificity to red blood cell antigens
Antibody identification	Identifies the specificity of red blood cell antibodies
Crossmatch	Determines serologic compatibility between donor and patient prior to transfusion
Antigen typing	Identifies a specific red blood cell antigen in a patient or donor

Table 1-5 Comparison of DAT and IAT Procedures

DAT	IAT
Detects IgG- and/or complement-coated red blood cells	Detects IgG- and/or complement-coated red blood cells
Sensitization has occurred within the patient's body	Sensitization has occurred as a result of performing a test procedure
One-stage procedure	Two-stage procedure
Patient's red blood cells are tested with antiglobulin reagent without an incubation step	Test requires an incubation step before the addition of antiglobulin reagent
Test for certain clinical conditions: hemolytic disease of the newborn, hemolytic transfusion reaction, and autoimmune hemolytic anemia	Used as a reaction phase of several tests in immunohematology

DAT, Direct antiglobulin test; *IAT,* indirect antiglobulin test.

Table 1-6 Common Sources of False Positive Error in Antiglobulin Testing

FALSE POSITIVE	POSSIBLE EXPLANATIONS
Red blood cells are agglutinated before washing step and addition of antihuman globulin reagent	Potent cold reactive antibody of patient origin
Use of dirty glassware	Particles or contaminants
Improper centrifugation: overcentrifugation	Red blood cell button packed so tightly on centrifugation that nonspecific clumping cannot be dispersed

Table 1-7 Common Sources of False Negative Error in Antiglobulin Testing

FALSE NEGATIVE	POSSIBLE EXPLANATIONS
Failure to wash cells adequately during the test procedure before the addition of AHG reagent	Unbound human serum globulins neutralize the AHG reagent
Testing is interrupted or delayed; AHG reagent is not added immediately after washing	Bound IgG or complement molecules may detach from the coated red blood cells
Failure to identify weak positive reactions	Technical error in testing
Loss of reagent activity	Improper reagent storage, bacterial contamination, or contamination with human serum
Failure to add AHG reagent	Technical error in testing
Improper centrifugation: undercentrifugation	Conditions for promoting agglutination are not optimal
Inappropriate red blood cell concentrations: red blood cell suspensions fall outside the optimal 2% to 5%	Concentration of red blood cells influences the reaction

AHG, Antihuman globulin.

test procedures, individuals who perform the AHG tests can avoid many of these false positive and false negative results. Common sources of error in antiglobulin testing are summarized in Tables 1-6 and 1-7.[3]

PRINCIPLES OF ANTIBODY POTENTIATORS

Antibody potentiators: reagents or methods that enhance or speed up the antibody-antigen reaction.
Enhancement media: reagents that enhance or speed up the antibody-antigen reaction.

Proteolytic enzymes: enzymes that denature certain proteins.

Antibody potentiators, or **enhancement media,** are reagents selected to adjust the in vitro test environment to promote agglutination. Potentiators are added to blood bank tests to enhance the detection of antigen-antibody complex formation. In this role, potentiators may enhance antibody uptake (first stage of agglutination), promote direct agglutination (second stage of agglutination), or serve both functions. The four major types of potentiators commonly used in the blood bank laboratory include low–ionic strength solution (LISS), bovine serum albumin (BSA), polyethylene glycol (PEG), and **proteolytic enzymes** (ficin and papain). These reagents are summarized in Table 1-8.

Low–Ionic Strength Solution

The incubation of serum and red blood cells in a reduced ionic environment increases the rate of antibody binding to specific antigen receptor sites on the red blood cells.[9] In physiologic saline, sodium and chloride ions cluster around the antigen and antibody molecules. As antigen-antibody complex formation is influenced by the attraction of opposite charges, the clustering of these free sodium and chloride ions hinders the complex formation. When the ionic strength is reduced, the antigen and antibody molecules are capable of combining at a faster rate.[10] In 1974 Löw and Messeter applied this principle in routine testing to detect unknown red blood cell antibodies by using an LISS as the suspending medium for red blood cells (the source of known antigens in the test).[11] Other investigators have also confirmed that LISS enhanced antibody reactions, especially in the indirect antiglobulin phases of testing.[12]

The low-ionic environment can be accomplished in several systems:

- Suspending red blood cells of the test in LISS reagent
- Using additive LISS reagent in conjunction with saline-suspended red blood cells

The LISS reagent contains sodium chloride, glycine, and salt-poor albumin. In addition, some low–ionic strength additive reagents may contain macromolecular additives to potentiate the direct agglutination of antigen-positive red blood cells by some antibodies. The reagent supplies a low-ionic environment to enhance antibody uptake and improve detection at antiglobulin phases of test-

Table 1-8 Summary of Antibody Potentiators

POTENTIATOR	MECHANISM OF ACTION
Low–ionic strength solution	Increases rate of antibody uptake
Bovine serum albumin	Affects the second stage of agglutination
Polyethylene glycol	Concentrates the antibody in the test environment in a low–ionic strength solution
Proteolytic enzymes (papain and ficin)	Removes negative charges from the red blood cell membrane, which reduces the zeta potential

ing. The final result is sensitization, or the potentiation of the first stage in the agglutination reaction.

Bovine Serum Albumin

BSA is prepared from bovine serum or plasma and is commercially available in either a 22% or a 30% concentration. This reagent is commonly used to potentiate the direct agglutination of red blood cells and IgG molecules. In contrast to LISS, albumin does not promote the antibody uptake stage of agglutination but influences the second stage by allowing antibody-sensitized cells to become closer together than is possible in a saline medium without additives. The addition of BSA to reaction tubes favors the direct agglutination of Rh antibodies and enhances the sensitivity of the indirect antiglobulin test for a wide range of antibody specificities.

Various theories have been proposed to explain BSA's enhancement properties. Pollack and his coworkers[13] suggested that albumin reduces the zeta potential by dispersing some of the positively charged ions surrounding each negatively charged red blood cell. In this theory, albumin increases the dielectric constant of the medium, defined as a measure of the ability to dissipate a charge. Other investigators believe that albumin bound to the cell membrane affects the degree of water hydration of the red blood cell membrane itself.[14]

Polyethylene Glycol Additive

PEG in a low–ionic strength test medium effectively concentrates antibody in the test mixture while creating a low–ionic strength environment that enhances the rate of antibody uptake. PEG has been reported to increase the sensitivity of the indirect antiglobulin test.[15] The PEG reagent removes water molecules in the test environment to allow a greater probability of collision between antigen and antibody molecules.[16] Since PEG can directly effect the aggregation of red blood cells, the reagent can be used only in indirect antiglobulin testing. Only anti-IgG specific AHG reagent is suitable for use with PEG because of reports of nonspecific agglutination with polyspecific AHG reagents.[17]

Proteolytic Enzymes

Proteolytic enzymes commonly used in the immunohematology laboratory include papain, ficin, and bromelin, all of which are commercially available. The term *proteolytic* refers to the breakdown of protein molecules. These enzymes possess the property to modify red blood cell membranes by removing the negatively charged molecules from the red blood cell membrane. The loss of these negatively charged molecules reduces the zeta potential and enhances the agglutination of some IgG molecules when suspended in a saline medium. Antibodies to red blood cell antigens in the Rh, Kidd, and Lewis blood group systems are enhanced in enzyme phases. Certain other red blood cell antigens are destroyed when exposed to these proteolytic enzymes. These red blood cell antigens include M, N, S, Xg^a, Fy^a, and Fy^b. Depending upon the red blood cell antibody, the use of enzymes in testing may enhance, depress, or entirely inhibit the antigen-antibody complex formation. A good knowledge of the blood group systems aids in the interpretation of these enzyme tests.

CHAPTER SUMMARY

1. Overview of the Immune System
   a. Innate or natural immunity is a nonspecific first line of defense against invading pathogens involving skin, mucosal linings, normal flora, and chemical secretions such as tears. The inflammatory response is a component of the body's natural line of defenses.
   b. Acquired or adaptive immunity is a specific immune response involving cells and mediators of the immune system.
   c. Phagocytes function in the internalization and killing of microorganisms as a first line of defense against infection. Macrophages are known as APCs as they process and present foreign materials to the lymphocytes to activate adaptive immunity.
   d. T cells play a major role in cellular immunity whereas B cells are crucial players in humoral immunity.
   e. Cellular immunity involves cell-mediated responses such as the killing by cytotoxic lymphocyte and the killing mediated by the natural killer cells.
   f. Humoral immunity is associated with a B cell response to antigen. Activated B cells, or plasma cells, manufacture antibody molecules that recognize a target antigen molecule. The clonal expansion of B cells generates memory B cells for lasting immunity to a particular antigen.
   g. T_H cells, or CD4 cells, recognize and interact with antigen and produce cytokines that activate other immune cells.
   h. T_C cells, or CD8 cells, are involved in the clearance of viral-infected cells, tumor cells, and cells of a foreign tissue graft.
   i. Cytokines have an important role in the cell-to-cell communications during an immune response.
   j. The complement system is a group of serum proteins with biologic roles in antigen clearance, cell lysis, and vasodilation.
2. Characteristics of Antigens
   a. An antigen is a foreign molecule that combines with an antibody.
   b. An immunogen describes the antigen in its role of eliciting an immune response in the body.
   c. All immunogens that lead to the production of antibodies are antigens. Not all antigens are immunogens.
   d. Different biologic materials have varying degrees of immunogenicity. Protein is the most immunogenic.
   e. The antigenic determinant is responsible for specificity.
   f. Red blood cell, HLA, and platelet antigens are important in immunohematology.
3. Characteristics of Antibodies
   a. Antibody molecules possess heavy chains and light chains, constant and variable regions, disulfide bonds, and a hinge region.
   b. The Fab fragment contains the portion of the molecule that binds to the antigenic determinant.
   c. The Fc fragment binds to receptors on immune cells to assist in the removal of antibody-coated red blood cells from the body.
   d. An immune response to a red blood cell antigen generates IgG and IgM antibodies.
   e. IgM molecules are pentameric in shape with 10 antigen-binding sites. They are very efficient in the activation of complement.

   f. IgG molecules possess two antigen binding sites and constitute about 80% of the total immunoglobulin concentration in serum. Four IgG subclasses exist and are designated IgG1, IgG2, IgG3, and IgG4.
4. Primary and Secondary Immune Response
   a. The primary immune response is elicited on first exposure to antigen and produces an IgM response initially.
   b. The secondary immune response, or anamnestic response, is elicited upon the second contact with the same antigen.
5. Antigen-Antibody Interactions
   a. The binding of an antigen and antibody follows the law of mass action and is reversible.
   b. The goodness of fit and the complementary nature of the antibody for its specific epitope determine the strength and rate of the reaction.
   c. The immune complex is held together by attractive forces, including electrostatic forces, hydrogen bonding, hydrophobic bonding, and Van der Waals forces.
6. Immunohematology: Antigen-Antibody Reactions in Vivo
   The exposure to foreign cellular antigens during transfusion may elicit an immune response in the patient receiving the transfusion. Likewise, the exposure to foreign fetal cellular antigens during pregnancy may elicit an immune response in the mother.
7. Immunohematology: Antigen-Antibody Reactions in Vitro
   a. Hemagglutination is a two-step process involving the antibody binding to red blood cells and the formation of lattices between sensitized red blood cells.
   b. The sensitization stage is affected by several variables such as serum to cell ratio, time, temperature, pH, and ionic strength.
   c. The lattice formation stage is influenced by the zeta potential and the optimal concentrations of antigen and antibody.
   d. Grading of agglutination reactions is a subjective qualitative measurement.
   e. In addition to agglutination, hemolysis in immunohematologic testing is an indicator of an antigen-antibody reaction.
8. Principles of the Antiglobulin Test
   a. The antiglobulin test detects IgG and complement proteins that have attached to red blood cells but have not resulted in a visible agglutination reaction.
   b. There are two types of antiglobulin tests performed in the immunohematology laboratory: the DAT and the IAT.
   c. The DAT detects antibody or complement that has sensitized red blood cells as a result of a clinical process or event within the body, such as a transfusion reaction or autoimmune hemolytic anemia.
   d. The IAT requires an incubation step in the test procedure for antigen-antibody interactions before the addition of the antiglobulin reagent.
   e. The antiglobulin test is prone to sources of error that result in either false negative or false positive results.
9. Principles of Antibody Potentiators
   a. Antibody potentiators or enhancement media are reagents that adjust the test environment to promote agglutination.
   b. Potentiators may function to enhance antibody uptake or promote direct agglutination.

CRITICAL THINKING EXERCISES

◆ ***EXERCISE 1-1***

Draw an IgG molecule and identify the following parts:

a. Antigen-binding site
b. Complement-binding region
c. Macrophage-binding site
d. Variable region on the light chain
e. Hinge region

◆ ***EXERCISE 1-2***

What are the differences between antigens and immunogens?

◆ ***EXERCISE 1-3***

How are antigen-antibody reactions observed in the blood bank laboratory? List four ways to enhance an antigen-antibody reaction. What forces keep red blood cells apart?

◆ ***EXERCISE 1-4***

Compare and contrast the primary and secondary immune response.

◆ ***EXERCISE 1-5***

The saline in an automated cell washer did not fill the test tubes consistently when the instrument was evaluated during a routine quality control check. Would this affect the AHG test?

◆ ***EXERCISE 1-6***

A physician ordered a DAT on a patient with a lowered hemoglobin level and no signs of bleeding. What is the purpose of the DAT test, and what is the physician investigating?

◆ ***EXERCISE 1-7***

Identify three sources of false negative errors in antiglobulin testing. How do these errors lead to false negative results in antiglobulin testing?

STUDY QUESTIONS

1. Antibodies are produced by:
   a. killer cells
   b. marrow stem cells
   c. mast cells
   d. B cells

2. Which of the following cells is capable of binding to and killing microorganisms?
   a. neutrophil
   b. lymphocyte
   c. erythrocyte
   d. eosinophil

3. Select the term that describes the unique configuration of the antigen that allows recognition by a corresponding antibody:
   a. immunogen
   b. epitope
   c. avidity
   d. clone

4. __________ molecules are usually not good antigenic substances.
   a. protein
   b. carbohydrate
   c. lipid
   d. glycoprotein

5. The chemical composition of an antibody is:
   a. protein
   b. lipid
   c. carbohydrate
   d. glycoprotein

6. In a hemagglutination test, the antigen is:
   a. on the red blood cell membrane
   b. secreted by the red blood cell
   c. in the red blood cell nucleus
   d. in the plasma or serum

7. Hemagglutination can be enhanced by:
   a. increasing the temperature above 37° C
   b. incubation time
   c. increasing antigen concentrations
   d. pH above 7

8. Molecules that promote the uptake of bacteria for phagocytosis are:
   a. opsonins
   b. cytokines
   c. haptens
   d. isotypes

9. An epitope is also termed a (an):
   a. binding site
   b. allotype
   c. antigenic determinant
   d. immunogen

10. Agglutination reactions characterized by many small agglutinates in a background of free cells would be graded in tube testing as:
    a. 1+
    b. 2+
    c. 3+
    d. 4+

11. Which of the following is an example of innate immunity?
    a. phagocytosis
    b. graft rejection
    c. allergic reaction
    d. antibody production

12. When C3 attaches to the cell, it:
    a. causes cell lysis
    b. enhances cell clearance
    c. attracts neutrophils
    d. generates vasoactive amines

13. Why are patient red blood cells washed before the addition of AHG reagents in the DAT?
    a. to remove traces of bacterial proteins
    b. to wash away traces of free hemoglobin
    c. to expose additional antigen sites
    d. to remove unbound serum proteins

14. The IAT requires incubation at 37° C. What is the purpose of this incubation step?
    a. allow time for IgM antibodies to attach to antigens on the red blood cells
    b. allow time for IgG antibodies to attach to antigens on the red blood cells
    c. allow time for the antiglobulin reagent to react with the red blood cells
    d. allow time for neutralization of AHG reagent

15. Select the antibody-potentiating reagent that functions by increasing the rate of antibody uptake:
    a. LISS
    b. BSA
    c. PEG
    d. ficin

16. How does PEG enhance the agglutination reaction?
    a. increases the dielectric constant of the medium
    b. reduces the net negative charge on the red blood cells
    c. concentrates the antibodies in the test environment
    d. reduces the pH of the test environment

17. How does ficin enhance the antigen-antibody complex formation?
    a. removes negative charges from the red blood cell membrane
    b. reduces the ionic strength of the test environment
    c. forms a bridge between sensitized red blood cells
    d. reduces the pH of the test environment

18. Select the blood group antibody that loses reactivity with ficin-treated panel cells:
    a. anti-D
    b. anti-B
    c. anti-K
    d. anti-M

For questions 19 through 25, match the characteristic with the correct immunoglobulin class.

Characteristic	Class
19. red blood cell alloantibodies	a. IgA
20. produced early in an immune response	b. IgD
21. found predominantly in secretions	c. IgE
22. cross the placenta	d. IgG
23. highest plasma-serum concentration	e. IgM
24. pentameric in shape	
25. fixes complement most efficiently	

REFERENCES

1. Kuby J: *Immunology*, ed 3, New York, 1997, WH Freeman.
2. Roitt I, Brostoff J, Male D: *Immunology*, ed 4, St Louis, 1996, Mosby.
3. Vengelen-Tyler V: *Technical manual*, ed 12, Bethesda, Md, 1996, American Association of Blood Banks.
4. Turgeon ML: *Immunology and serology in laboratory medicine*, St Louis, 1996, Mosby.
5. Issitt PD, Anstee D: *Applied blood group serology*, ed 4, Durham, NC, 1998, Montgomery Scientific Publications.
6. Sheehan C: *Clinical immunology: principles and laboratory diagnosis*, ed 2, Philadelphia, 1997, Lippincott-Raven.
7. Stevens CD: *Clinical immunology and serology: a laboratory perspective*, Philadelphia, 1996, FA Davis.
8. Coombs RRA, Mourant AE, Race RR: A new test for the detection of weak and "incomplete" Rh agglutinins, *Br J Exp Pathol* 26:255, 1945.
9. Hughes-Jones NC, Polley MJ, Telford R: Optimal conditions for detecting blood group antibodies by the antiglobulin test, *Vox Sang* 9:385, 1964.
10. Elliot M, Bossom E, Dupuy ME, et al: Effect of ionic strength on the serologic behavior of red blood cell isoantibodies, *Vox Sang* 9:396, 1964.
11. Löw B, Messeter L: Antiglobulin test in low ionic strength salt solution for rapid antibody screening and crossmatching, *Vox Sang* 26:53, 1974.

12. Wicker B, Wallas CH: A comparison of a low ionic strength saline medium with routine methods for antibody detection, *Transfusion* 16:469, 1976.
13. Pollack W, Hager HJ, Reckel R, et al: A study of forces involved in the second stage of hemagglutination, *Transfusion* 5:158, 1965.
14. Steane EA: Red cell agglutination: a current perspective. In Bell CA, editor: *Seminar on antigen-antibody reactions revisited,* Arlington, Va, 1982, American Association of Blood Banks.
15. Nance SJ, Garratty G: A new potentiator of red blood cell antigen-antibody reactions, *Am J Clin Pathol* 87:633, 1987.
16. de Man AJ, Overbeeke MA: Evaluation of the polyethylene glycol antiglobulin test for detection of red blood cell antibodies, *Vox Sang* 58:207, 1990.
17. *Polyethylene glycol additive for antibody detection tests,* Product insert (rev), Houston, Tex, 1993, Gamma Biologicals.

BLOOD BANKING REAGENTS
Overview and Applications in Immunohematology

2

Paula R. Howard

CHAPTER OUTLINE

LEARNING OBJECTIVES

Upon completion of this chapter, the reader should be able to:

1. Describe the basic principles of routine testing in the immunohematology laboratory.
2. Identify sources of antigen and antibody used in testing.
3. List several routine tests performed in the immunohematology laboratory.
4. Describe the relationship of potency and specificity to blood banking reagents.
5. Compare and contrast polyclonal and monoclonal antisera.
6. Compare and contrast the composition and appropriate uses of polyspecific and monospecific antiglobulin reagents.
7. Discuss the different types of antisera available for ABO typing.
8. Discuss the different types of antisera available for D-typing.
9. Define the Rh control and describe its purpose.
10. Define and identify common lectins used in blood banking.
11. Discuss the different types and purposes of reagent red blood cells.
12. Describe the principles of gel technology, microplate techniques, and solid phase red blood cell adherence techniques.

This chapter demonstrates how the basic principles of antigen-antibody reactions in vitro are applied in the immunohematology laboratory and introduces the basic procedures and the major reagents used in the testing of patient and donor samples. A section on gel testing and solid phase red blood cell adherence is included to introduce the techniques that use technologies different from traditional tube testing in the detection of antigen-antibody reactions.

INTRODUCTION TO ROUTINE TESTING IN IMMUNOHEMATOLOGY

The basic procedures in immunohematology are based on the principle of placing a source of antigen and a source of antibody into a testing environment to detect an antigen-antibody reaction (Fig. 2-1). The evidence for the formation of an antigen-antibody reaction in vitro has traditionally been the visualization of agglutinates or the presence of hemolysis within the test tube. Recently, newer techniques for the detection of antigen-antibody reactions have been marketed based on detection systems using gel and solid phase adherence technology. These methods all share common denominators: a source of antigen and a source of antibody added to a testing environment. The selection of the appropriate source of either antigen or antibody for inclusion in the procedure depends on the purpose or intent of the test. Is the purpose of testing directed toward detecting the presence or absence of a particular red blood cell antigen? Or is it directed toward detecting the presence or absence of a particular red blood cell antibody? In either situation, no matter what variable is unknown in testing, the other variable must be obtained from a known source. For example, if the procedure meant to detect the presence of the A antigen on a patient's red blood cells, the patient's red blood cells are combined with a commercial source of anti-A reagent. If the A antigen is present on the red blood cells, agglutination is observed in the test tube. If the A antigen is absent on the red blood cells, no agglutination is observed in the test tube (Fig. 2-2).

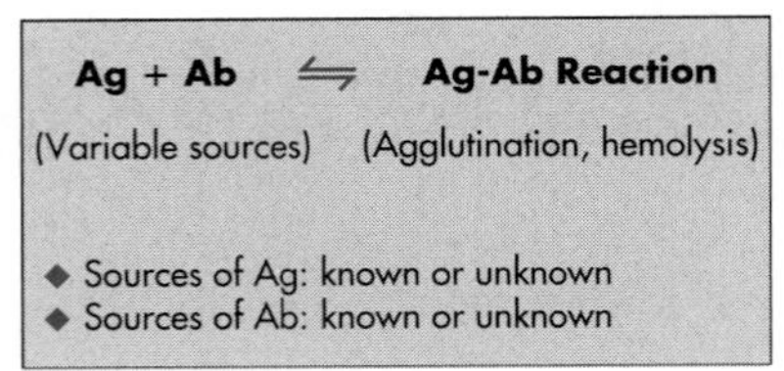

Fig. 2-1 Routine testing in the immunohematology laboratory. Sources of antigen and antibody vary depending on the test procedure. *Ag,* Antigen; *Ab,* antibody.

Sources of Antigen for Testing

Sources of antigen for immunohematologic testing include reagent red blood cells or a patient's red blood cells. Reagent red blood cells are commercially prepared cell suspensions. The manufacturer has previously identified many of the red blood cell antigens. Therefore these reagent red blood cells are known sources of red blood cell antigens. By use of a known antigen source, an unknown antibody can be identified or detected.

When using patient red blood cell suspensions, the red blood cell antigens are usually unknown. The patient's red blood cells are considered the unknown

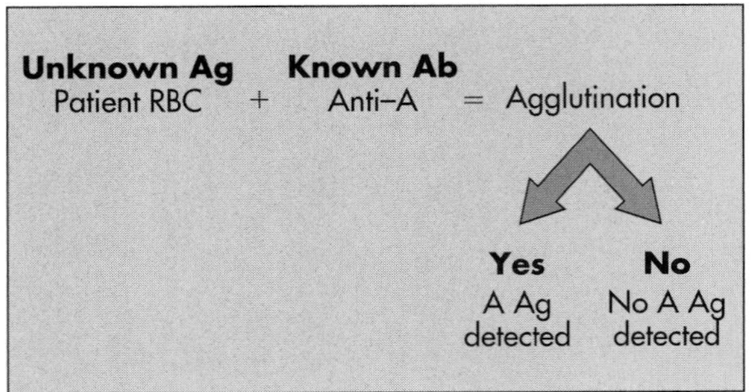

Fig. 2-2 Example of a routine test in immunohematology: detection of A antigens on red blood cells. *RBC,* Red blood cells; *Ag,* antigen; *Ab,* antibody.

variable and are tested with a known antibody source to determine the antigen identity. When a known antibody source is used, the unknown antigens on the patient's red blood cells can be identified (Fig. 2-2).

Table 2-1 Sources of Antigen and Antibody in Immunohematologic Procedures

	Known source	Unknown source
Antigen	Reagent red blood cells	Patient red blood cells
Antibody	Commercial antisera	Patient serum/ plasma

Sources of Antibody for Testing

Sources of antibody for immunohematologic testing include commercial antisera or a patient's serum or plasma. Commercial antisera contain known red blood cell antibodies. In this case a known source of antibody such as commercial antisera is used to identify unknown antigens.

Another potential source of antibodies is the patient's serum or plasma. Similar to patient antigens, the antibodies made by patients are usually unknown. Patient serum or plasma samples are tested for the presence of red blood cell antibodies using a known antigen source for identification or detection (Table 2-1).

Routine Testing Procedures in the Immunohematology Laboratory

Several universal procedures in immunohematology apply these principles in the testing of patient samples before transfusion with blood products containing red blood cells or in the testing of donor samples. These procedures are outlined as follows:

- ABO/Rh typing for the detection of the A, B, and D antigens
- Determination of the presence or absence of red blood cell antigens from other blood group systems in patient and donor samples (e.g., testing a donor unit for the E antigen of the Rh blood group system)
- Antibody screen (antibody detection) for the detection of preformed antibodies to red blood cell antigens as a result of previous exposure to red blood cells through transfusion and pregnancy
- **Antibody identification**, which determines the specificity of red blood cell antibodies after they are detected with the antibody screen
- **Crossmatch**, which provides the serologic check of donor unit and patient compatibility before transfusion

The sources of antigen and antibody used in these tests are outlined in Table 2-2.

Antibody identification: procedure that determines the identity of a red blood cell antibody detected in the antibody screen by reacting serum with commercial panel cells.

Crossmatch: procedure that combines donor's red blood cells and patient's serum to determine the serologic compatibility between donor and patient.

Table 2-2 Routine Procedures in the Immunohematology Laboratory

PROCEDURE	PURPOSE	SOURCE OF AG	SOURCE OF AB
ABO/Rh typing	Detects A, B, and D antigens	Patient's RBCs	Commercial anti-A, anti-B, and anti-D
Antibody screen	Detects antibodies with specificity to RBC antigens	Screening cells	Patient's serum
Antibody identification	Identifies the specificity of RBC antibodies	Panel cells	Patient's serum
Crossmatch	Determines serologic compatibility between donor and patient before transfusion	Donor's RBCs	Patient's serum

RBCs, Red blood cells.

INTRODUCTION TO BLOOD BANKING REAGENTS

Reagents may be grouped into four basic categories:

- Reagent red blood cells possessing known red blood cell antigens
- Antisera containing known red blood cell antibodies
- Antiglobulin reagents that detect IgG immunoglobulins and complement
- Potentiators that enhance the detection of antibodies (discussed in Chapter 1)

As introduced in the previous section, known sources of blood banking reagents are routinely used in the blood bank to detect antigen-antibody reactions. These reagents are the tools of blood banking, allowing the provision of safe and viable blood products.

An understanding of these reagents enhances the ability to interpret the results from patient and donor testing. A discussion of the composition, sources, uses, and limitations of reagents is presented following an overview of the regulatory aspects of reagent manufacturing.

Regulation of Reagent Manufacture

Food and Drug Administration: agency responsible for the regulation of the blood banking industry and other manufacturers of products consumed by humans.

Code of Federal Regulations: FDA publication outlining the legal requirements of blood banking facilities.

Specificity: unique recognition of an antigenic determinant and its corresponding antibody molecule.

Potency: strength of an antigen-antibody reaction.

Commercial antisera and reagent red blood cell products are licensed by the Center for Biologics Evaluation and Research of the **Food and Drug Administration** (FDA). The publication ***Code of Federal Regulations*** outlines the FDA's criteria for the licensure of reagents in conjunction with other regulations for the manufacture of blood and blood components.[1] The FDA has established minimum standards for blood banks and transfusion services relating to product **specificity** and **potency** before a license is assigned to a commercial reagent. Specificity reflects the unique recognition of the antigenic determinant and its corresponding antibody molecule. For example, commercial D antibodies react with red blood cells possessing D antigens and do not react with red blood cells lacking D antigens. Potency addresses the strength of the antigen-antibody reaction. For example, commercial anti-A reagents are prepared to agglutinate strongly (3+ to 4+) with red blood cells possessing the A antigen. Once a manufacturer has demonstrated that a product has met the FDA's specificity and potency requirements, the reagent is assigned a product license number that is displayed on the product's label. Each product is also labeled with a manufacturer's expiration date. According to FDA regulations, routine blood banking reagents cannot be used in testing after the expiration date. Exceptions to this rule can be made for rare antisera and red blood cells if the reagent demonstrates acceptable quality control results. If reagents are produced for in-house use (within the facility), a license is not required, but the FDA's requirements for specificity and potency must be met and documented.

Standard operating procedures: written procedures to help ensure the complete understanding of a process and achieve consistency in performance from one individual to another.

Each manufacturer provides a package or product insert to the consumer that details the reagent's description, the procedures for proper use, the specific performance characteristics, and the reagent's limitations. Laboratory **standard operating procedures** (SOPs) are written to reflect the procedures outlined in these product inserts. As new lots of reagents are received in the blood bank, the product inserts must be reviewed for any procedural changes. Any revisions must be incorporated into the SOPs before the introduction of the reagent in routine testing. The total compliance with the manufacturer's circular of directions cannot be overstressed, since that document details the appropriate procedures and recommends the appropriate reagent controls for accurate interpretation of test results.

Reagent Quality Control

Quality control: testing to determine the accuracy and precision of the equipment, reagents, and procedures.

Quality control is the term assigned to technical procedures designed to determine if the analytical testing phase is working properly. It includes checks on blood banking reagents and equipment before their use in tests on patient or donor samples. Each laboratory establishes quality control protocols for the validation and documentation of reagent and equipment function. The quality control of reagents is performed daily on reagent red blood cells and antisera. These reagents are tested to determine whether they meet preset acceptable performance criteria.

Components of a quality control program for blood banking reagents include the following items:

1. A statement of the criteria for acceptable reagent performance

   Requirements for the acceptable performance of a reagent are outlined in the facility's SOP. Typically, the potency of the agglutination reaction defines the acceptability of the reagent performance when challenged with the corresponding red blood cell antigen. For example, anti-A is tested against reagent red blood cells known to possess the A antigen. When the anti-A reagent and group A red blood cells are combined, a 3+ to 4+ reaction is expected for optimal antisera performance. When anti-A is reacted with group B red blood cells, no agglutination is expected. If agglutination results are less than 3+ in strength with group A red blood cells (e.g., 2+ or less), the anti-A reagent may be deteriorating in potency. The loss of agglutination strength over time is an indicator of a loss of potency, and the ability to detect A antigens in patient samples is potentially compromised.
2. The documentation of reagent use

   Reagents are tested, and the results of quality control testing are recorded and reviewed. Records of quality control testing must be maintained, including results, interpretations, date of testing, and identity of personnel performing the testing.
3. Appropriate corrective actions for reagents that do not meet the performance requirements must be outlined in the SOP.[2]

In addition to quality control testing of reagents, inspections should be performed on antisera for any evidence of bacterial contamination. Any turbidity or cloudiness in the reagent bottles raises suspicion of a contaminated product.

COMMERCIAL REAGENT ANTISERA: POLYCLONAL VERSUS MONOCLONAL PRODUCTS

An ideal reagent antiserum contains a concentrated suspension of highly specific, well-characterized, and uniformly reactive immunoglobulin molecules. Commercially prepared antibody reagents can be either polyclonal or monoclonal antibody–based products. If several clones of B cells secrete antibodies in an immunologic response to a foreign antigen, the antiserum produced is called polyclonal. If the antibody is the product of a single clone of B cells, the antiserum produced is called monoclonal.

Until the recent introduction of monoclonal antibody-based blood banking reagents, commercial antisera were derived from polyclonal sources as a result of the immunization of animals and humans with purified antigens. Time-consuming separation techniques were used to produce the polyclonal antisera. In **polyclonal antisera** several different clones of B cells secrete antibodies (Fig. 2-3). The product contains multiple antibody specificities directed toward different antigens in the immunization injection or toward different parts of a purified antigen injected for an immune response.

Polyclonal antisera: several different clones of B cells that secrete antibodies.

In contrast to polyclonal antisera, **monoclonal antisera** production creates an immortal clone that manufactures a single antibody of a defined specificity

Monoclonal antisera: single clones of B cells that secrete one antibody.

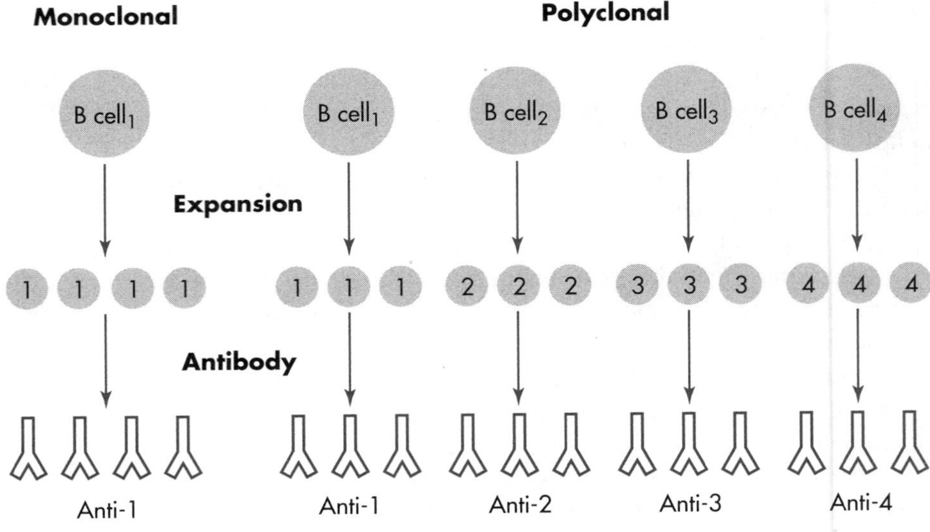

Fig. 2-3 Comparison of monoclonal and polyclonal antisera.

(Fig. 2-3). These antibodies have the advantage of being manufactured in vitro. Monoclonal antibody–based reagents were introduced into the blood bank to replace polyclonal-based reagents because of necessity and desirability. Currently, FDA-approved monoclonal antisera include anti-A, anti-B, anti-A,B, anti-D, anti-C, anti-E, anti-c, anti-e, anti-IgG, anti-C3b, anti-C3d, and other blood group system antibodies.[3] Box 2-1 summarizes the advantages and disadvantages of the practice of monoclonal-based reagents in the blood bank.[4]

BOX 2-1

Advantages and Disadvantages of Monoclonal Antibody–Based Reagents

ADVANTAGES

- Unlimited production
- Standardized reagents
- Small variations between batches
- No human/animal source materials
- No contaminating antibodies
- Direct agglutination/shorter time because of IgM antibodies
- Can be used to type RBCs from positive direct antiglobulin test

DISADVANTAGES

- Specificity may be relative, since an antigenic determinant may be shared by several RBC antigens
- Single specificity antibodies may not react with all antigen-positive RBCs, since RBCs may not express every antigenic determinant

RBCs, Red blood cells.

Monoclonal-based reagents are correctly employed in serologic testing by following these guidelines:

- Careful review of the package inserts
- Adherence to the manufacturer's directions
- Recognition of the relevant characteristics of the **hybridoma** clone
- Review of the manufacturer's formulation

Protein concentrations in the formulation of products produced by different manufacturers may vary. The majority of these monoclonal-based products possess a low concentration (3% to 8%) of protein.

Hybridoma: hybrid cell formed by the fusion of a myeloma cell and an antibody-producing cell; used in the production of monoclonal antibodies.

ANTISERA FOR ABO TYPING

Anti-A and anti-B commercial antisera are used to determine whether an individual's red blood cells possess the A or B antigens of the ABO blood group system. Donor or patient red blood cells (unknown antigen) are combined with commercial antisera (known antibodies) and observed for the presence or absence of agglutination. Agglutination indicates the presence of antigen; no agglutination indicates the absence of antigen on the red blood cells tested (Table 2-3). Based on the testing results, an ABO blood type is assigned to the patient or donor. Four major blood types in the ABO blood group system exist: A, B, AB, and O. Group A individuals possess the A antigen and lack the B antigen. Group B individuals possess the B antigen and lack the A antigen. Group AB individuals possess both the A and B antigens, while group O individuals lack both the A and B antigens. The procedure to determine this ABO blood group system

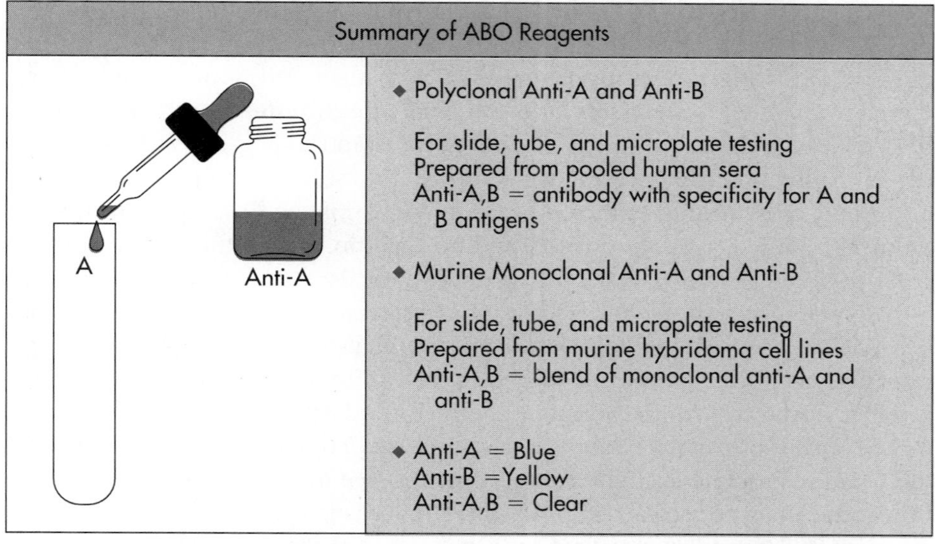

Fig. 2-4 Summary of ABO reagents.
Modified from Gamma Biologicals, Houston, Tex.

Table 2-3 ABO Red Blood Cell Testing (Forward Grouping)

ABO Blood group	Anti-A	Anti-B
A	+	0
B	0	+
AB	+	+
O	0	0

+, Agglutination; *0*, no agglutination.

assignment has been referred to as ABO grouping, ABO forward grouping, front typing, and ABO red blood cell testing. The most recent edition of the ***Technical Manual*** of the **American Association of Blood Banks** (AABB) refers to the act of typing, or determining the ABO of an individual's red blood cells as a type rather than a group.[5] This textbook adopts the AABB terminology and refers to the determination of an individual's ABO *type*, not an ABO *group*. Many other references still retain the terminology of ABO grouping. For instance, the FDA name for these reagents remains "ABO grouping reagents."

Technical Manual: publication of the American Association of Blood Banks that provides a reference to current acceptable practices in blood banking.

American Association of Blood Banks: professional organization that accredits and provides educational and technical guidance to blood banks and transfusion services.

Since the discovery of the ABO blood group system, routine testing has been performed with polyclonal antisera derived from human plasma sources. In the past 5 years the blood banking community has been phasing out these reagents. Two events have contributed to this trend: the emergence of murine monoclonal ABO antisera in 1985 and the shortage of injectable A and B substances for polyclonal antibody production.[6] Reagent manufacturers cite many benefits to the adoption of murine monoclonal reagents, including the recognition of weaker A and B antigens, the removal of contaminating antibodies, cost-effectiveness, and the availability of a reagent source not dependent on human sources.

The murine monoclonal ABO products are tested to meet FDA potency and specificity requirements before licensure. The antibodies are suspended in a diluent that usually does not exceed a 6% bovine albumin concentration and is considered a low-protein medium. Testing is performed in **immediate spin phases.** Manufacturers recommend that testing be confirmed by checking for expected **ABO antibodies** using reagent red blood cells. Anti-A always contains a blue dye, whereas anti-B is always yellow. These dyes have been added to reduce potential errors in testing. A summary of ABO reagents is presented in Fig. 2-4.

Immediate spin phases: source antigen and source antibody used in immunohematologic testing are combined, immediately centrifuged, and observed for agglutination.

ABO antibodies: anti-A, anti-B, and anti-A,B; patients possess the ABO antibody to the ABO antigen lacking on their red blood cells (e.g., group A individuals possess anti-B).

ANTISERA FOR Rh TYPING

Of the antigens within the Rh blood group system, the D antigen is the most important in routine blood banking. The D antigen has been linked to adverse consequences in patients, including hemolytic transfusion reactions and hemolytic disease of the newborn. Because of its increased immunogenicity as a blood group antigen, D antigen typing of all patient and donor samples is required by the AABB's ***Standards for Blood Banks and Transfusion Services***.[7] This requirement enables the distinction of D-positive and D-negative individuals. In the Rh typing procedure, commercial anti-D is combined with patient or donor red blood cells. Agglutination indicates presence of the D antigen on the red blood cells tested (e.g., D-positive), and no agglutination in these tests indicates absence of the D antigen (e.g., D-negative) (Table 2-4).

Standards for Blood Banks and Transfusion Services: publication of the American Association of Blood Banks that outlines the minimal standards of practice in areas relating to transfusion medicine.

Table 2-4 Typing for the D Antigen with Patient or Donor Red Blood Cells

D type	Anti-D	Rh control
D-positive	+	0
D-negative	0	0
Cannot interpret typing	+	+

+, Agglutination; *0*, no agglutination.

Several reagent product classifications exist to accomplish D typing. They can be divided into several categories, including high-protein reagents, saline IgM reagents, chemically modified IgG reagents, and monoclonal reagents. Each product is labeled with the antibody specificity and a phrase that specifies how it can be used. For instance, a bottle of anti-D may contain the phrase "for slide, tube, and microplate testing." This statement specifies the test method in which the product may be used according to its FDA licensure. The detailed methods are provided in the product insert along with the unique characteristics of each product. Chemically modified IgG antisera and saline IgM reagents are available, but monoclonal-based products have replaced them in many laboratories (Fig. 2-5 summarizes these reagents). In addition to D typing, similar products are available for the phenotyping of other antigens within the Rh blood group system, such as C, E, c, and e.

One of the most confusing aspects of Rh reagents is the negative, or diluent, control in Rh typing procedures. The negative control is referred to as the Rh control. Rh controls are added to the Rh typing procedure to aid in the detection of several false positive reactions in routine testing for D antigen. The Rh control is needed in routine D typing when commercial antisera with high-protein concentrations are selected as reagents. Commercial antisera with high protein concentrations contain anti-D and macromolecular additives in a high-protein diluent to enhance agglutination. Because it serves as the negative control, the Rh control reagent contains *only* the macromolecular additives in a high-protein diluent unique to each manufacturer. No D antibodies are present in the Rh control reagent. In essence, the Rh control tests the effects of suspending the patient or donor red blood cells in the manufacturer's reagent diluent. Because the Rh control does not contain D antibodies, it should not demonstrate any agglutination in the tube (Fig. 2-6). It is the negative control in Rh typing.

Why is the negative control important? It can detect several situations that may demonstrate false positive reactions in routine testing for the D antigen if high-protein reagents are used. These false positive reactions lead to error in assigning correct D antigen typing to patients and donors. Situations demonstrating agglutination of the Rh control reagent irrespective of the individual's actual D typing status may include the following:

Autoantibodies: antibodies to self-antigens.

- A patient's red blood cells have been sensitized in vivo with **autoantibodies.** In other words, the patient's red blood cells have a positive direct antiglobulin test (DAT) because of autoantibodies attached to the patient's red blood cells. Suspension of these red blood cells in a high-protein diluent promotes an agglutination reaction.
- Red blood cells obtained from a patient or donor whose serum contains abnormal protein concentrations. **Rouleaux,** or pseudoagglutination, may be observed in testing when using unwashed patient samples.

Rouleaux: aggregation of red blood cells that may result from the presence of abnormal proteins in the patient; red blood cells appear as stacked coins.

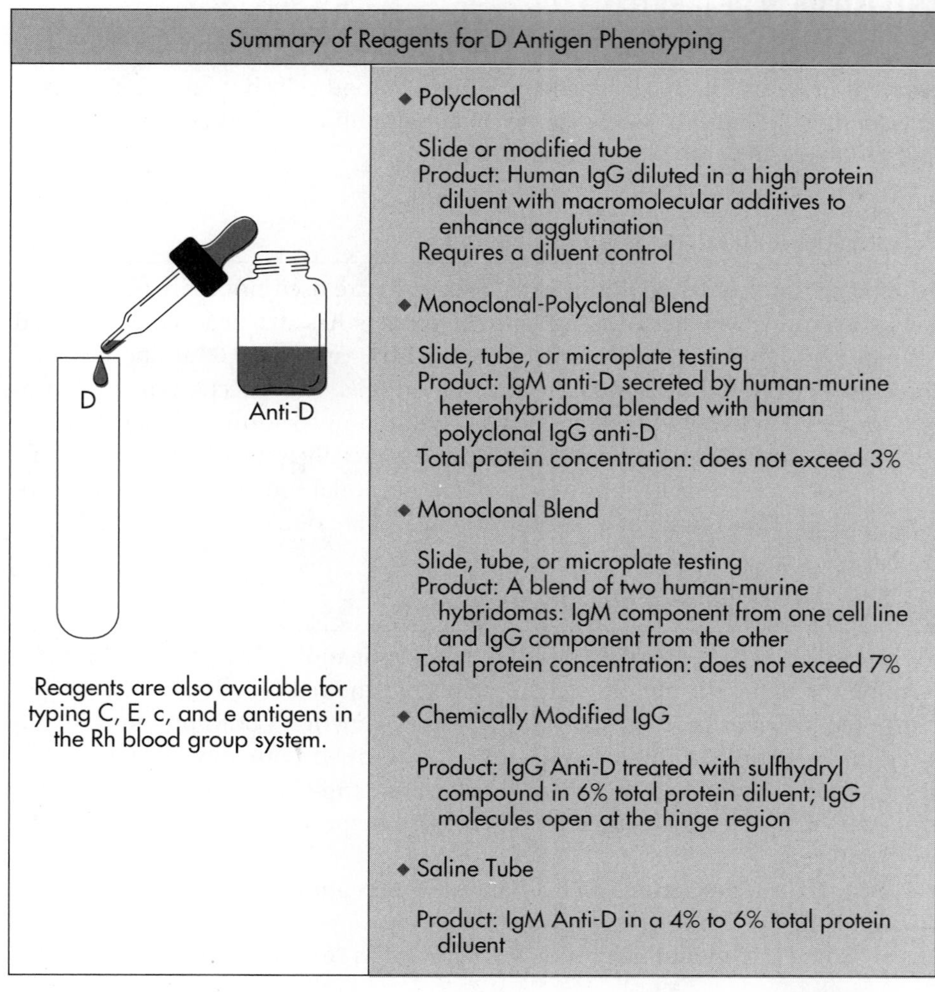

Fig. 2-5 Summary of reagents for D antigen phenotyping.
Modified from Gamma Biologicals, Houston, Tex.

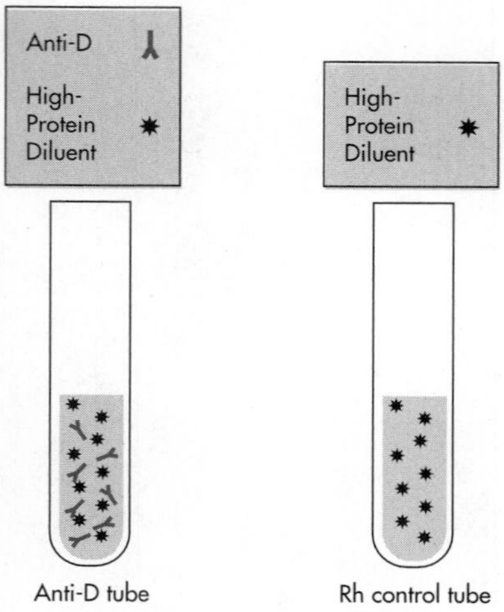

Anti-D
High-Protein Diluent
High-Protein Diluent
Anti-D tube
Rh control tube

Fig. 2-6 Anti-D and Rh control tubes. The anti-D tube contains anti-D antibodies suspended in the high-protein diluent. The Rh control contains diluent and no anti-D antibodies.

In these situations the test diluent is promoting the agglutination that may lead to possible errors in antigen typing for D or other Rh antigens (e.g., C, c, E, e). Any positive reaction in the Rh control test negates an interpretation of a D typing. An investigation of the positive Rh control must be completed before the assignment of the D antigen.

Monoclonal anti-D reagents possess a low-protein diluent formulation similar in protein concentration to the diluent of the ABO reagents. The low-protein diluent does not promote the agglutination of immunoglobulin-coated red blood cells. However, a false positive test result may occur if strong cold autoantibodies or protein abnormalities are present. Such phenomena would probably be demonstrated in the ABO reactions also. Therefore a control in D typing is not essential if the patient or donor red blood cells show no agglutination with either anti-A or anti-B in ABO red blood cell testing. If the test sample shows definite or doubtful agglutination with both anti-A and anti-B, an Rh control should be performed with appropriate control reagents specified by the manufacturer when using the monoclonal anti-D reagent.

ANTIGLOBULIN REAGENTS

The antiglobulin test is important for the detection of IgG antibodies and complement proteins that have attached to the red blood cells but have not resulted in visible agglutination. Two categories of antiglobulin reagents exist: polyspecific and monospecific antiglobulin reagents.

Polyspecific Antihuman Globulin Reagents

Polyspecific antihuman globulin (AHG) reagents are used primarily in DAT testing to determine whether either IgG or complement has attached to the red blood cells in vivo. This reagent contains both anti-IgG and anti-C3 antibodies, and therefore detects both IgG and C3 on red blood cells. The detection of either protein implies that red blood cell antigen-antibody complex formation has clinically occurred. Several reagent preparations are commercially available for polyspecific products derived from either polyclonal or monoclonal sources. All of these products meet the FDA requirements for licensure and are outlined in Fig. 2-7.

Monospecific Antihuman Globulin Reagents

Differential DAT: Immunohematologic test that uses monospecific anti-IgG and monospecific anti-C3 reagents to determine the cause of a positive DAT with polyspecific antiglobulin reagents.

Monospecific AHG reagents are used in the investigation of a positive DAT to determine the nature of the molecules attached to the red blood cells. Are the patient's red blood cells sensitized with IgG, complement, or both proteins? To answer this question, a **differential DAT** is performed with monospecific AHG reagents using individual sources of anti-IgG and anti-C3 (Table 2-5). Monospecific AHG reagents are prepared by separating the specificities of the polyspecific AHG reagents.

Anti-IgG monospecific AHG products contain antibodies to human gamma chains. They are commercially available as either polyclonal- or monoclonal-based products. Often these products are labeled as "heavy chain specific," mean-

Table 2-5 Differential Direct Antiglobulin Test Procedure

Interpretation	Monospecific anti-IgG	Monospecific anti-C3
Patient RBCs sensitized with IgG only	+	0
Patient RBCs sensitized with IgG and C3	+	+
Patient RBCs sensitized with C3 only	0	+

RBCs, Red blood cells; +, agglutination; *0,* no agglutination.

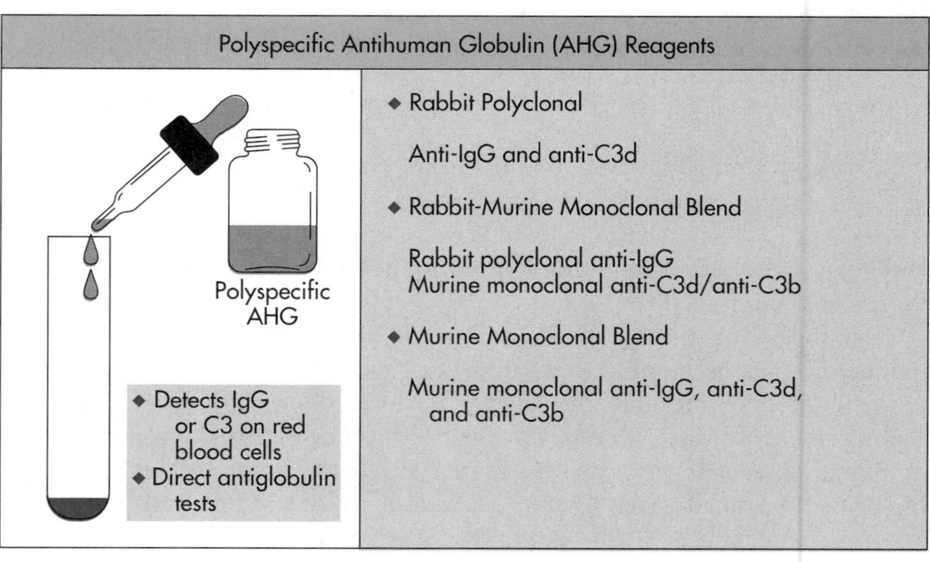

Fig. 2-7 Polyspecific antihuman globulin reagents.

Data from *Code of federal regulations,* 21CFR 660.55, Washington, DC, 1997, US Government Printing Office. Illustration modified from Gamma Biologicals, Houston, Tex.

ing that the antiserum contains antibodies specific for the gamma heavy chains of the IgG molecule. Products without this label may contain antibodies that react with immunoglobulin light chains. From the immunology discussion in Chapter 1, recall that immunoglobulin light chains (kappa and lambda) are common to all immunoglobulin classes (e.g., IgG, IgM, IgA). In addition to their use in the investigation of a positive DAT, anti-IgG reagents are used in many laboratories for antibody detection, antibody identification, and crossmatching procedures. Fig. 2-8 summarizes monospecific anti-IgG products.

Anti-C3b and anti-C3d monospecific reagents contain no reactivity to human immunoglobulin molecules. These reagents specifically detect complement proteins that have been attached to the red blood cell surface as a result of the activation of complement's classical pathway. The activation of the complement pathway can lead to red blood cell destruction in vivo through either **intravascular hemolysis** or **extravascular hemolysis.** For the detection of any complement proteins bound in vivo, a product requires specificity for the C3d fragment. This fragment of complement is usually the only protein that remains attached to the patient's red blood cells. Anti-C3 is commercially available as either polyclonal- or monoclonal-based products (Fig. 2-9).

Intravascular hemolysis: destruction of red blood cells and release of hemoglobin within the vascular compartment through immune or nonimmune mechanisms; antibodies of the ABO system can cause this type of hemolysis.

Extravascular hemolysis: removal of red blood cells from circulation by the phagocytic cells of the reticuloendothelial system (liver and spleen).

Check Cells (Coombs' Control Cells)

The AABB *Standards for Blood Banks and Transfusion Services* requires a control system for antiglobulin tests interpreted as negative.[7] The control system consists of red blood cells that have been commercially prepared with IgG antibodies attached. This control is often referred to as "check cells" or "Coombs' control cells." Since antiglobulin testing has its own set of test limitations that may affect the interpretation of results, check cells were designed as an additive system for negative antiglobulin tests to control the possibility of false negative reactions.

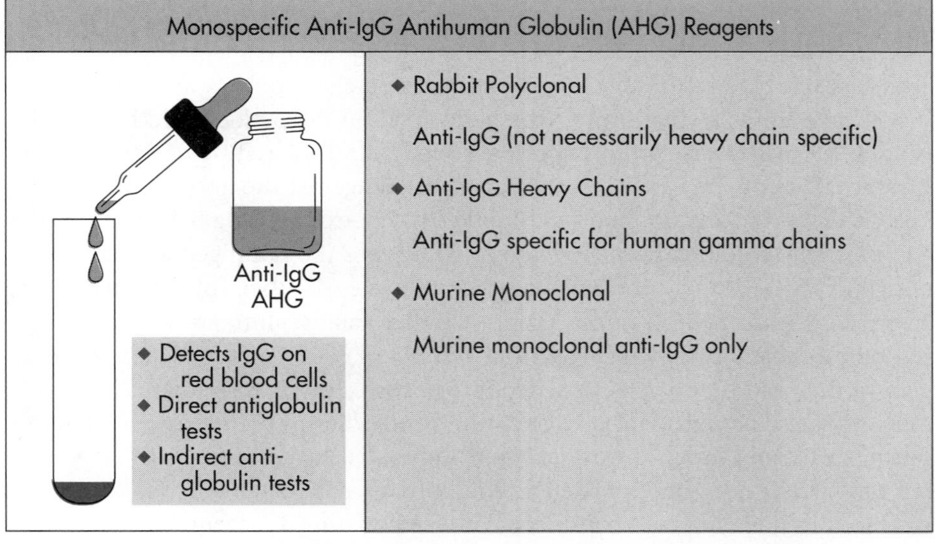

Fig. 2-8 Monospecific anti-IgG antihuman globulin reagents.

Text from *Code of federal regulations*, 21CFR 660.55, Washington, DC, 1997, US Government Printing Office. Modified from Gamma Biologicals, Houston, Tex.

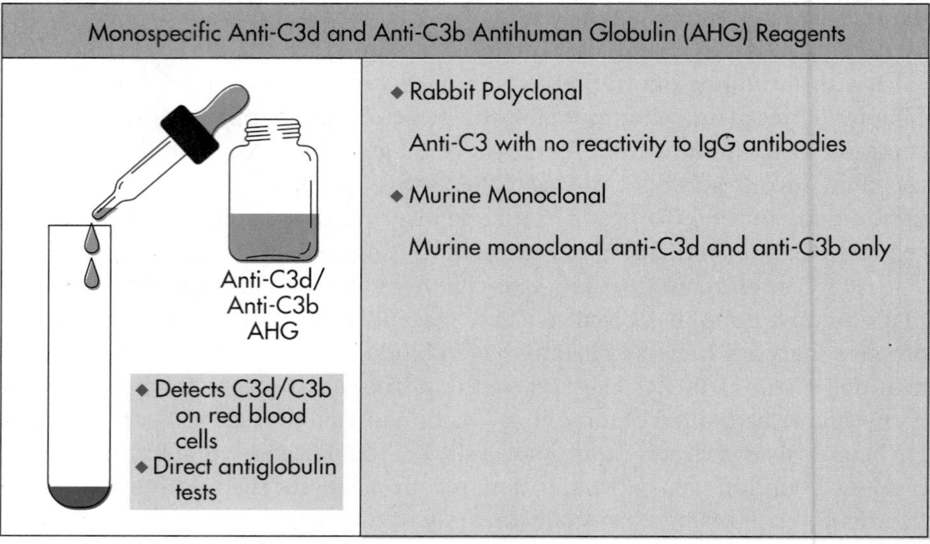

Fig. 2-9 Monospecific anti-3d and anti-C3 antihuman globulin reagents.
Text from *Code of federal regulations*, 21CFR 660.55, Washington, DC, 1997, US Government Printing Office. Modified from Gamma Biologicals, Houston, Tex.

Unfortunately, check cells cannot provide assurance that all causes of false negative reactions are controlled. The following are three potential reasons for a false negative result detected by the use of check cells in an antiglobulin test:

- Failure to add the antiglobulin reagent to the test
- Failure of the added antiglobulin reagent to react
- Failure to adequately wash red blood cells

REAGENT RED BLOOD CELLS

A_1 and B Cells for ABO Serum Testing

Testing a patient's serum or plasma with commercial group A_1 and group B red blood cells confirms the ABO typing performed on the patient's red blood cells. Known as ABO reverse grouping or back typing, this procedure detects ABO antibodies. Patients possess the antibody directed against the antigen of the ABO system that is lacking on their red blood cells. For example, patients with A antigen on their red blood cells (e.g., group A) possess the A antigen and lack the B antigen. These patients possess anti-B antibodies in their plasma. Therefore serum or plasma samples from group A individuals agglutinate with reagent B red blood cells but not with reagent A_1 red blood cells. Patients with the B antigen on their red blood cells (e.g., group B) possess the B antigen and lack the A antigen. These patients will possess anti-A antibodies in their plasma. Therefore serum or plasma samples from group B individuals agglutinate with reagent A_1 red blood cells but not with reagent B red blood cells. When compared with the red blood cell testing with commercial anti-A and anti-B reagents, the ABO antibody results provide an additional confirmation or check of the assigned ABO typing (Table 2-6).

Table 2-6 ABO Serum Testing (Reverse Grouping)

ABO blood group	A cells	B cells
A	0	+
B	+	0
AB	0	0
O	+	+

+, Agglutination; *0*, no agglutination.

Reagent red blood cells for serum testing are obtained from selected human donors and are manufactured in several optional packages. The most commonly used package consists of a two-vial set of A_1 and B red blood cells. Depending on the manufacturer, the red blood cell source may be obtained from either a single donor or a pool of several donors.

During the manufacturing process, all reagent red blood cells are washed to remove blood group antibodies and resuspended to a 2% to 5% concentration in a buffered preservative solution to minimize hemolysis and loss of antigenicity during the dating period. These red blood cell preparations are usually negative for the Rh antigens D, C, and E. Each reagent lot is tested to meet the FDA standards of specificity; however, no potency standard requirement exists for this reagent. Reagent red blood cells should not be used if the red blood cells darken in color, spontaneously agglutinate in the reagent vial, or exhibit significant hemolysis.[8]

Screening Cells

Screening cells are used in antibody screen tests. This procedure looks for antibodies with specificity to red blood cell antigens in patient and donor samples. Patients and donors may have preformed antibodies to red blood cell antigens as a result of exposure to foreign red blood cell antigens from previous transfusions or pregnancies. For transfusion purposes, the detection of these preformed red blood cell antibodies in patient and donor samples is an important step in the provision of red blood cell products. The reagent red blood cells are obtained from group O donor sources and are commercially available as two- or three-vial sets. Why are group O donors selected? Since the group O phenotype lacks A and B antigens, these red blood cells do not react with ABO antibodies present in patient or donor serum or plasma. Therefore serum or plasma from any ABO type may be used in the antibody screen test without interference from the ABO antibodies. Each vial in these sets represents the red blood cells harvested from a single donor. In addition, a product with pooled screening cells is commercially available and contains group O red blood cells derived from two donors in equal proportions.

According to AABB's *Standards for Blood Banks and Transfusion Services*, tests for antibodies performed on **recipient** specimens (e.g., those of a patient who may be receiving a transfusion) require unpooled screening cells.[7] Recipient testing must maximize sensitivity to detect the presence of weakly reactive antibodies. Since a pooled red blood cell reagent decreases the ability to detect a weakly reactive antibody, this reagent is not recommended for recipient samples. Pooled screening cells are acceptable in screening donors for red blood cell antibodies. Each lot of reagent screening cells arrives with an accompanying antigenic profile, or **antigram**, of each donor. Screening cells licensed by the FDA require an antigenic profile capable of detecting most clinically significant red blood cell antibodies. Blood group antigens that must be expressed on the screening cells include D, C, E, c, e, M, N, S, s, P_1, Le^a, Le^b, K, k, Fy^a, Fy^b, Jk^a, and Jk^b.[5] Diminished reagent reactivity may be observed as the screening cells approach the end of their dating period. Because of the danger of antigen deterioration, these screening cells should not be used beyond their expiration date.[9] Any signs of significant hemolysis, discoloration, or agglutination might indicate contamination.

Recipient: patient receiving the transfusion.

Antigram: profile of antigen typings of each donor used in the manufacturing of commercially supplied screening and panel cells.

Panel Cells

Red blood cell panels are required to determine the specificity of a red blood cell antibody in a blood banking procedure called antibody identification (discussed in Chapter 7). These reagent red blood cells possess the same sources as the

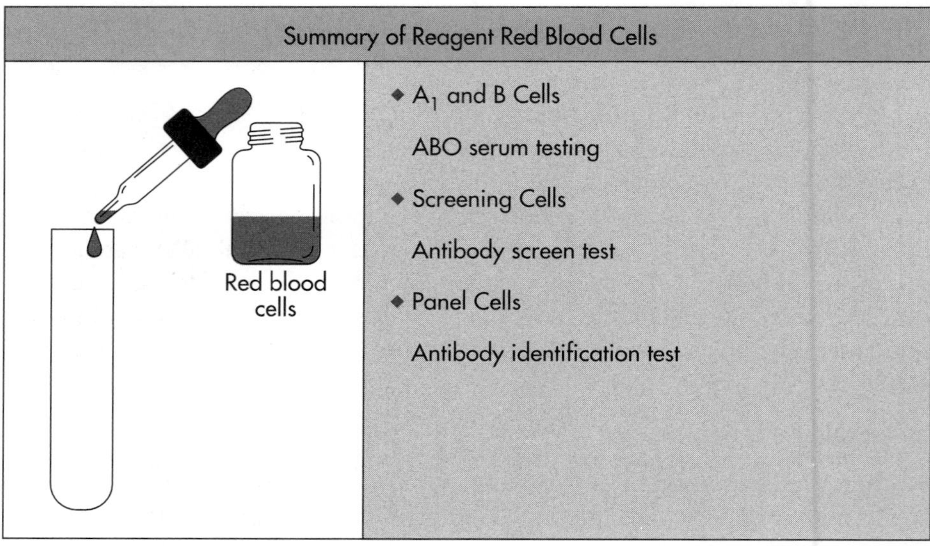

Fig. 2-10 Summary of reagent red blood cells.
Modified from Gamma Biologicals, Houston, Tex.

screening cells (individual group O donors). However, antibody identification panels are packaged in sets of 10 or more depending on the individual manufacturer. The selected donors for the identification panels possess the majority of the most frequently inherited red blood cell antigens. An antigenic profile of each donor is provided with each lot number of panel cells. A laboratory often will have several indated panels to help resolve antibody problems. Since panels are selected for problem resolution, the correct panel sheet and lot numbers must be verified when selected. Fig. 2-10 summarizes the various types of reagent red blood cells.

LECTINS

Lectins: plant extracts useful as blood banking reagents; they bind to carbohydrate portions of certain red blood cell antigens and agglutinate the red blood cells.

Lectins are useful alternatives to antisera for blood typing purposes in blood group serology. Some extracts of seeds known as lectins have specificity toward certain red blood cell antigens. These extracts contain proteins that behave in an identical manner to antibodies but are not immunoglobulin in nature. The lectins bind specifically to the carbohydrate determinants of certain red blood cell antigens with resultant agglutination. Although no antibodies exist in these reagents, lectins can be useful in identifying antigens present on patient or donor red blood cells. Table 2-7 reviews the major lectins used in blood group serology.

Table 2-7 Summary of Common Lectins in the Blood Bank

Lectin	Antigen specificity
Dolichos biflorus	A_1
Ulex europaeus	H
Vicia graminea	N
Iberis amara	M

OTHER METHODS OF DETECTING ANTIGEN-ANTIBODY REACTIONS

Blood bank reagents have been used in testing designed to detect agglutination in test tubes. Recent advances in technology have introduced other methods for detecting antigen-antibody reactions, such as placing the reagents mentioned in this chapter in gel-filled plastic cards and microtiter plates. This section presents a brief overview of these techniques.

Gel Technology Methods

Gel technology is a new and unique method introduced into the blood bank. Developed by Lapierre in 1985, the technology uses dextran acrylamide gel particles combined with diluent or reagent in prefilled plastic cards.[10] Each gel card contains six microtubes for six tests to allow for possible sample batching. The porous gel particles are spherical beads that function as a reaction medium and filter. They serve to trap red blood cell agglutinates and create a new way to observe agglutination endpoints. Anti-IgG cards are commercially available for performance of DATs and indirect antiglobulin tests (IATs) for antibody screening, antibody identification, and crossmatch procedures. ABO and Rh typing cards are also available.

The following outline illustrates the application of gel technology in antibody screening:

1. A measured volume of diluted screening cells is added to anti-IgG gel cards.
2. A measured volume of patient serum is then added to the gel card.
3. The gel card is incubated at 37° C for a predetermined time and centrifuged.
4. Following centrifugation, the test results are read and graded. No washing step is required for antiglobulin testing.

Larger agglutinates are trapped at the top of the gel microtubes and do not travel through the gel during the centrifugation process. Smaller agglutinates travel through the gel microtubes and may be trapped in either the top or bottom half of the microtubes. Unagglutinated screening cells travel unimpeded through the length of the microtube and form a pellet at the tip after centrifugation (Fig. 2-11).

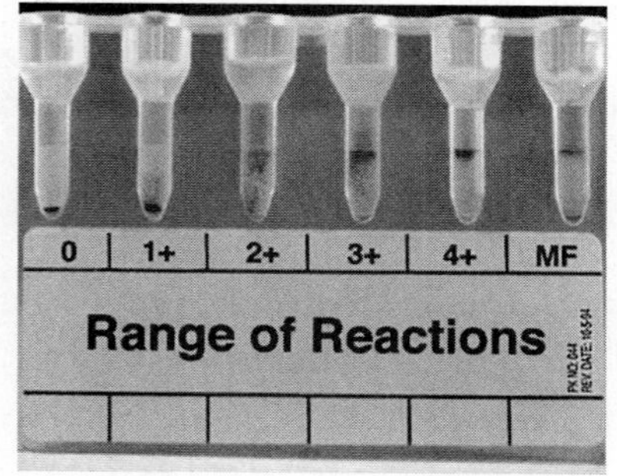

Fig. 2-11 Range of reactions in gel testing.

Courtesy Ortho Clinical Diagnostics, Raritan, NJ, and Micro Typing Systems, Pompano Beach, Fla.

Another variation of gel technology takes advantage of the principle of affinity chromatography.[11] This technology is based on the adherence of red blood cells to an immunologically active matrix. In this system, recombinant protein G with a high affinity and specificity for IgG antibodies is bound to agarose in a microcolumn format. Red blood cells sensitized with IgG adhere to the immunoreactive matrix and form a band of red blood cells on top of the microcolumn upon centrifugation. Red blood cells with no attached IgG collect at the bottom of the microcolumn after centrifugation.

Microplate Testing Methods

Since the late 1960s microplate methods have been used for routine processing in blood donor centers. A microtiter plate with 96 wells serves as the substituted test tubes to which the principles of blood banking are applied. The microplate technique can be adapted to red blood cell antigen testing or serum testing for antibody detection. Small quantities of red blood cells and antisera are added to the microtiter wells followed by centrifugation of the microtiter plates. The cell buttons are resuspended by manually tapping the plate or with the aid of a mechanical shaker. A concentrated button of red blood cells is indicative of antigen-antibody reactions whereas the red blood cells in a negative result are dispersed throughout the well. Automated photometric devices are available to read and interpret the reactions on the plates. Alternatively, the microtiter plates may be observed for a streaming pattern of red blood cells when the plate is placed on an angle.[5]

Solid-Phase Red Blood Cell Adherence Methods

Another serologic method for the blood bank is solid-phase red blood cell adherence.[12] Commercial solid-phase test procedures have been available for the

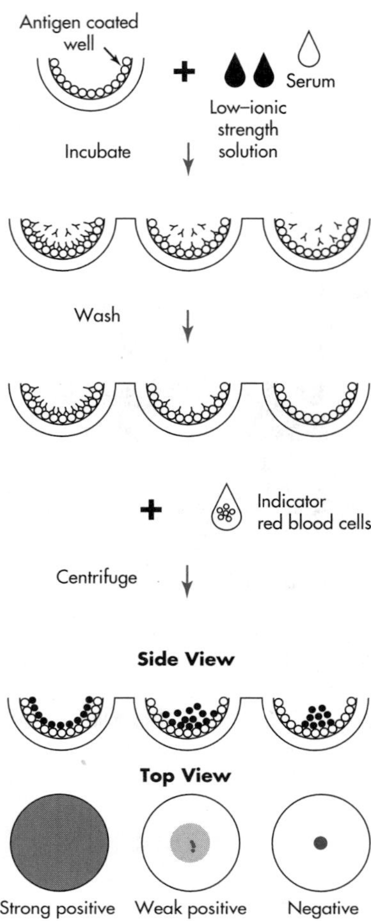

Fig. 2-12 Solid-phase red blood cell adherence procedure.
Courtesy Immucor, Norcross, Ga.

detection of both red blood cell and platelet antibodies since the late 1980s. An overview of the procedure for red blood cell antibody detection follows:

1. Red blood cell membranes (screening cells) are bound to the surface of polystyrene microtiter plates.
2. When patient or donor serum is added to these wells, the red blood cell membranes capture IgG antibodies during an incubation phase.
3. The plates are washed to remove unbound antibodies.
4. Indicator cells (anti-IgG–coated red blood cells) are added to the wells.
5. The microtiter plates are centrifuged, thus bringing indicator cells in contact with bound antibody.

A negative reaction appears as a red blood cell button on the bottom of the wells. A positive reaction is indicated by the attachment of indicator cells to the sides and bottom of the wells. The red blood cells are said to have adhered to the wells (Fig. 2-12).

CHAPTER SUMMARY

1. The reagents used in the immunohematology laboratory provide the tools to detect antigen-antibody reactions. Principles of routine testing are based on the combination of a source of antigen and a source of antibody in a test environment. Agglutination or hemolysis is indicative of antigen-antibody recognition.
2. Blood banking reagents are categorized into four basic groups:
   a. Reagent red blood cells that possess antigens of known specificity
   b. Antisera that possess antibodies of known specificity
   c. Antiglobulin reagents that detect IgG and complement attachment to red blood cells
   d. Potentiators that enhance the detection of antibodies
3. The purposes of reagents used in the immunohematology laboratory are to:
   a. Determine the ABO/Rh type of donors and patients
   b. Detect antibodies produced by patients or donors that have been exposed to red blood cells through transfusion or pregnancy
   c. Identify the specificity of antibodies detected in the antibody screen procedure
   d. Determine the presence or absence of additional antigens on the red blood cells in addition to the A, B, and D antigens
   e. Perform crossmatches to evaluate serologic compatibility of donor and patient before transfusion
4. An awareness of the proper use and limitations of reagents enhances the ability of laboratory personnel to provide accurate interpretations of results generated in testing and ultimately affects overall transfusion safety.

CRITICAL THINKING EXERCISES

◆ ***EXERCISE 2-1***

The quality control procedure for commercial anti-A and anti-B is performed by reacting each antiserum with A_1 and B cells. The results of the daily quality control for ABO reagents for your facility are represented in the chart at the top of page 53. Do the quality control results meet acceptable performance criteria, or are they unacceptable for the commercial antisera? Discuss your answer.

Antisera	Antisera with Reverse Cells	
	A_1 Cells	B Cells
Anti-A	3+	0
Anti-B	0	3+

◆ ***EXERCISE 2-2***

The results of anti-D quality control for the past week are presented in the following chart. What are the implications of these results regarding reagent potency and specificity?

Days	Anti-D Quality Control for Red Blood Cells	
	D-positive	D-negative
Day 1	3+	0
Day 2	3+	0
Day 3	2+	0
Day 4	2+	0
Day 5	1+	0

◆ ***EXERCISE 2-3***

Using several product inserts as resources, what are the visible signs of possible reagent deterioration in both reagent red blood cells and antisera outlined by the manufacturers?

◆ ***EXERCISE 2-4***

Using a product insert for a commercial source of antisera, identify the manufacturer's limitations placed on the product.

◆ ***EXERCISE 2-5***

Read a reagent quality control procedure from a transfusion service and identify the criteria for acceptable performance for each reagent and the action plan if reagents do not meet acceptable criteria.

STUDY QUESTIONS

1. What is the most common reason for a positive Rh control tube when using a high-protein anti-D reagent?
   a. bacterial contamination
   b. hypotonic saline solution
   c. positive DAT
   d. overreading of agglutination

2. Monospecific AHG reagents:
   a. increase the dielectric constant in vitro
   b. contain either anti-IgG or anti-C3 antibody specificities
   c. are not useful in identifying the protein causing a positive DAT
   d. contain human IgG or complement molecules

3. You have added Coombs' control cells (check cells) after performing an IAT on a patient. You observe agglutination in the tube. What situation was NOT controlled for in testing by adding these check cells?
   a. addition of patient serum
   b. addition of AHG reagent
   c. adequate washing of cell suspension
   d. potency of AHG reagent

4. Part of the daily quality control in the blood bank laboratory is the testing of reagent antisera with corresponding antigen-positive and antigen-negative red blood cells. What does this procedure ensure?
   a. antibody class
   b. antibody titer
   c. antibody specificity
   d. antibody sensitivity

5. Group O red blood cells are used as a source for commercial screening cells because:
   a. anti-A is detected using group O cells
   b. anti-D reacts with most group O cells
   c. weak subgroups of A react with group O cells
   d. ABO antibodies do not react with group O cells

6. Information regarding reagent limitations is located in the:
   a. standard operating procedures
   b. blood bank computer system
   c. product inserts
   d. product catalogs

7. What regulatory agency provides licensure for blood banking reagents?
   a. American Association of Blood Banks
   b. Food and Drug Administration
   c. American Red Cross
   d. College of American Pathologists

8. What antibodies are present in polyspecific AHG reagent?
   a. anti-IgG
   b. IgG and C3
   c. anti-IgG and anti-C3
   d. anti-C3

9. In which source are the regulations regarding the manufacturing of blood banking reagents published?
   a. *Code of Federal Regulations*
   b. AABB *Standards for Blood Banks and Transfusion Services*
   c. AABB *Technical Manual*
   d. AABB *Accreditation Requirements Manual*

10. After the addition of monoclonal-based anti-D to a patient's red blood cell suspension, agglutination was observed. What is the interpretation of this result?
    a. patient is D-negative
    b. patient is D-positive
    c. cannot interpret the test
    d. invalid result

11. What reagent would be selected to detect the presence of unexpected red blood cell antibodies in a patient's serum sample?
    a. A_1 and B cells
    b. panel cells
    c. Coombs' control cells
    d. screening cells

12. Select the method that uses the principle of sieving to separate larger agglutinates from smaller agglutinates in antigen-antibody reactions.
    a. gel technology
    b. solid phase adherence
    c. microplate
    d. none of the above

13. To determine the presence of a red blood cell antigen in a patient sample, what source of antibody is selected?
    a. commercial reagent red blood cells
    b. commercial antisera
    c. patient serum
    d. patient plasma

14. To determine the presence of a red blood cell antibody in a patient sample, what source of antigen is selected?
    a. commercial reagent red blood cells
    b. commercial antisera
    c. patient serum
    d. patient's red blood cells

15. What reagents are derived from plant extracts?
    a. panel cells
    b. commercial anti-B
    c. lectins
    d. antiglobulin reagents

REFERENCES

1. Food and Drug Administration: *Code of federal regulations,* 21 CFR 211-800, Washington, DC, 1996, US Government Printing Office.
2. Sazama K: *Accreditation requirements manual,* ed 6, Bethesda, Md, 1995, American Association of Blood Banks.
3. Lomas-Francis C: *The potential of monoclonal antibodies to Rh, MNS, and other blood group antigens: the compendium,* Arlington, Va, 1997, American Association of Blood Banks.
4. Walker PS: *Using FDA-approved monoclonal reagents: the compendium,* Arlington, Va, 1997, American Association of Blood Banks.
5. Vengelen-Tyler V, editor: *Technical manual,* ed 12, Bethesda, Md, 1996, American Association of Blood Banks.
6. Beck ML, Kirkegaard JR: Annotation—monoclonal ABO blood grouping reagents: a decade later, *Immunohematology* 11:67, 1995.
7. Mentitove JE, editor: *Standards for blood banks and transfusion services,* ed 18, Bethesda, Md, 1997, American Association of Blood Banks.
8. *Referencells,* Product Insert (rev), Norcross, Ga, 1989, Immucor.
9. *Reagent red cells for the detection of unexpected antibodies,* Product Insert (rev), Houston, Tex, 1996, Gamma Biologicals.
10. Lapierre Y, Rigal D, Adam J, et al: The gel test: a new way to detect red blood cell antigen-antibody reactions, *Transfusion* 30:109, 1990.
11. Champagne K, Spruell P, Chen J, et al: Comparison of affinity column technology and LISS tube tests, *Immunohematology* 14:149, 1998.
12. Plapp FV, Rachel JM, Beck ML, et al: Blood antigens and antibodies: solid phase adherence assays, *Lab Med* 22:39, 1984.

SUGGESTED READINGS

Harmening D: *Modern blood banking and transfusion practices,* ed 4, Philadelphia, 1999, FA Davis.

Issitt PD, Anstee DL: *Applied blood group serology,* ed 4, Durham, NC, 1998, Montgomery Scientific Publications.

3 GENETIC PRINCIPLES IN BLOOD BANKING

Kathy D. Blaney
William W. Safranek

CHAPTER OUTLINE

LEARNING OBJECTIVES

Upon completion of this chapter, the reader should be able to:

1. Define the term *blood group system* with regard to genetic terms.
2. Differentiate *phenotype* from *genotype*.
3. Define the following terms: gene, allele, haplotype, and polymorphic.
4. Distinguish *homozygous* from *heterozygous* and provide an example using blood group system alleles.
5. Define the *dosage effect* and explain its significance in testing.
6. Explain the difference between *cis* and *trans* and their effect on gene interactions.
7. Differentiate among recessive, dominant, and codominant inheritance.
8. Explain phenotype frequency and how it is used to find compatible red blood cell units.
9. Describe the application of the Hardy-Weinberg law in population genetics.
10. Explain the Mendelian Laws of independent assortment and independent segregation and how they apply to blood group antigen inheritance.
11. Define the terms *linkage* and *crossing over* and explain how they affect independent assortment.
12. Discuss the effects of suppressor genes and amorphic genes.
13. Differentiate direct and indirect exclusion in parentage testing.
14. Compare and contrast the polymerase chain reaction and restriction fragment length polymorphism molecular testing methods.
15. List applications of molecular testing methods to the field of blood banking.

The concept of an antigen as a molecule that can elicit an immune response was introduced in Chapter 1. In the study of immunohematology the antigens of interest are part of the red blood cell membrane. These antigens are inherited characteristics or traits categorized into **blood group systems** based on their genetic and serologic properties.

Blood group systems: groups of antigens on the red blood cell membrane that share related serologic properties and genetic patterns of inheritance.

The study of blood group systems requires an understanding of certain genetic principles and terminology. What makes each blood group system unique are the structure and location of the antigens present on the red blood cells, the antibodies they elicit, and the genetic control of antigen expression. Since these properties can be demonstrated by serologic and molecular genetic methods, each blood group system is said to be serologically and genetically defined. Classification of some blood group systems has been modified because of enhanced knowledge regarding the molecular structure of the genes producing the antigens.

In later chapters describing the blood group systems the reader will be introduced to the specific genetic pathways that create each antigen. In some systems, such as the Rh blood group system, the gene directly encodes a protein on the red blood cell, which is recognized by the immune system as an Rh antigen. With other blood group systems several interacting genes encode a particular antigen on the red blood cell. For example, the expression of the ABO antigens requires the interaction of the *ABO, Hh,* and *Se* genes. Appreciating that each blood group system is the product of a gene or group of genes assists in their classification and further enhances the understanding of their related serologic properties.

This section includes a review of molecular genetics that apply to the field of immunohematology. Molecular genetics have enhanced the understanding of the molecular basis of blood group antigens, provided more sensitive methods for viral antigen testing in donors, and contributed to more accurate paternity and forensic analysis. This section describes the procedures for deoxyribonucleic acid (DNA) testing used in research and clinical diagnostic testing.

BLOOD GROUP GENETICS

Genetic Terminology

Genes are units of inheritance that encode certain traits or visible characteristics. Genetic information is carried on double strands of DNA known as **chromosomes**. Humans have 23 pairs of chromosomes: 22 pairs of autosomes and one pair of sex chromosomes.

Chromosomes: structures within the nucleus that contain DNA.

Cell division allows the genetic material in cells to be replicated so that identical chromosomes can be transmitted to the daughter cells. This occurs during a process called **mitosis** in somatic cells and through **meiosis** in gametes.

Mitosis: cell division in somatic cells that results in the same number of chromosomes.

Meiosis: cell division in gametes that results in half the number of chromosomes present in somatic cells.

Before the knowledge of genes and DNA, the inheritance patterns of certain detectable traits were observed, and theories of inheritance were established. These theories are applicable to the study of blood group genetics. In the following section genetic terms are described as they pertain to red blood cell antigen inheritance patterns and as products of specific genes.

Phenotype versus Genotype

Serologic testing determines the presence or absence of antigens on the red blood cells. The **phenotype**, or the physical expression of inherited traits, is determined

Phenotype: observable expression of inherited traits.

by reacting red blood cells with known antisera and observing for the presence or absence of hemagglutination. Reagents used for this purpose were described in the preceding chapter. For example, testing cells with anti-A or anti-B reagents can determine if a person has the A or B antigen. If neither anti-A nor anti-B demonstrates agglutination, the cells are classified as type O. This determination is called the phenotype.

Genotype: actual genetic makeup; determined by family studies.

The **genotype,** or the actual genes inherited from each parent, can only be inferred from the phenotype. Family studies are required to determine the actual genotype. For example, if an individual's phenotype is *A*, the genotype may be *A/A* or *A/O*. *A/A* indicates that both parents contributed the *A* gene. The *A/O* genotype indicates that one parent contributed the *A* gene and the other contributed the *O* gene. Since the *O* gene has no detectable product, only the A antigen is expressed when the *A/O* genotype is inherited. If the *A/O* individual has a type O child, it becomes evident that the individual carried the *O* gene. Thus two people with group A red blood cells have the same phenotype but can have different genotypes.

Predicting the genotype from the phenotype is important in paternity studies or when determining a fetus's probable phenotype. In text the gene is italicized to differentiate it from the phenotype or antigen.

Pedigree chart: diagrammatic method of illustrating the inheritance patterns of traits in a family study.
Punnett square: square used to calculate the frequencies of different genotypes and phenotypes among the offspring of a cross.

Pedigree Charts and the Punnett Square

Examination of family history is an important component in the investigation of inheritance patterns. A **pedigree chart** allows the important elements of the patterns to become more visibly apparent, and it can illustrate the difference between genotype and phenotype. Fig. 3-1 illustrates and defines some of the standard symbols used to denote sex, mating, zygosity, affected individuals, and carrier status. Figs. 3-2 and 3-3 are examples of genotypes and phenotypes for the ABO system and another blood group system, the MNS system. The MNS system is a collection of antigens expressed on the red blood cell membrane that are encoded by genes unrelated to the ABO genes. The pedigree chart demonstrates the inheritance patterns of each family member.

A **Punnett square** illustrates the probabilities of phenotypes from known or inferred genotypes. It visually portrays the potential offspring's genotypes or the

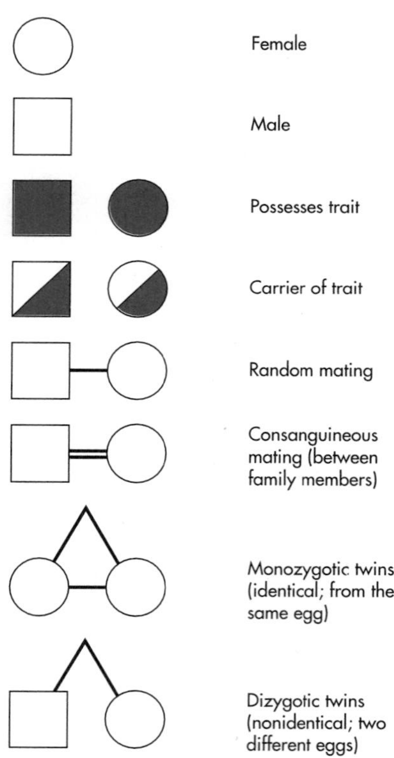

Fig. 3-1 Pedigree chart symbols.

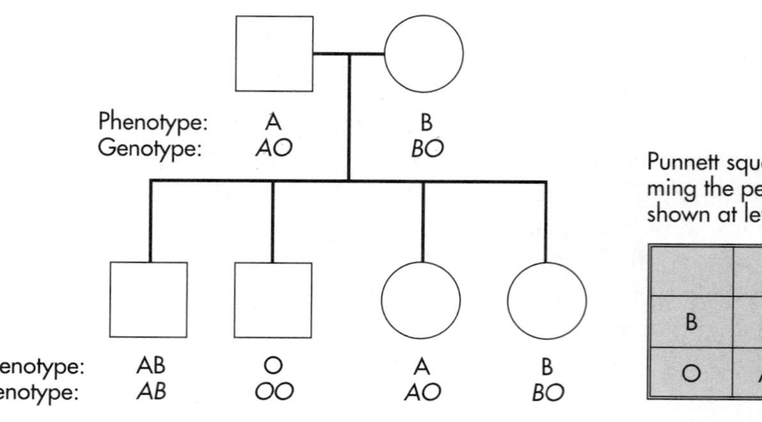

	A	O
B	AB	BO
O	AO	OO

Fig. 3-2 Pedigree chart: ABO inheritance patterns.

probable genotypes of the parents. Fig. 3-4 shows possible ABO system gene combinations through the use of Punnett squares. From this figure it would be easy to determine that two group A parents can have a group O child. The geneticist could also illustrate that the parents of an AB child can be A, B, or AB, but not group O.

Genes, Alleles, and Polymorphism

Genes, the basic units of inheritance on a chromosome, are located in specific places called **genetic loci**. Several different forms of a gene, called **alleles**, may exist for each locus (Fig. 3-5). For example, *A, B,* and *O* are alleles on the *ABO* gene locus. The term **antithetical**, meaning *opposite*, is sometimes used when referring to antigens produced by allelic genes. For example, the Kp^a antigen is antithetical to the Kp^b antigen. The term **polymorphic** refers to having two or more alleles at a given locus, as with the ABO blood group system. Some blood group systems are more polymorphic than others; in other words, many more alleles exist at a given locus. The Rh system is highly polymorphic compared with the ABO system because of the greater number of alleles. The frequency of a particular phenotype in a population depends on how polymorphic a blood group system is. A highly polymorphic system makes it less likely to find two identical individuals. An example of a highly polymorphic system is one involving the genes that encode the human leukocyte antigens (HLAs). Since bone marrow and organ transplants require HLA matching, the HLA polymorphism contributes to the challenge of finding suitable donors. If several polymorphic systems are used to determine a phenotype of an individual, finding two identical individuals becomes increasingly difficult. For this reason the blood group system antigens and the HLA system are useful in excluding or predicting parentage in paternity studies.

Inheritance Patterns

In most cases blood group antigens are inherited with **codominant** expression, or the equal expression of both inherited alleles. The product of each allele can be identified when inherited as a codominant trait. If one parent passed on an *A* gene and the other parent passed on a *B* gene, both the A and B antigens would be

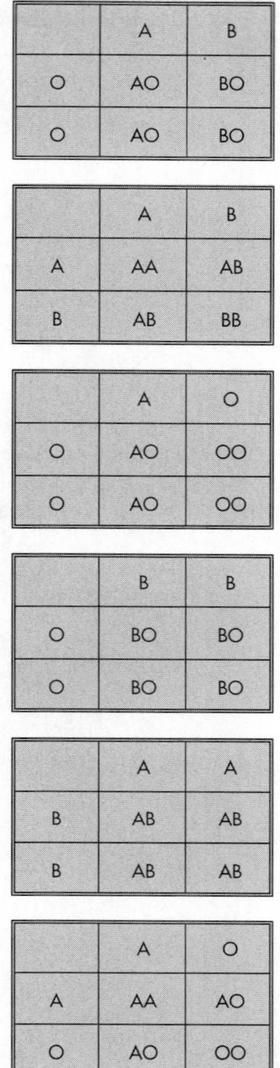

	A	B
O	AO	BO
O	AO	BO

	A	B
A	AA	AB
B	AB	BB

	A	O
O	AO	OO
O	AO	OO

	B	B
O	BO	BO
O	BO	BO

	A	A
B	AB	AB
B	AB	AB

	A	O
A	AA	AO
O	AO	OO

Fig. 3-4 Punnett squares showing ABO inheritance.

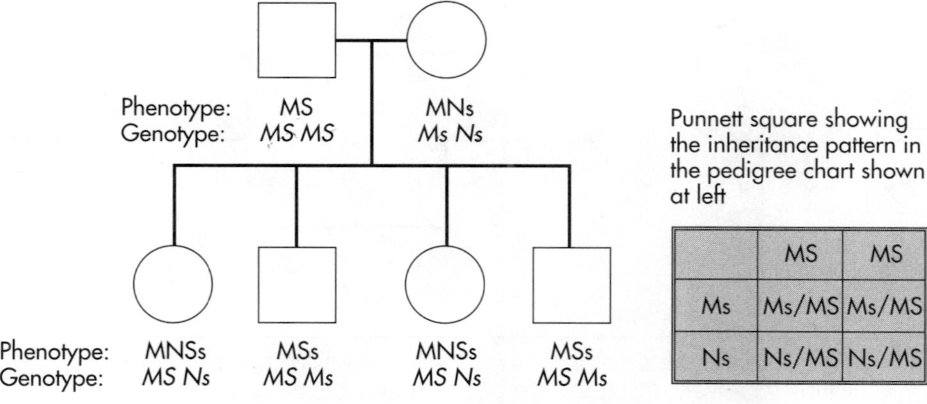

Fig. 3-3 Pedigree chart: MNS inheritance patterns.

Gene: basic unit of inheritance on a chromosome.
Genetic loci: sites of a gene on a chromosome.
Alleles: alternate forms of a gene at a given locus.
Antithetical: opposite allele.
Polymorphic: genetic system that expresses two or more phenotypes.
Codominant: equal expression of two different inherited alleles.

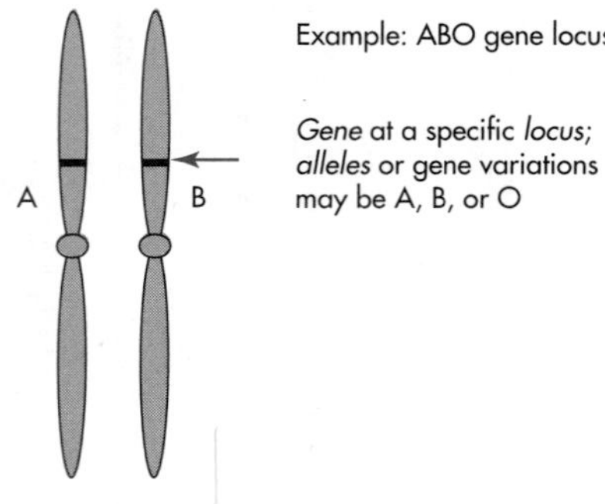

Fig. 3-5 Terminology.

Recessive: gene product expressed only when inherited by both parents.
Dominant: gene product expressed over another gene.
Amorphic: describes a gene that does not express a detectable product.

expressed equally on the red blood cells. **Recessive** or **dominant** inheritance patterns are uncommon to blood group system genetics. A recessive inheritance would require that the same allele from both parents be inherited to demonstrate the trait, whereas a dominant expression would require only one form of the allele to express the trait. Describing traits as dominant and recessive also depends on the method used to detect the product of the gene. It would appear that the *O* gene is recessive, since it is expressed only when both parents contribute the *O* allele. The product of an *O* gene, however, does not affect the membrane proteins.[1] Its expression is termed **amorphic** rather than recessive. Dominant, recessive, and codominant traits are illustrated and summarized in Table 3-1 and Fig. 3-6.

Table 3-1 Characteristics of Patterns of Inheritance

INHERITANCE PATTERN	CHARACTERISTIC
Autosomal dominant	The trait appears whenever the allele is present; can be found in each generation if the allele is present in a family; equal frequency in males and females
Autosomal recessive	Must be homozygous for the alleles to express the trait; equal frequency in males and females; both parents who do not express the trait must be "carriers" or heterozygous for the recessive allele
Sex-linked dominant	Absence of father-to-son transmission of the trait; will be expressed if passed from father to daughter; an example includes the Xg^a blood group system
Sex-linked recessive	Males inherit the trait from carrier mothers; children of an affected male and a female who lacks the allele will have sons who are normal and daughters who are carriers; trait is exhibited almost exclusively in males; an example is hemophilia A
Codominant	Heterozygotes express the product of both alleles; an example is the inheritance of the blood group systems

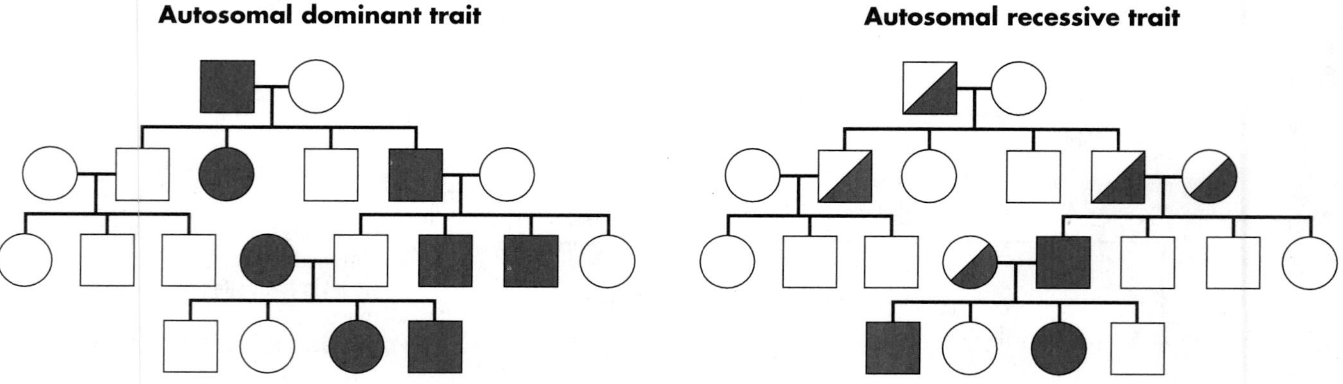

Fig. 3-6 Inheritance patterns. The autosomal dominant trait can be found in each generation if the allele is present. In the autosomal recessive trait two carriers (heterozygous) can pass on the trait. To express the trait in successive generations, the mating of two recessive individuals or a recessive and a carrier must occur.

Mendelian Principles

Gregor Mendel observed certain hereditary patterns in his early genetic experiments that have subsequently been applied to the study of blood group system genetics. His law of **independent segregation** refers to the transmission of a trait in a predictable fashion from one generation to the next.[2] This concept was described previously with the Punnett square by using the ABO blood group system genes. It illustrates that each parent has a pair of genes for a particular trait, either of which can be transmitted to the next generation. The genes "segregate" and allow only one gene from each parent to be passed on to each child. Another important law, **independent assortment**, is demonstrated by the fact that blood group antigens, inherited on different chromosomes, are expressed separately and discretely. Fig. 3-7 illustrates that the ABO blood group system genes, located on chromosome 1, and the Kell blood group system genes, located on chromosome 7, are inherited independent of each other.

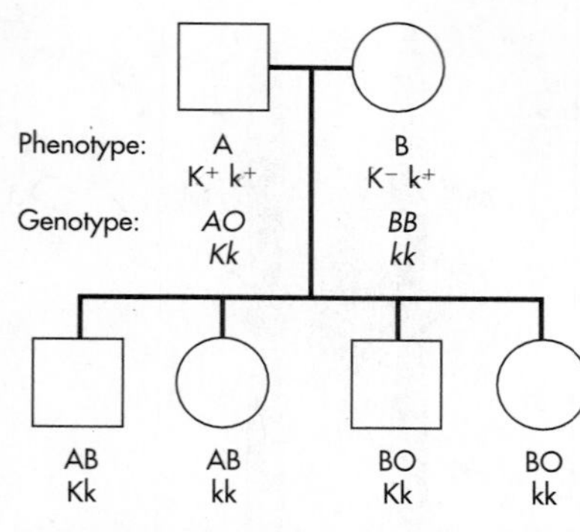

Fig. 3-7 Independent assortment. The ABO system genes are sorted independently from the Kell system genes.

Chromosomal Assignment

The genetic loci of most of the blood group system genes have been determined. Table 3-2 shows the chromosomal assignment for common blood group systems.[1] Most of the blood group–associated genes are on **autosomes**, with a few exceptions of linkage to sex chromosomes in the Xg[a] and Xk blood group systems.

Table 3-2 Blood Group System Chromosomal Assignment of Genes

Blood Group System	Chromosome
Rh	1
Duffy	1
Gerbich	2
MNS	4
Chido/Rodgers	6
Kell	7
ABO	9
Diego	17
Kidd	18
Lewis	19
Landsteiner-Wiener	19
Lutheran	19
Hh	19
P	22

Heterozygosity and Homozygosity

An individual whose genotype is made up of identical genes, such as *AA*, *BB*, or *OO*, is called **homozygous**. An individual who has inherited different alleles from each parent, such as *AO*, *AB*, or *BO*, is called **heterozygous** (Fig. 3-8).

In serologic testing the concept of homozygous and heterozygous inheritance is important with some blood group antigens. As discussed in the previous chapters, agglutination reactions vary in strength. This variation can be due to the strength of the antibody or the density of the antigens on the red blood cells. When antigen density varies between cells of different individuals, it is often due to the inheritance of the antigen expression. An individual who inherits different blood group system alleles from each parent (Kk) has a "single dose" of that antigen on the red blood cells. The agglutination reaction may demonstrate a weaker antigenic expression, or lower antigen density, on the red blood cells,. If the same allele was inherited from both parents (*KK* or *kk*), a stronger red blood cell antigen would be apparent because a "double dose" of the K or k antigen was present on the red blood cells. The variation in antigen expression because of the number of alleles present is called the **dosage effect** (Table 3-3). Not all blood group system antigens demonstrate the dosage effect.

Independent segregation: passing of one gene from each parent to the offspring.
Independent assortment: random behavior of genes on separate chromosomes during meiosis that results in a mixture of genetic material in the offspring.
Autosomes: chromosomes other than the sex chromosomes.
Homozygous: two alleles for a given trait are identical.
Heterozygous: two alleles for a given trait are different.
Dosage effect: stronger agglutination when a red blood cell antigen is expressed from homozygous genes.

Table 3-3 Dosage Effect

GENOTYPE	DOSAGE EFFECT ON ANTIGEN EXPRESSION
Homozygous: MM	Red blood cells tested with anti-M: 4+
Heterozygous: MN	Red blood cells tested with anti-M: 2+

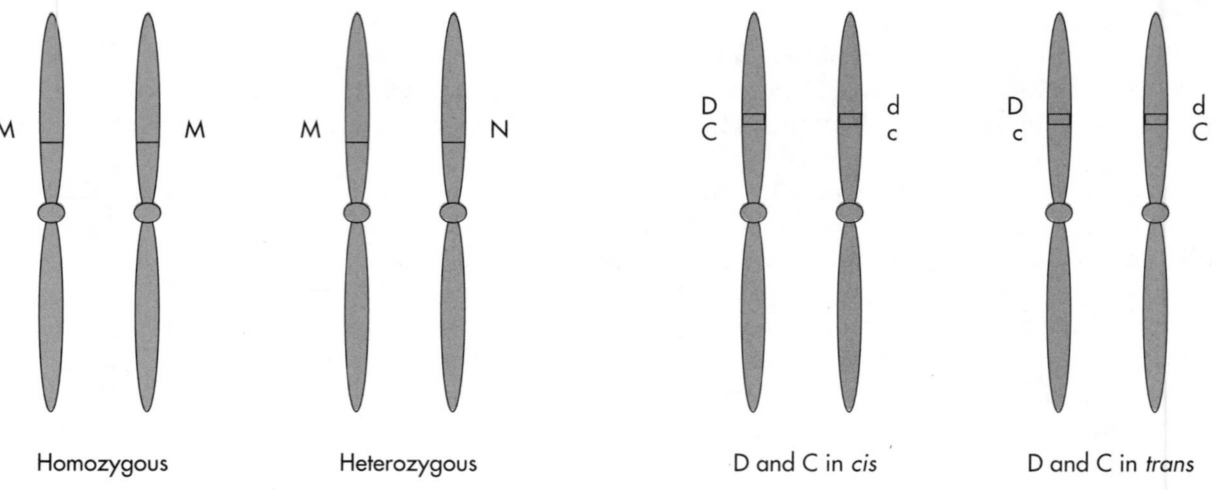

Fig. 3-8 Homozygosity and heterozygosity.

Fig. 3-9 *Cis* and *trans* position genes.

Cis: two or more genes on the same chromosome of a homologous pair.
Trans: genes inherited on opposite chromosomes of a homologous pair.
Linked: when two genes are inherited together by being very close on a chromosome.
Haplotype: linked set of genes inherited together because of their close proximity on a chromosome.
Linkage disequilibrium: occurrence of a set of genes inherited together more often than would be expected by chance.

Genetic Interaction

Sometimes genes can interact with each other depending on whether they are inherited on the same chromosome ***(cis)*** or on the opposite chromosome ***(trans)***. This interaction may weaken the expression of one of the antigens encoded by the genes. For example, the *C* and *D* genes of the Rh system are inherited on different genetic loci. When *C* is inherited in *trans* to *D*, it will weaken the D antigen expression on the red blood cell (Fig. 3-9).

Linkage and Haplotypes

Gregor Mendel described the principle of independent assortment from experiments with plant hybridization. His theories were based on statistical distributions of various characteristics of pea plants. He observed that many traits are inherited independent of each other, and the statistical probability that these traits do not occur together confirmed this. It is now understood that independent assortment is most often observed with traits inherited on different chromosomes.

In some blood group systems the antigens are encoded by two or more genes on the same chromosome. When genes are very close together, they are inherited from each parent as a unit. Genes that are so close together on a chromosome that they are inherited as a unit are **linked**. Independent assortment does not occur when genes are linked. These gene units are called **haplotypes**. For example, in the MNSs blood group system, *M* and *N* are alleles on one gene while *S* and *s* are alleles on another gene. Since the genes are close, they are inherited as haplotypes: *MS, Ms, NS,* or *Ns* (Fig. 3-10). Haplotypes occur in the population at a different frequency than would be expected if the genes were not linked. **Linkage disequilibrium** refers to the phenomenon of antigens occurring at a different frequency in the population depending on whether they were inherited by linked or unlinked genes. In other words, if the *M* and *S* gene were not linked, the expected frequency of the M and S antigen in the population would be 17%, according to calculated frequency probabilities.[2] Because of linkage disequilibrium the observed frequency of the MS haplotype is actually 24%.[2]

M
S
N
s
Phenotype: MNSs
Genotype: *MS, Ns*

Fig. 3-10 Haplotypes.

Linkage between the A and B loci in the HLA system occurs because these genetic loci are very close. The HLA genes are inherited as haplotypes of one A and one B locus. Each sibling shares at least one haplotype with the other and has one from each parent. Fig. 3-11 illustrates this concept. For this reason siblings are likely matches when organ or bone marrow transplants are required.

Crossing over: exchange of genetic material during meiosis between paired chromosomes.
Suppressor genes: genes that suppress the expression of another gene.

Crossing Over

Another exception to Mendel's law of independent assortment occurs if two genes on the same chromosome recombine. **Crossing over** is the exchange of genetic material during meiosis after the chromosome pairs have replicated (Fig. 3-12). The resulting genes are exchanged during this process but not lost. The recombination results in two new and different chromosomes. Crossing over can be observed with genes on the same chromosome but does not usually occur when the genes are close together. Since the genes expressing blood group systems are either close (linked) or on different chromosomes, crossing over rarely affects the inheritance of the blood group system. Crossover frequencies are used to map the relative locations of genes on a chromosome because the closer the genes, the rarer the possibility for the genes to be separated. The low rate of crossing over has permitted the use of blood group determinations as a reliable method of paternity testing.

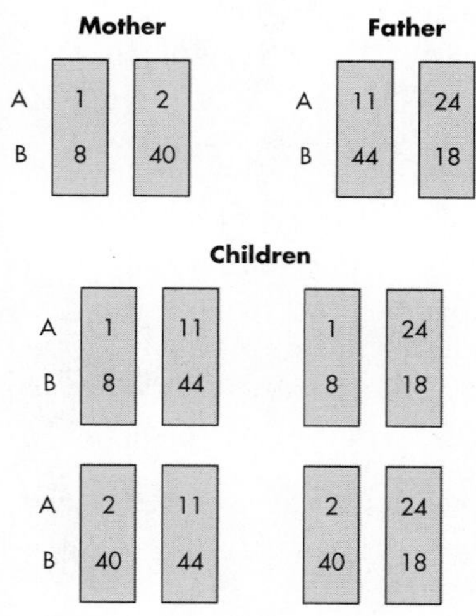

Fig. 3-11 Linkage in the HLA system. Inheritance of the A and B genes in the HLA system occurs as a set or a haplotype.

Silent Genes

In some blood group systems genes do not produce a detectable antigen product. These "silent" genes are called amorphs. Amorphs can result in an unusual phenotype if passed on by both parents (Table 3-4). The phenotypes are often called "null" types because expressions of the blood group system antigens are not apparent. For example, an Rh_{null} individual lacks the presence of all Rh system antigens. Rare genes must be inherited from both parents (homozygous) to produce a null phenotype. For this reason null types caused by amorphic genes are rare.

Unusual phenotypes may also result from the action of **suppressor**, or regulator, **genes**. These genes act to inhibit the expression of another gene and, like amorph genes, must be inherited in the homozygous state to create this effect. The occurrence of suppressor genes that affects the blood group antigen expression is rare. Null phenotypes therefore can be a result of either an amorphic or a suppressor gene.

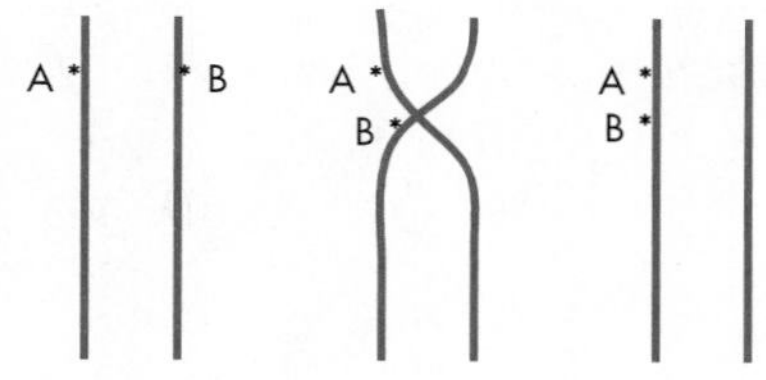

Fig. 3-12 Unequal crossing over during meiosis.

POPULATION GENETICS

Population genetics is the statistical application of genetic principles to determine genotype and phenotype occurrence, which is dependent on the gene frequency.[3] Two types of calculations are applicable in the study of blood group population genetics. The first calculation involves combined phenotype frequencies, and the second involves gene or allele frequency estimates.

Table 3-4 Amorphs and Suppressor Genes in Blood Groups

Blood Group System	Amorph/ Regulator Gene	Phenotype When Homozygous
H	*h*	Bombay
Rh	*r* / *X°r*	Rh null
Kell	*K°*	Kell null
Lutheran	*Lu* / *In(Lu)*	Lu(a-b-)
Kidd	*Jk*	Jk(a-b-)
Duffy	*Fy*	Fy(a-b-)

Combined Phenotype Calculations

Determining the frequency of a particular phenotype in the population enables finding a unit of red blood cells with certain antigen characteristics. For example, patients with multiple antibodies may require red blood cells that are negative for several different antigens. The calculation of combined phenotype frequencies provides an estimate of the number of units that may need to be tested to find the unit with the desired antigens.

The frequency of multiple traits inherited independently is calculated by multiplying the frequency of each trait. If a patient produced red blood cell antibodies from exposure to previous transfusions or pregnancies, red blood cells that were negative for the corresponding antibodies would be required for transfusion. For example, if a patient produced antibodies such as anti-C, anti-E, and anti-S, red blood cell units that are negative for the antigens C, E, and S would be required for transfusion. The percentage of donors negative for the individual antigens is expressed as a decimal point and then multiplied.

70% C positive	30% C negative:	= 0.30
30% E positive	70% E negative	= 0.70
55% S positive	45% S negative	= 0.45

$$0.30 \times 0.70 \times 0.45 = 0.0945 \text{ or } 0.10$$

Therefore 10% of the population, or 1 in 10 units of red blood cells, is negative for the combined antigens. The percentages used are established antigen frequencies and can be found in Chapter 6, the AABB *Technical Manual*, and package inserts for the corresponding antisera. Antigen frequencies vary with race. The predominant race found in the donor population for the area should be used when calculating antigen frequencies. The frequency of an antigen in the population is the occurrence of the positive phenotype. Subtracting the frequency from 100 yields the percentage that is negative. Another example follows: If a patient has an anti-Fy^a, an anti-Jk^b, and an anti-K, how many units must be tested to find 2 units of the appropriate phenotype?

66% Fy^a positive	34% Fy^a negative
72% Jk^b positive	28% Jk^b negative
9% K positive	91% K negative

$$0.34 \times 0.28 \times 0.91 = 0.087 \text{ or } 9\%$$

$$\frac{9}{100} = \frac{2}{X}$$

If nine out of 100 units are negative for the combined phenotypes, solving for X shows that 22 units would be required to find 2 units that are negative.

Gene Frequencies

The concept of genetic equilibrium was developed independently in 1908 by the English mathematician G. Hardy and the German physician W. Weinberg. Their theories led to the formulation of the Hardy-Weinberg law. The statistical formulas derived from these principles are used to estimate the frequency of genetic diseases and establish probability tables for forensic and paternity calculations. The formula is based on the principle that the sum of the gene frequencies when expressed as a decimal is equal to one. By observing phenotypes or traits in a large number of individuals, a percentage of occurrences of that trait is established. The Hardy-Weinberg formula can be used to calculate a determination of the gene frequencies that produced that trait. The probability of heterozygous and homozygous expression for each of the genes in a system can be predicted. The use of this formula in the routine blood bank setting is uncommon. Readers are encouraged to refer to the works by Vengelen-Tyler[2] and Wilson[3] for more information on this topic.

Parentage Testing

Because red blood cell and HLA antigens are easily identifiable and follow Mendelian laws of inheritance, they are useful in paternity analysis. Although molecular methods are being used more frequently in paternity testing because they provide a higher calculation for the probability of paternity, paternity studies using red blood cell and white blood cell markers are included in this text because they are useful in illustrating genetic principles. The blood groups with the greatest number of alleles (greatest polymorphism) are most useful in determining parentage. Since the HLA system is highly polymorphic, it is possible to identify over 700 haplotypes and approximately 180,000 phenotypes.[4] The more polymorphic the system, the less likely it is to find two people who are identical. Including more "markers" or genetic traits in the analysis also increases the likelihood of establishing paternity.

The primary goal of genetic marker testing in cases of disputed parentage is to identify a falsely accused person.[4] By eliminating or excluding the men who are not the father, failure to exclude determines paternity. Exclusion can occur directly or indirectly. In a **direct exclusion** (as shown in the following example) the child possesses a marker that is absent in both the mother and the **alleged father**.

Direct exclusion: exclusion of paternity when a child has a trait that neither parent demonstrates.

Alleged father: man accused of being the biologic father; the putative father.

	Mother	Alleged Father	Child
Phenotype	Group O	Group A	Group B
Genotype	*O/O*	*A/A* or *A/0*	*B/0*

The child inherited a *B* allele, which was not present in the alleged father. Since the child did not inherit the *B* allele from the mother, the *B* gene is called the **obligatory** paternal **gene**, or the gene that had to be passed on by the father.

Obligatory gene: gene that should be inherited from the father to prove paternity.

In the HLA system the A and B loci are inherited as a haplotype. The example below shows an exclusion of the alleged father in the HLA system.

Mother	Alleged Father	Child
A 3, 30	A 1, 31	A 3, 31
B 18, 35	B 8, 39	B 35, 51

Although the alleged father shares the A 31 antigen with the child, the haplotype that the child did not get from his mother (A 30, B 18) was not contributed by the tested man. This haplotype represents the obligate genes for the HLA system in this example.

In an **indirect exclusion** the child lacks a genetic marker that the father should have transmitted to all of his offspring. The failure to find an expected genetic marker in the child when the father is homozygous for the gene is not as obvious as a direct exclusion.

Indirect exclusion: failure to find an expected marker in a child when the alleged father is apparently homozygous for the gene.

	Mother	Alleged Father	Child
Phenotype	Jk(a+b−)	Jk(a−b+)	Jk(a+b−)
Genotype	Jk^a / Jk^a	Jk^b / Jk^b	Jk^a / Jk^a

The alleged father appears to be homozygous for the Jk^b allele, but the child did not inherit Jk^b. The presence of an undetectable, silent (amorph) allele or null allele can make the conclusion of an indirect exclusion incorrect. In this case the father may not have been homozygous Jk^bJk^b; he may have possessed the amorph *Jk* allele that does not express a detectable product. His genotype in that case would be Jk^bJk. For this reason indirect exclusions are not used as the only marker to exclude paternity. The finding of an indirect exclusion in two independent systems is usually sufficient evidence to reach a conclusion of nonpaternity.

Paternity index: chance that the alleged father is the biologic father compared to the chance that an untested man is the father.
Random man: untested man whose phenotype is unknown; the gene frequency is the same as that of the general population of the same race.

If no exclusions are found in a paternity analysis, a calculation to determine the probability of paternity is made.[5] Gene frequency tables are used to calculate a **paternity index**. The probability that the alleged father transmitted the obligatory genes is divided by the probability that a **random man** in the population from the same racial background could have transmitted those genes. The paternity index can be expressed as a percentage as well. For example, a paternity index of 210 indicates that the alleged father is 210 times more likely to be the father of the tested child than is a random man in the population. When this is translated to a percentage, the alleged father has a 99% chance of being the father. Regardless of the testing performed, a 100% chance of paternity cannot be established.

MOLECULAR GENETICS

Fundamentals of DNA Testing

Restriction fragment length polymorphism: variation of size of the fragments within a gene, for a given population, produced by restriction enzymes.
Polymerase chain reaction: technique for the amplification of a specific targeted DNA sequence.

Procedures based on the detection or analysis of DNA and ribonucleic acid (RNA) have made important contributions to biologic science in general and to blood banking regarding tissue typing and paternity testing. The following section describes the two most commonly used techniques for analyzing nucleic acids: **restriction fragment length polymorphism** (RFLP) and **polymerase chain reaction** (PCR). RFLP analysis has been a common feature of tissue typing and paternity testing in the blood bank setting. The PCR is a relatively new procedure in routine testing applications. PCR is destined to play an important role in all areas of nucleic-acid–based testing, especially in the detection of agents of infectious diseases. Since an appreciation of nucleic acid structure is important for the discussion of RFLP analysis and PCR, a brief review follows.

Structure of Nucleic Acids

Nucleotide: phosphate, sugar, and base that constitute the basic monomer of the nucleic acids DNA and RNA.

The basic building blocks of nucleic acids are the five **nucleotides**: adenine, cytosine, guanine, thymine, and uracil (abbreviated A, C, G, T, and U, respectively) (Fig. 3-13). Each nucleotide is composed of three parts: a phosphate group, a sugar group (ribose for RNA, deoxyribose for DNA) composed of a ring of five atoms, and a base. The nucleotides of DNA include A, C, G, and T whereas those of RNA include A, C, G, and U.

In its "native" or natural state a DNA molecule is a double helix composed of two intertwined polynucleotide chains, each thousands or millions of nucleotides long (Fig. 3-14). The backbone of each polynucleotide chain is formed by the phosphate groups linking the fifth (5-prime) carbon of one atom of one nucleotide's deoxyribose to the third (3-prime) carbon atom of the adjacent nucleotide's deoxyribose. This 5′ to 3′ linkage gives directionality to the DNA molecule, because it creates a 5′ end with an exposed phosphate group and a 3′ end with an unlinked 3′ carbon.

The nucleotide bases of a DNA molecule are oriented into the interior of the helix where they form hydrogen bonds with the adjacent bases of the other DNA polynucleotide chain. The hydrogen bonds formed between the paired bases are relatively weak interactions, but the cumulative effect of these bonds is strong and serves to bind the complementary chains together under normal conditions found in the cell. Because of the spatial relationships between the bases, A can pair and bond only with T, and G can pair and bond only with C. A consequence

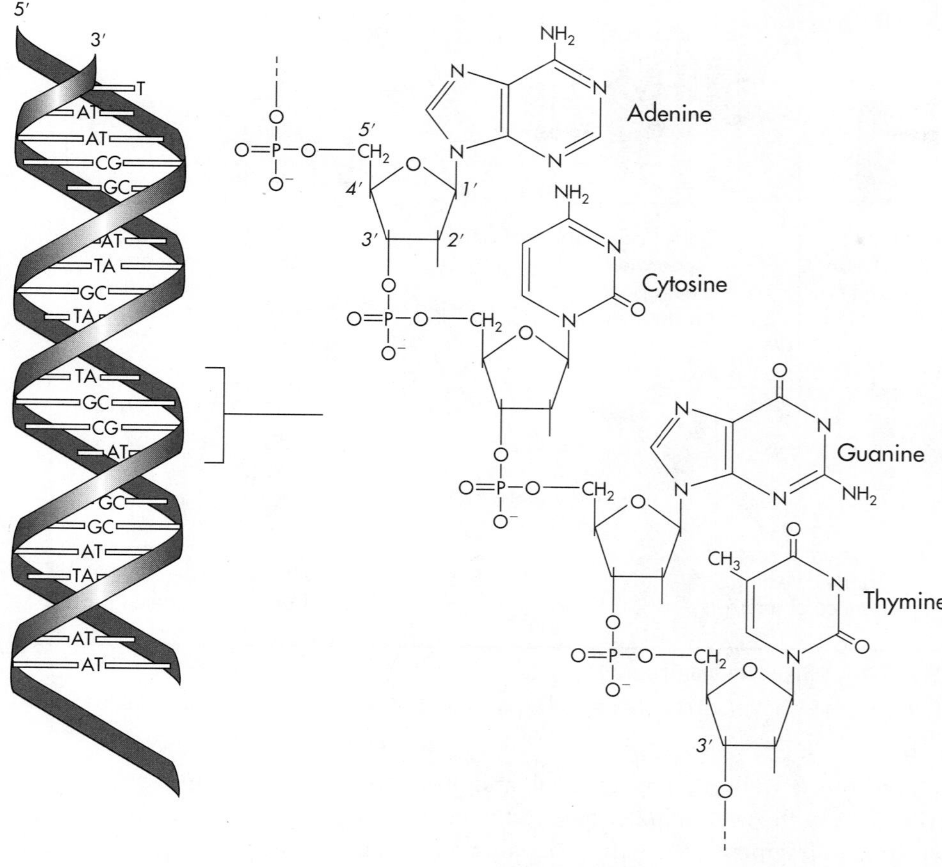

Fig. 3-13 The structure of DNA.
From Gelehrter TD: *Principles of medical genetics*, Baltimore, 1990, Williams & Wilkins.

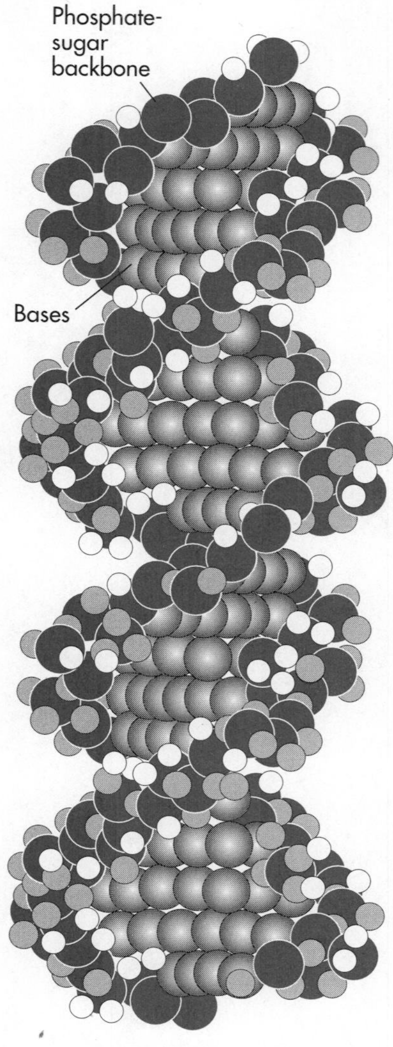

Fig. 3-14 DNA double helix model.
From Gelehrter TD: *Principles of medical genetics*, Baltimore, 1990, Williams & Wilkins.

of these base-pairing rules is that the nucleotide sequence of each polynucleotide chain is complementary to the sequence of the other chain. This means that the nucleotide sequence of one chain can be determined if the sequence of the complementary chain is known.

Restriction Fragment Length Polymorphism Analysis

RFLPs are differences in the patterns of fragments produced by cutting a length of DNA with **restriction endonuclease** (RE). An RE is an enzyme of bacterial origin that cuts DNA at a specific nucleotide sequence referred to as a recognition site. An RFLP is typically four to six nucleotides long. Dozens of REs have been isolated, and each will usually produce a different fragment pattern when cutting the same piece of DNA. RFLP analysis, which uses Southern blotting, is diagrammed in Fig. 3-15. RFLP analysis provides a relatively simple way of comparing the nucleotide sequence similarity of two different sources of DNA, since the difference in the number and size of the restriction fragments produced is related to natural sequence variations or mutations in the DNA. Southern blotting is used to detect specific DNA sequences. Labeled probes specific to the sequence of interest are used after the restriction-enzyme fragments are transferred onto a polymer sheet.

Restriction endonuclease: bacterial enzyme that recognizes and cleaves at specific DNA nucleotide sequences.

In an RFLP procedure DNA of interest is cut with an restriction endonuclease in an appropriate buffer. A portion of the restriction reaction product is then

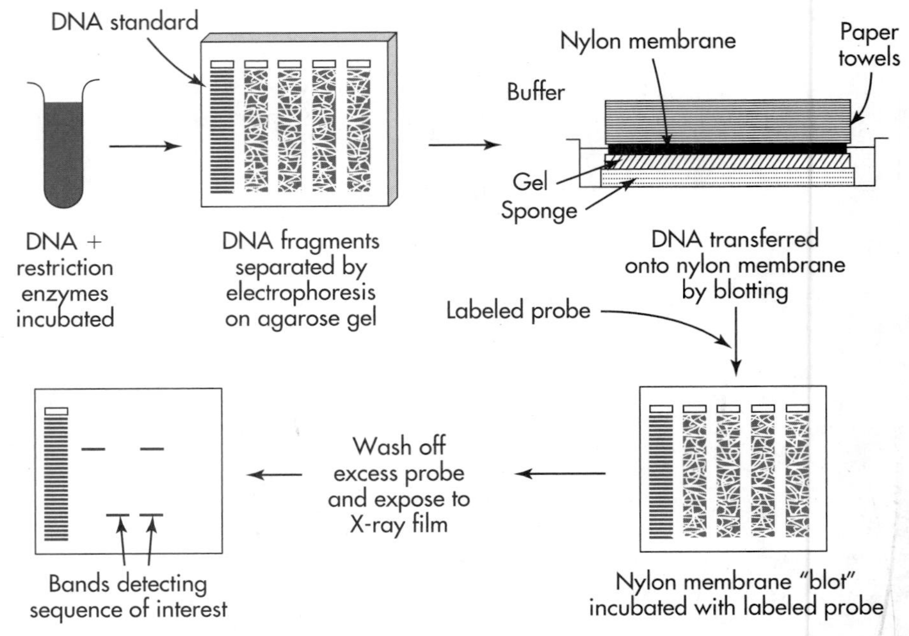

Fig. 3-15 Southern blotting.

From Vengelen-Tyler V: *Technical manual*, ed 13, Bethesda, Md, 1999, American Association of Blood Banks.

placed in the well of an agarose gel, and an electric current is applied to the gel. The DNA in the well migrates toward the positive electrode and separates itself according to fragment size, with the smaller fragments migrating farther into the gel. The DNA can then be detected by staining the gel with ethidium bromide, which causes the DNA fragments to appear light pink under ultraviolet light. If the source DNA is complex, many fragments are created, thus making it difficult to interpret the results. In these cases the restriction fragments can be transferred from the gel to a membrane. The membrane can then be tested, or "probed," with a DNA probe. DNA probes are lengths of single-stranded DNA with nucleotide sequences complementary to the sequence of the DNA fragments or the sequence being sought. During a probing procedure the DNA probe binds to its complementary sequence. Detecting fluorescent or enzymatic reporter molecules incorporated into the probe confirms the presence of the complementary sequence.

Polymerase Chain Reaction

The PCR[6] is a biochemical technique that can synthesize millions of copies of a target DNA sequence in just a few hours, theoretically starting with only one copy of the target sequence. This ability to synthesize large quantities of specific DNA sequences from a small number of starting copies has revolutionized the biologic sciences by providing new ways for researchers and applied scientists to work with and detect nucleic acids.

The PCR is a relatively simple biochemical reaction consisting of the five components listed in Table 3-5. The target DNA is typically a known DNA sequence selected by the analyst for study and is usually 50 to 1000 nucleotides long. This target sequence may be selected from thousands of gene sequences maintained in Internet-accessible sequence data banks. Target sequences for any particular organism's unsequenced genes may be determined directly by manual

Table 3-5 Polymerase Chain Reaction Components

COMPONENT	DESCRIPTION
Target DNA	This potentially could be from any mammalian, plant, or microbial source; usually the DNA must be extracted from the source cells; the extraction process can be as simple as boiling cells in water, as is done for many bacteria to expose the DNA to the PCR reagents, or it may involve more complex procedures that purify the DNA using organic solvents
Taq DNA polymerase	This is the enzyme that synthesizes the new strands of DNA; isolated from the bacterium *Thermus aquaticus* (*Taq*), which lives in hot thermal spring water; *Taq* polymerase can tolerate the high temperatures of the PCR without significant loss of activity
Primers	These are short pieces of single-stranded DNA that are complementary to the end sequences of the target DNA; the primers mark out the sequence to be amplified and provide the initiation site on each DNA strand for the *Taq* polymerase
Nucleotides	These are building blocks incorporated into the newly synthesized DNA by the *Taq* polymerase
Magnesium	Required for the function of *Taq* polymerase

DNA, Deoxyribonucleic acid; *PCR*, polymerase chain reaction.

or automated sequencing techniques. Once the target sequence has been selected, the primer sequence that marks out the target can be identified and then ordered from a primer synthesis service. Most PCR-based procedures have three parts: the extraction of the DNA source containing the target sequence, the PCR itself, and a method for detecting the product of the PCR.

Each step of the PCR (Fig. 3-16) is controlled by temperature. The reaction is performed in a thermal cycler—a computer-controlled heating-cooling block—which can rapidly heat or cool the PCR reaction vessel to the temperatures required for each step of the reaction. Depending on the application anywhere from 20 to 40 cycles of PCR may be performed in a PCR test. The increase in the concentration of target DNA in the reaction is exponential and doubles with each PCR cycle. When the PCR is completed the amplified target sequence, or **amplicon**, must be detected.

Amplicon: amplified target sequence of DNA produced by the PCR.

Amplicon detection can be accomplished by a number of techniques. The two most common are gel electrophoresis, as previously described for RFLP analysis, and DNA capture probes. DNA capture probes are lengths of single-stranded DNA with nucleotide sequences complementary to the sequence of at least one strand of the amplified PCR product. The capture probes are usually attached to a solid support, such as a membrane or a plastic microwell. Amplicon detection is accomplished by denaturing the double-stranded amplicons to separate the individual DNA strands. The denatured amplicons are then exposed to the capture probe, which hybridizes to the complementary amplicon sequence. The presence of the captured amplicon can be confirmed by detecting fluorescent or enzymatic reporter molecules that are incorporated into the amplicons during the PCR.

In recent years important variations of the basic PCR have been developed. These modified reactions have extended the range of PCR to the testing of RNA

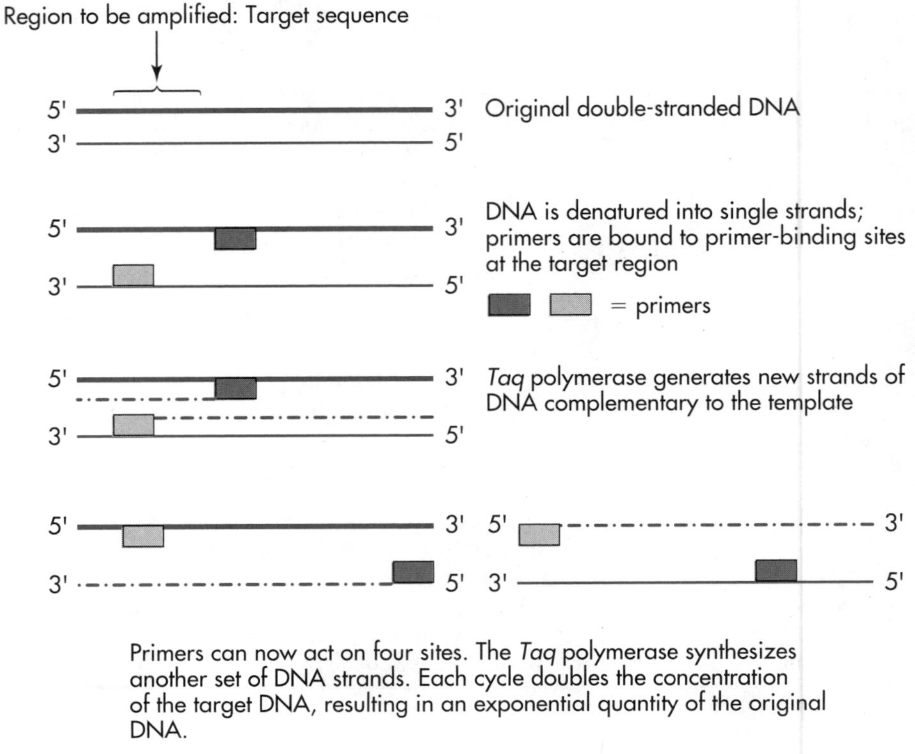

Fig. 3-16 Polymerase chain reaction.

(reverse transcriptase PCR), the detection or analysis of multiple nucleic acid targets (multiplex PCR), and the determination of the initial copy number of target nucleic acid in a sample (quantitative PCR).

Users of PCR must be aware of several important limitations that can adversely affect the results of a PCR-based test. Sampling variation, which is the inconsistent presence of a rare target sequence in multiple aliquots of a positive specimen, will cause a false negative test result if the specimen aliquot does not contain the target sequence. A typical sample volume for a PCR is between 5 and 10 μl. It is possible for a rare target sequence to be present in the sample but not in the aliquot taken for analysis. Another cause of false negative PCR results is the introduction of inhibitors of the polymerase into the PCR reaction from the sample. The use of adequate extraction techniques that eliminates inhibitor carryover is essential, as is the use of internal positive controls in the PCR reaction mix to detect the presence of inhibitors. False positive reactions may be caused by amplicon contamination of negative specimens. Because they are produced by the millions, amplicons created in previous PCR tests may escape into the laboratory environment and be inadvertently introduced into specimens in the next round of testing if proper containment techniques are not observed. Amplicon contamination may be prevented by controlling aerosol production of amplified specimens, providing for the physical separation of the reagent preparation, specimen extraction, amplification, and amplicon detection steps of a PCR-based procedure, and using "chemical sterilization" techniques such as the uracil N′-glycolsylase procedure. This procedure eliminates contaminating amplicons from the next group of specimens before PCR testing.

Application of Molecular Genetics to Blood Banking

RFLP analysis is currently a common analytic technique for DNA testing in blood bank settings, primarily in the areas of paternity testing and determining HLA profiles in transplantation studies. The use of RFLP analysis is slowly being replaced with PCR techniques for these applications, since the PCR is usually faster to perform, requires smaller amounts of DNA, is less labor intensive, and offers a greater potential for automation.

PCR is being integrated into the testing of donor blood for infectious agents, thus eliminating the reliance on antibody response to a virus. This methodology further reduces the window period in viral detection. Developers of PCR methods for donor screening are working on the challenges of designing a test that is not cost prohibitive and provides a timely completion.

CHAPTER SUMMARY

Red blood cell antigens and HLAs are easily identifiable traits that are inherited in a predictable Mendelian fashion. Various forms of genes called alleles encode the blood group antigens. They segregate randomly and independently and are expressed as codominant traits. A homozygous or heterozygous inheritance of the genes can sometimes affect the expression of the antigen, thus causing agglutination reactions to be stronger or weaker. The testing of red blood cell antigens or antibodies results in the phenotype. Inferences regarding the genotype or genetic makeup are often made, but family studies are required to conclusively determine inheritance. Each blood group system is unique in its serologic properties and inheritance. Unusual red blood cell antigen expression or nonexpression occurs in many of the systems, which often has a genetic basis. Techniques of molecular genetics, such as RFLP and the PCR, have made possible significant improvements in HLA tissue typing and paternity testing. Molecular techniques are also being used to screen donated blood for infectious agents, since automated systems geared to the needs of the blood-banking community are now available. Being familiar with genetic terms and concepts enhances the understanding of blood group systems' antigen properties in the following chapters.

CRITICAL THINKING EXERCISES

◆ ***EXERCISE 3-1***

Given the following pedigree for a family study involving the ABO system, determine the phenotype and the probable genotype of the father:

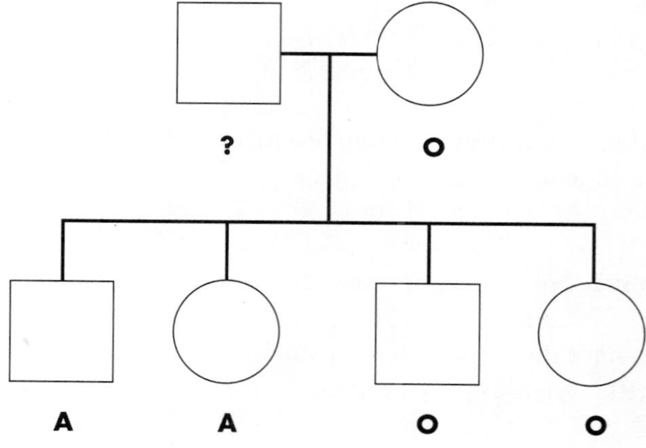

◆ ***EXERCISE 3-2***

While working in the blood bank you receive a call from a father who wants to know if his group O son could possibly belong to him, since he knows that he is group B and the mother is group A. Provide an explanation in terms understandable to a person without a background in basic genetics.

◆ ***EXERCISE 3-3***

Is a person who is typed as M+, N− homozygous or heterozygous for the *M* gene? Would you expect reactions with this person's red blood cells to be stronger or weaker than those of someone who tested M+, N+?

◆ ***EXERCISE 3-4***

Given the following paternity results (phenotype) using the MNS system (inherited as a haplotype), determine which of the children cannot have the same father as the rest. The mother's phenotype is MNSs, and the alleged father is NSs.

1. Child 1: MNSs
2. Child 2: Ns
3. Child 3: MNS
4. Child 4: MSs

◆ ***EXERCISE 3-5***

A patient's antibodies are identified to be anti-K, anti-Jk^a, and anti-E. How many units will be needed to find two antigen-negative units? The antigens occur in the population with the following frequency: E: 30%; K: 9%; Jk^a: 77%.

◆ ***EXERCISE 3-6***

HLA testing on a mother, child, and alleged father produced the following results:

Mother	Child	Alleged Father
A 2, 24	A 2, 24	A 2, 25
B 18, 55	B 44, 18	B 8, 18

Is the alleged father excluded? Explain your interpretation.

STUDY QUESTIONS

1. Which of the following describes the expression of most blood group inheritance?
   a. dominant
   b. recessive
   c. sex-linked
   d. codominant

2. With which of the following red blood cell phenotypes would anti-Jk^a react most strongly?
   a. Jk(a−b+)
   b. Jk(a+b−)
   c. Jk(a+b+)
   d. Jk(a−b−)

3. A gene that produces no detectable product is referred to as:
   a. a regulator gene
   b. an allele
   c. a null gene
   d. an amorph

4. Which of the following is important as a useful genetic marker for paternity testing?
   a. all races have the same gene frequencies
   b. the genetic system is polymorphic

c. there are no amorphic genes
d. recombination is common

5. The term used when two of the same forms of a gene are inherited from each parent is:
   a. homozygous
   b. allele
   c. heterozygous
   d. syntenic

6. When the child does not inherit a trait from an alleged father that should have been passed on, the exclusion is:
   a. direct
   b. indirect
   c. an error, and testing would need to be repeated
   d. a result of a weak reagent

7. Alternate forms of a gene at given genetic loci are called:
   a. alleles
   b. amplicons
   c. nucleotides
   d. amorphs

8. The technique that uses a small amount of DNA and amplifies it for identification is called:
   a. restriction fragment length polymorphism
   b. a DNA probe
   c. polymerase chain reaction
   d. gene mapping

9. A gene that can inhibit the expression of another gene is called:
   a. an amorph
   b. a *cis* gene
   c. a null gene
   d. a suppressor gene

10. The phosphate, sugar, and base that constitute DNA and RNA are called:
    a. amplicons
    b. polymerases
    c. nucleotides
    d. anticodons

11. Sections of single-stranded DNA used to identify certain sections of complementary DNA are called:
    a. amplicons
    b. target DNA
    c. DNA probes
    d. *Taq* polymerases

12. Genes located far apart on the same chromosome are more likely to:
    a. be inherited as a haplotype
    b. cross over
    c. be linked
    d. suppress each other

13. In a pedigree, a square is a standard symbol for:
    a. males
    b. females
    c. twins
    d. stillbirths

14. When a trait is passed from a father to all of his daughters but none of his sons, the trait is said to be:
    a. X-linked dominant
    b. X-linked recessive
    c. autosomal dominant
    d. codominant

15. A gene inherited in a *cis* position to another gene is:
    a. on an opposite chromosome
    b. on a different chromosome number
    c. on the same chromosome
    d. antithetical

REFERENCES

1. Hultgren D: *Biology, an appreciation of life*, Del Mar, Calif, 1972, CRM Books.
2. Vengelen-Tyler V, editor: *Technical manual*, ed 12, Bethesda, Md, 1996, American Association of Blood Banks.
3. Wilson JK, editor: *Genetics for blood bankers*, Washington, DC, 1980, American Association of Blood Banks.
4. Polesky HF: Application of genetic marker testing in disputed parentage cases. In Rossi EC, Simon TL, Moss GS, editors: *Principles of transfusion medicine*, Baltimore, 1991, Williams & Wilkins.
5. Walker RH: Probability in the analysis of paternity test results. In *Paternity testing*, Washington, DC, 1978, American Association of Blood Banks.
6. Watson J, Gilman M, Witkowski J, Zoller M: *Recombinant DNA*, ed 2, New York, 1992, Scientific American Books.

Overview of the Major Blood Groups

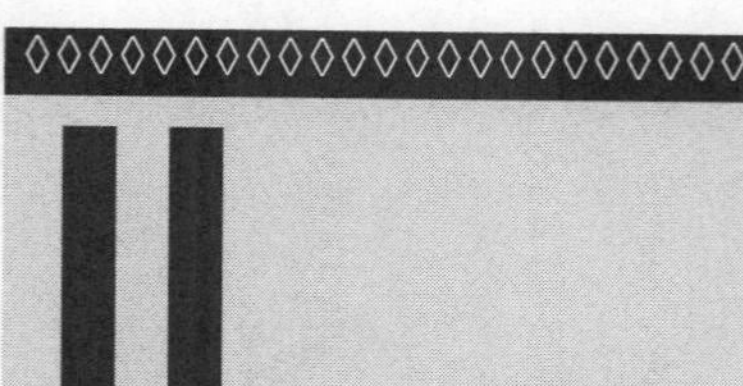

ABO AND H BLOOD GROUP SYSTEMS AND SECRETOR STATUS

4

Paula R. Howard

CHAPTER OUTLINE

LEARNING OBJECTIVES

Upon completion of this chapter, the reader should be able to:

1. Define a blood group system with regard to blood group antigens and their inheritance.
2. Explain Landsteiner's rule.
3. List the cells, body fluids, and secretions where ABO antigens can be located.
4. Describe the relationship among the *ABO, H,* and *Se* genes.
5. Differentiate between type 1 and type 2 oligosaccharide structures and state where each is located.
6. Describe the formation of the H antigen from the gene product and its relationship to ABO antigen expression.
7. List the glycosyltransferases and the immunodominant sugars for the *A, B, O,* and *H* alleles.
8. Compare and contrast the A_1 and A_2 phenotypes with regard to antigen structure and serologic testing.
9. Describe how to differentiate among A_3, A_x, and A_{el} subgroups by serologic testing.
10. Determine the possible ABO genotypes with an ABO phenotype.
11. Describe the ABO system antibodies with regard to immunoglobulin class, clinical significance, and in vitro serologic reactions.
12. Discuss the selection of whole blood, red blood cell, and plasma products for transfusions.
13. Define the terms *universal donor* and *universal recipient* as they apply to red blood cell and plasma products.
14. List the technical errors that may result in an ABO discrepancy.
15. Define the acquired B and the B(A) phenotypes; discuss the ABO discrepancies that would result from these phenotypes and methods used in resolving these discrepancies.
16. List reasons for missing or weakly expressed ABO antigens and the test methods used to resolve these discrepancies.
17. Describe ABO discrepancies caused by extra reactions in serum testing and how they can be resolved.
18. Discuss the Bombay phenotype with regard to genetic pathway, serologic reactions, and transfusion implications.
19. Define the terms *secretor* and *nonsecretor.*

This chapter begins a section of the textbook dedicated to the basic understanding of blood group systems and their significance in the practice of transfusion medicine. A blood group system is composed of antigens that are produced by alleles at a single genetic locus or at loci so closely linked that genetic crossing-over rarely occurs.[1] Blood group antigens are molecules primarily located on the red blood cell membrane. These molecules can be classified biochemically as proteins and as carbohydrates linked to either a lipid (glycolipid) or a protein (glycoprotein). With adequate immunologic exposure a blood group antigen may elicit the production of its corresponding antibody in individuals who lack the antigen. Exposure to many blood group antigens occurs during transfusions. Patients receiving transfusions may produce antibodies in response to the exposure to blood group antigens not present on their own red blood cells.

Because the terminology for red blood cell antigens is inconsistent, the International Society of Blood Transfusion (ISBT) created a Working Party on Terminology for Red Cell Antigens in 1980 to standardize blood group systems and antigen names. The committee's goal was to provide additional terminology suitable for use with computer software rather than create replacement terminology. The ISBT Working Party has assigned genetically based numerical designations for red blood cell antigens and has defined 23 blood group systems (Table 4-1).[2,3] According to ISBT criteria genetic studies and serologic data are required before an antigen is assigned to a blood group system. The ABO system has been assigned the ISBT number 001 and includes four antigens, whereas the H system is number 018 with one antigen. This textbook addresses blood group systems with commonly used names and includes ISBT symbols and numbers.

Table 4-1 ISBT Blood Group System Assignments

BLOOD SYSTEM NAME	ISBT SYMBOL	ISBT NUMBER
ABO	ABO	001
MNS	MNS	002
P	P1	003
Rh	RH	004
Lutheran	LU	005
Kell	KEL	006
Lewis	LE	007
Duffy	FY	008
Kidd	JK	009
Diego	DI	010
Cartwright (Yt)	YT	011
Xg	XG	012
Scianna	SC	013
Dombrock	DO	014
Colton	CO	015
Landsteiner-Wiener	LW	016
Chido/Rodgers	CH/RG	017
Hh	H	018
Kx	XK	019
Gerbich	GE	020
Cromer	CROM	021
Knops	KN	022
Indian	IN	023

ISBT, International Society of Blood Transfusion.

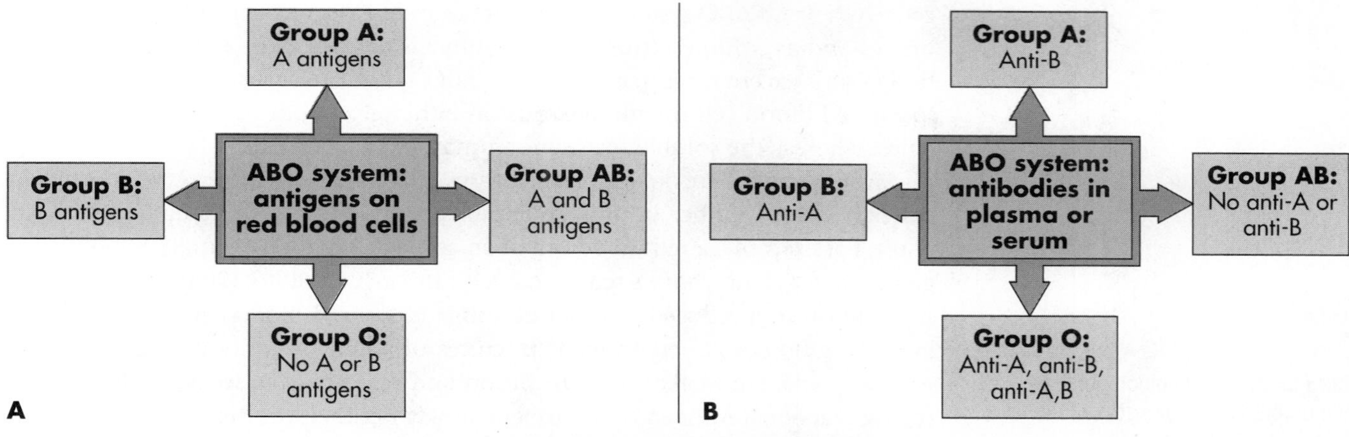

Fig. 4-1 ABO antigens *(A)* and antibodies *(B)*.

HISTORICAL OVERVIEW OF THE ABO SYSTEM

The discovery of the ABO system by Karl Landsteiner in 1900 marked the beginning of modern blood banking and transfusion medicine.[4] In a series of experiments designed to demonstrate serologic incompatibilities between humans, Landsteiner recognized different patterns of agglutination when human blood samples were mixed in random pairings. He described the blood groups as A, B, and O. Landsteiner's associates, von Decastello and Sturli, added group AB to the original observations several years later.[5] In his investigations Landsteiner noted the presence of agglutinating antibodies in the serum of individuals who lacked the corresponding ABO antigen. He observed that group A red blood cells agglutinated with the serum from group B individuals. This observation has been termed **Landsteiner's rule** (or Landsteiner's law). Landsteiner's rule established that normal, healthy individuals possess ABO antibodies to the ABO antigens lacking on their red blood cells. For example, individuals with group A red blood cells possess the A antigen and lack the B antigen. Therefore these individuals possess anti-B antibodies. Individuals with group B red blood cells, however, possess the B antigen and lack the A antigen. Therefore these individuals possess anti-A antibodies. Antigens and antibodies associated with each ABO phenotype are illustrated in Fig. 4-1. Four major phenotypes are derived from the two major antigens (A and B) of the system. These phenotypes are group A, group B, group AB, and group O.

Landsteiner's rule: rule stating that normal, healthy individuals possess ABO antibodies to the ABO antigens absent from their red blood cells.

Even though it was the first blood group system described, the ABO system remains the most important blood group system for transfusion purposes. Accurate donor and recipient ABO types are fundamental to transfusion safety because of the presence of ABO antibodies in individuals with no exposure to human red blood cells. The transfusion of ABO-incompatible blood to a recipient may result in intravascular hemolysis and other serious consequences of an **acute hemolytic transfusion reaction**.

Acute hemolytic transfusion reaction: complication of transfusion associated with intravascular hemolysis characterized by rapid onset with symptoms of fever, chills, hemoglobinemia, and hypotension; major complications include irreversible shock, renal failure, and disseminated intravascular coagulation.

ABO AND H SYSTEM ANTIGENS

General Characteristics of the ABO Antigens

ABO antigens are widely distributed and located on red blood cells, lymphocytes, platelets, tissue cells, bone marrow, and organs such as the kidneys. Soluble forms of the ABO system antigens can also be synthesized and secreted by tissue cells. As a result ABO system antigens are found in association with cellular membranes and as soluble forms. Soluble antigens are detected in secretions and all body fluids except cerebrospinal fluid.[6] ABO system antigens, which are intrinsic to the red blood cell membrane, exist as either glycolipid or glycoprotein molecules, whereas the soluble forms are primarily glycoproteins.

ABO antigens are detectable as early as 5 to 6 weeks in utero. A newborn possesses a lower number of antigen copies per red blood cell compared with an adult. For example, a red blood cell of an adult carries 610,000 to 830,000 B antigens, whereas a newborn's red blood cell carries 200,000 to 320,000 B antigens.[7] In addition to a reduced number of antigens, the red blood cells of a newborn lack the fully developed antigen structures of adults' red blood cells. Therefore ABO antigens are weaker on **cord blood** and may result in weaker ABO phenotyping reactions. Antigen development slowly occurs until the full expression of adult levels is reached at approximately 2 to 4 years of age.

Cord blood: whole blood obtained from the umbilical vein or artery of the fetus.

The worldwide frequency of ABO phenotypes within the White population has been well documented. Group O and group A individuals constitute 45% and 40% of the White population, respectively. These two blood groups are the most common ABO phenotypes followed by group B with an 11% frequency and group AB with a 4% frequency.[8] ABO phenotype frequencies differ in selected populations and ethnic groups. For example, the group B phenotype has a higher frequency in the Black and Asian populations than in the White population (Table 4-2).

Table 4-2 Frequency Distributions of ABO Phenotypes (U.S. Population)

ABO phenotype	White (%)	Black (%)	Asian (%)
A	40	27	28
B	11	20	27
AB	4	4	5
O	45	49	40

Inheritance and Development of the A, B, and H Antigens

A discussion of the inheritance and formation of ABO antigens requires an understanding of the H antigen, inherited independent of the ABO system antigens. The production of H antigen is genetically controlled by the *H* gene, located on a different chromosome from the ABO genetic locus. In addition to the *ABO* and *H* genes the expression of soluble ABO antigens is influenced by inheritance of the *Se* gene (see the Secretor Status section in this chapter). The *Se* gene genetically influences the formation of ABO antigens in saliva, tears, and other body fluids. Consequently the occurrence and location of the ABO antigens are influenced by three genetically independent loci: *ABO*, *H*, and *Se*.

ABO antigens are assembled on a common carbohydrate structure that also serves as the base for the formation of the H, Lewis, I/i, and P_1 antigens. Consequently this common carbohydrate structure is capable of antigen expression for more than one blood group system (Fig. 4-2). This common structure is analo-

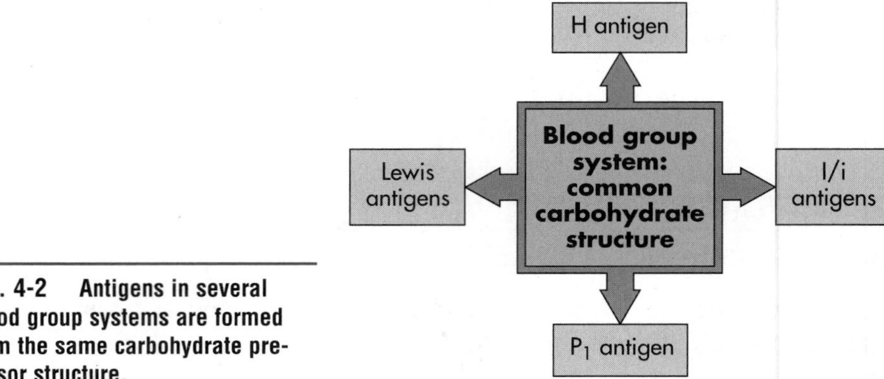

Fig. 4-2 Antigens in several blood group systems are formed from the same carbohydrate precursor structure.

gous to an antigen building block. Because of the interrelationship between the common antigen building block and multiple blood group systems, it is important to recognize that the action of genes of one blood group system may affect the expression of antigens in another system.

Common Structure for A, B, and H Antigens

The common structure (antigen building block) for A, B, and H antigens is an **oligosaccharide chain** attached to either a protein or lipid carrier molecule. The oligosaccharide chain comprises four sugar molecules linked in simple linear forms or in more complex structures with a high degree of branching. The two terminal sugars, D-galactose and *N*-acetylglucosamine, may be linked together in two different configurations. When the number 1 carbon of D-galactose is linked with the number 3 carbon of *N*-acetylglucosamine, the linkage is described as $\beta 1 \rightarrow 3$. Type 1 oligosaccharide chains are formed. When the number 1 carbon of D-galactose is linked with the number 4 carbon of *N*-acetylglucosamine, the linkage is described as $\beta 1 \rightarrow 4$. Type 2 oligosaccharide chains are formed (Fig. 4-3). Type 2 structures are primarily associated with glycolipids and glycoproteins on the red blood cell membrane, and type 1 structures are associated primarily with body fluids. Some type 2 glycoprotein structures are located in body fluids and secretions.[9]

Oligosaccharide chain: compound formed by a small number of simple carbohydrate molecules.

Development of the H Antigen

The H antigen is the only antigen in the H blood group system. This blood group system has been assigned to a locus on chromosome 19 and is closely linked with the *Se* locus. The *H* locus has two significant alleles: *H* and *h*. The *H* allele is a dominant allele with high frequency (greater than 99.99%), whereas the *h* allele is classified as an amorph with rare frequency. Genes encode for the production of proteins, and the gene product of the *H* allele is a protein classified biochemically as a **transferase** enzyme. Transferase enzymes promote the transfer of a biochemical group from one molecule to another. A **glycosyltransferase** enzyme catalyzes the transfer of glycosyl groups (simple carbohydrate units) in biochemical reactions. In the formation of H antigen a glycosyltransferase enzyme transfers a sugar molecule, L-fucose, to either type 1 or type 2 common oligosaccharide chains. The biochemical name for this enzyme is L-fucosyltransferase. The L-fucose added to the terminal galactose of the type 1 and type 2 chain is called the **immunodominant sugar** for H antigens, since the sugar confers H specificity (Fig. 4-4).[10] The formation of the H antigen, therefore, is the end product of an

Transferase: class of enzymes that catalyzes the transfer of a chemical group from one molecule to another.
Glycosyltransferase: enzyme that catalyzes the transfer of glycosyl groups (simple carbohydrate units) in biochemical reactions.

Immunodominant sugar: sugar molecule responsible for specificity.

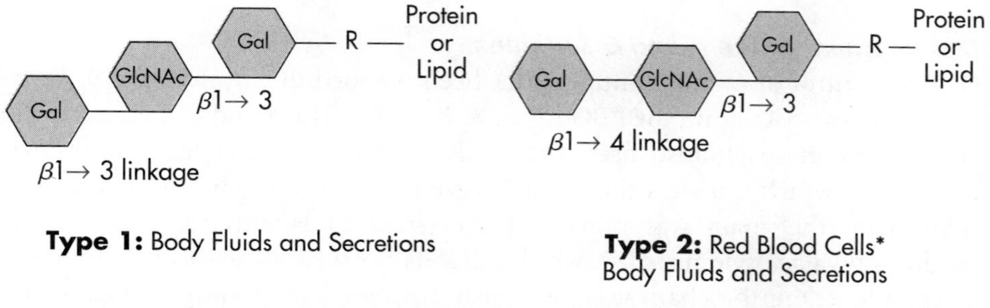

Fig. 4-3 Type 1 and type 2 oligosaccharide chain structures. *Gal,* Galactose; *GlcNAc, N*-acetylglucosamine. *Majority of type 2 chains are located on the red blood cells.

Modified from Vengelen-Tyler V, editor: *Technical manual,* ed 12, Bethesda, Md, 1996, American Association of Blood Banks.

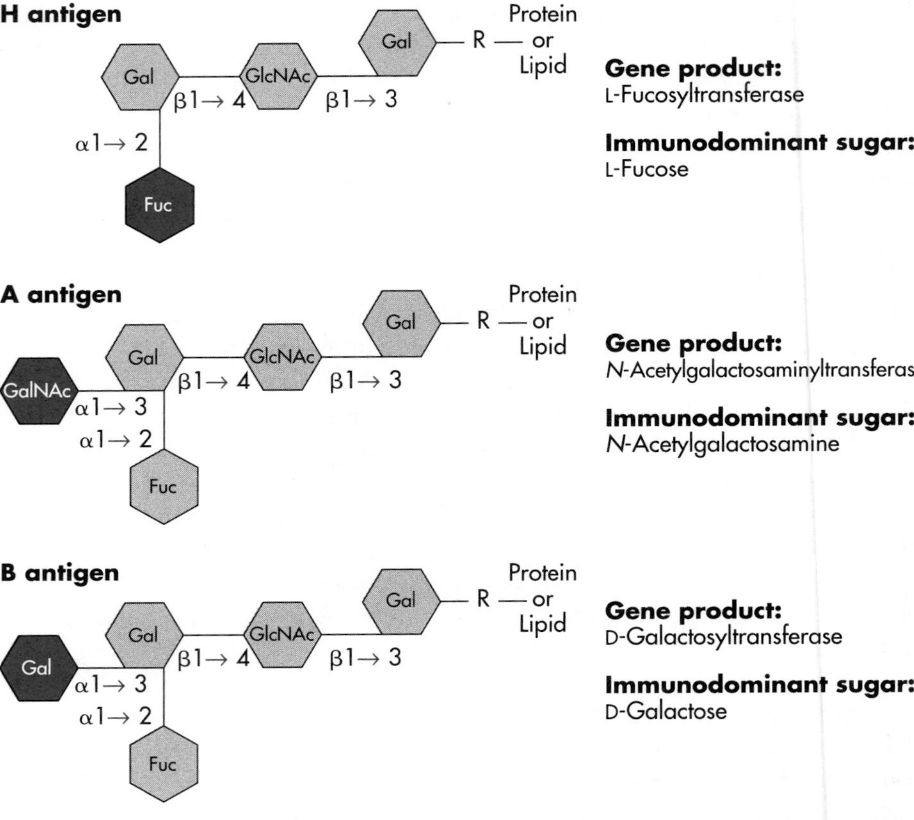

Fig. 4-4 Biochemical structures of the H, A, and B antigens. *Gal,* D-Galactose; *GlcNAc, N*-acetylglucosamine; *Fuc,* L-fucose; *GalNAc, N*-acetylgalactosamine.

Modified from Vengelen-Tyler V, editor: *Technical manual,* ed 12, Bethesda, Md, 1996, American Association of Blood Banks.

enzymatic reaction. This formation is critical to the expression of A and B antigens, since the gene products of the *ABO* alleles require that the H antigen be the acceptor molecule.

This section previously described the *h* allele as an amorph with no detectable gene product. The red blood cells from an *h* homozygote (*hh*) are classified as the **Bombay phenotype.** These rare individuals lack both H antigen and ABO antigen expression on their red blood cells. A more detailed discussion of the Bombay phenotype is presented at the end of this chapter.

Bombay phenotype: rare phenotype of an individual who genetically has inherited *h* allele in homozygous manner; individual's red blood cells lack H and ABO antigens.

Development of the A and B Antigens

Genetic control of A and B antigens has been mapped to chromosome 9. Three major alleles exist within the *ABO* locus: *A, B,* and *O.* The *A* and *B* alleles, like the *H* allele, are glycosyltransferases. The *A* allele produces *N*-acetylgalactosaminyltransferase, which transfers the sugar *N*-acetylgalactosamine to an oligosaccharide chain; the chain was previously converted to H antigen. The *B* allele produces D-galactosyltransferase, which transfers the sugar D-galactose to an oligosaccharide chain; the chain was previously converted to H antigen (Fig. 4-4).[10] Therefore *N*-acetylgalactosamine is the immunodominant sugar for A specificity, and D-galactose is the immunodominant sugar for B specificity.

The *O* allele is considered nonfunctional, since the resulting gene product is an enzymatically inactive protein. As a result group O red blood cells carry no A

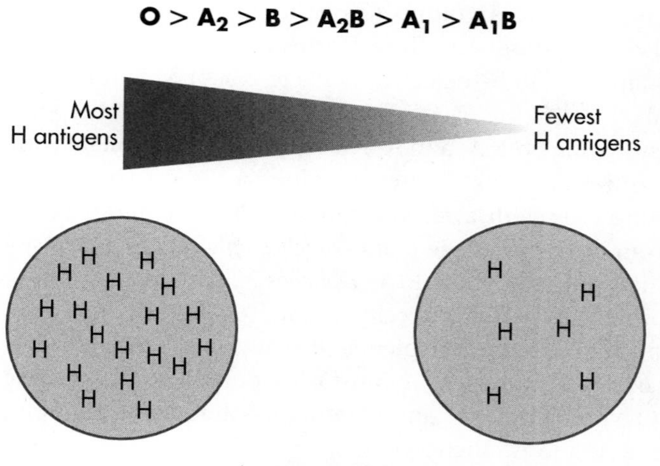

Fig. 4-5 Variation of H-antigen concentrations in ABO phenotypes.

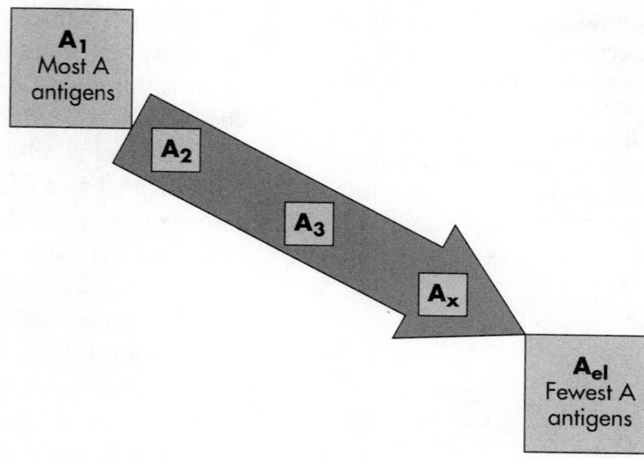

Fig. 4-6 Gradient of the subgroups of A: number of A antigen sites per red blood cell.

or B antigens but are rich in unconverted H antigens. Adult group O red blood cells have approximately 1.7 million H-antigen copies per red blood cell and possess the greatest concentration of H antigens per red blood cell.[6] Other ABO phenotypes have fewer copies of H antigens, since the H antigen is the acceptor molecule for the A and B enzymes. Group A_1B phenotype possesses the lowest number of unconverted H sites. Fig. 4-5 illustrates the variation of H-antigen concentration in ABO phenotypes.

Yamamoto and associates[11] have recently defined the molecular basis of the ABO phenotypes. These investigators have shown that a small number of mutations exist in the glycosyltransferase gene at the ABO locus. On the molecular level the A and B glycosyltransferases differ slightly in their nucleic acid compositions. Additionally the nucleic acid composition of the O allele has revealed that it does not produce an enzymatically active protein capable of acting on the H-antigen precursors. Readers are encouraged to review the suggested reading list for greater detail on the molecular basis of the ABO phenotypes.

ABO Subgroups

Comparison of the A_1 and A_2 Phenotypes

The ABO phenotypes can be divided into categories, or subgroups. Subgroups differ in the amount of antigen expressed on the red blood cell membrane, representing a quantitative difference in antigen expression (Fig. 4-6). Some evidence also exists to support the theory of qualitative differences in antigen expression. Some subgroups possess more highly branched, complex antigenic structures, whereas others have simplified linear forms of antigen.[12]

The group A phenotype is classified into two major subgroups: A_1 and A_2. These glycosyltransferase gene products, which are genetically controlled by the A^1 and A^2 genes, respectively, differ slightly in their ability to convert H antigen to A antigen. The A_1 phenotype, encoded by the A^1 gene, exists in approximately 80% of group A individuals. In the A_1 phenotype, A antigens are highly concentrated on branched and linear oligosaccharide chains. The A^1 gene effectively acts on the H antigens in the production of A antigens. The A_2 phenotype, encoded by the A^2 gene, constitutes approximately 20% of group A individuals. In the A_2

Dolichos biflorus: plant lectin with specificity for the A_1 antigen.
Ulex europaeus: plant lectin with specificity for the H antigen.
Mixed field: agglutination pattern where a population of the red blood cells has agglutinated and the remainder of the red blood cells is unagglutinated.

phenotype A antigen copies are fewer in number than in the A_1 phenotype. This phenotype is assembled on the simplified linear forms of the oligosaccharide chains. An alloantibody, anti-A_1, can be detected in 1% to 8% of A_2 and in 22% to 35% of A_2B individuals.

In routine ABO phenotyping both A_1 and A_2 red blood cells agglutinate with commercially available anti-A reagents. These red blood cells can be distinguished in serologic testing only with a reagent called ***Dolichos biflorus*** lectin. This lectin is extracted from the seeds of the plant *Dolichos biflorus* and possesses an anti-A_1 specificity. When properly diluted the *Dolichos biflorus* lectin (anti-A_1 lectin) agglutinates A_1, but not A_2, red blood cells. The anti-A_1 lectin is not used in the routine ABO testing of donors and recipients, since it is unnecessary to distinguish between the A_1 and A_2 phenotypes for transfusion purposes. This reagent is useful in resolving ABO typing problems and identifying infrequent subgroups of A. Fig. 4-7 compares the A_1 and A_2 phenotypes.

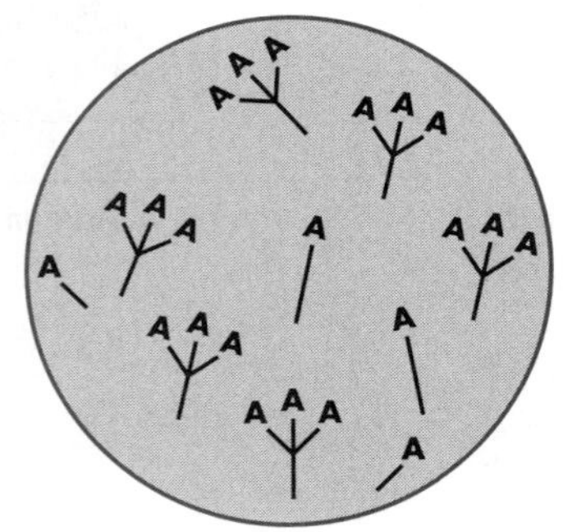

A_1 Phenotype

Branched A antigens
2 million A antigens/adult red blood cells*
Positive with anti-A
Positive with anti-A_1 lectin

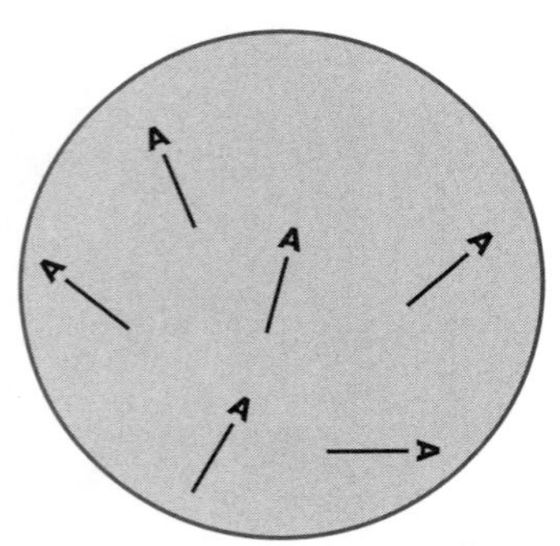

A_2 Phenotype

Linear A antigens
500,000 A antigens/ adult red blood cells*
Positive with anti-A
Negative with anti-A_1 lectin

Fig. 4-7 Comparison of the A_1 and A_2 red blood cells.

*From Issitt PD, Anstee DJ: *Applied blood group serology*, ed 4, Durham, NC, 1998, Montgomery Scientific Publications.

Additional Subgroups of A and B

Although more infrequent than A_1 and A_2 other A subgroups have been described that involve reduced expression of A antigens. These A subgroups have been classified as A_{int}, A_3, A_x, A_m, A_{end}, A_{el}, and A_{bantu}, based on the reactivity of red blood cells with reagent anti-A and anti-A,B. Human polyclonal-based anti-A,B reagent contains an antibody with specificity toward both the A and B antigens that cannot be separated into anti-A and anti-B components. One unique feature of this reagent is its enhanced ability to detect weaker subgroups compared with anti-A. The subgroups are genetically controlled by the inheritance of rare alleles at the *ABO* locus and collectively occur at less than 1% frequency. For the purposes of this book the discussion is limited to the A_3, A_x, and A_{el} subgroups. For an in-depth presentation of the other subgroups the reader is referred to the suggested readings at the end of the chapter.

The classification of the rare A subgroups is determined by the following:

- Degree of red blood cell agglutination with anti-A and human anti-A,B commercial reagents (polyclonal based)
- Presence or absence of anti-A_1 in the serum

Weak or no agglutination with commercial anti-A is a key factor in recognizing a subgroup in this category. Recent murine monoclonal blends of commercial anti-A have been formulated to enhance the detection of these weaker subgroups in ABO phenotyping. Saliva studies for the detection of soluble forms of A and H antigens and testing with anti-H lectin ***(Ulex europaeus)*** may provide additional information. However, these techniques are not performed routinely. Refer to Fig. 4-8 for a simplified approach to use in the problem solving of a subgroup.

A_3 SUBGROUP. An agglutination pattern characteristic of A_3 red blood cells is called **mixed field.**[13] Mixed field reactions of A_3 red blood cells with human polyclonal anti-A and human polyclonal anti-A,B are seen as small agglutinates in a mass of unagglutinated red blood cells. A_3 red blood cells are negative with anti-A_1 lectin. Serum studies have demonstrated the presence of anti-A_1 in some A_3 individuals.

A_x SUBGROUP. A_x red blood cells typically show weak or no agglutination with human polyclonal anti-A and stronger agglutination with human polyclonal anti-A,B reagents.[14] Some murine monoclonal antibody preparations of anti-A agglutinate with A_x red blood cells. These red blood cells do not react with anti-A_1 lectin. Serum from A_x individuals almost always contains anti-A_1.[10]

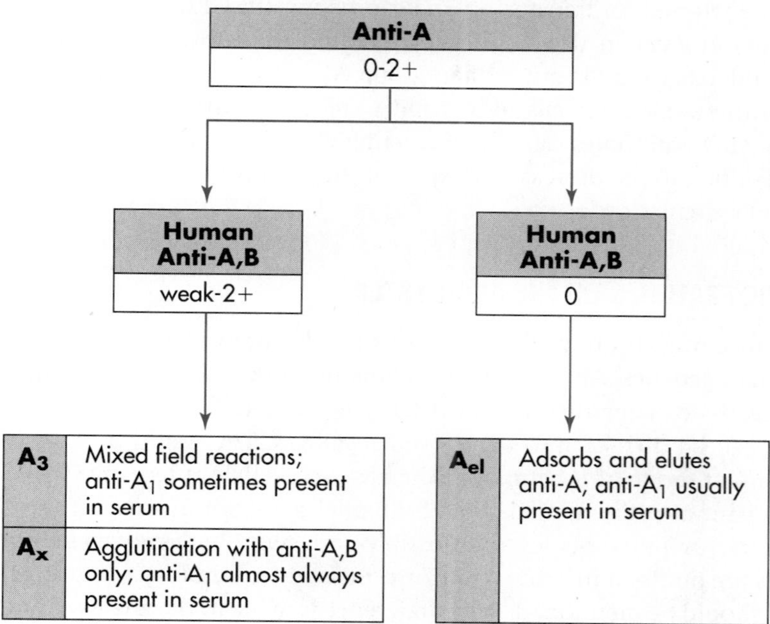

Fig. 4-8 **Practical application: recognition and resolution of rare A subgroups.**

Table 4-3 Serologic Characteristics of A_3, A_x, and A_{el} Subgroups

	RED BLOOD CELL AGGLUTINATION WITH					
SUB-GROUP	ANTI-A	HUMAN ANTI-A,B	ANTI-H LECTIN*	ANTI-A_1 LECTIN†	SOLUBLE ANTIGENS IN SALIVA‡	ANTI-A IN SERUM
A_3	++mf	++mf	+++	0	A and H	Less frequent
A_x	weak/0	+/++	++++	0	H	More frequent
A_{el}	0	0	++++	0	H	Frequent

mf, Mixed field; ++++, 4+; +++, 3+; ++, 2+; +, 1+.
**Ulex europaeus.*
†*Dolichos biflorus.*
‡If secretor.

A_{el} SUBGROUP. Human polyclonal and monoclonal anti-A and human polyclonal anti-A,B do not agglutinate A_{el} red blood cells. Special techniques of **adsorption** and **elution** are necessary to demonstrate the presence of the A antigen. Serum from A_{el} individuals usually contains anti-A_1.[10] A summary of these rare A subgroups is presented in Table 4-3.

SUBGROUPS OF B. Subgroups of B are rarer than the A subgroups previously discussed. The criteria for the recognition and differentiation of these subgroups are similar to those of the A subgroups. Typically these subgroups demonstrate weak or no agglutination of red blood cells with anti-B.

Adsorption: immunohematologic technique that uses red blood cells (known antigens) to remove red blood cell antibodies from a solution (plasma or antisera); group A red blood cells can remove anti-A from solution.
Elution: process that dissociates antigen-antibody complexes on red blood cells; freed IgG antibody is tested for specificity.

Importance of Subgroup Identification in Donor Testing

Although subgroups of A and B are considered of academic interest, the failure to detect a weak subgroup could have serious consequences. If a weak subgroup is missed in a recipient (the individual receiving the transfusion), the recipient would be classified as group O. Classification as a group O rather than a weak subgroup would probably not harm the recipient, since group O red blood cells would be selected for transfusion and can be transfused to any ABO phenotype. However, an error in donor phenotyping and the subsequent labeling of the donor unit as group O (rather than group A) might result in the decreased survival of the transfused cells in a group O recipient. Group O recipients would possess ABO antibodies capable of reacting with the weak subgroup antigens in vivo, resulting in the decreased survival of these transfused red blood cells in the recipient's circulation.

GENETIC FEATURES OF THE ABO SYSTEM

Inheritance of genes from the *ABO* locus on chromosome 9 follows the laws of Mendelian genetics. An individual inherits two *ABO* genes (one from each parent). The three major alleles of the ABO system are *A*, *B*, and *O*. Subsequently the *A* gene can be divided into the A^1 and A^2 alleles. The *A* and *B* genes express a codominant mode of inheritance, whereas the *O* allele is recessive. The A^1 allele is dominant over the A^2 allele, and both alleles are dominant over the *O* allele. The major ABO phenotypes and possible corresponding genotypes for the phenotypes are outlined in Table 4-4. Correct use of terminology regarding the ABO system should be mentioned. When reference is made to the alleles A^1 and A^2, the numbers are always indicated as superscripts. However, in references to the A_1 and A_2 phenotypes, the numbers are always indicated in a subscript format.

Table 4-4 ABO Phenotypes and Possible Genotypes

Phenotype	Possible genotypes
A_1	A^1A^1
	A^1A^2
	A^1O
A_2	A^2A^2
	A^2O
B	*BB*
	BO
A_1B	A^1B
A_2B	A^2B
O	*OO*

Because the *O* allele is recessive, it is not always possible to determine the ABO genotype from the corresponding phenotype without family studies. Red blood cells can only be phenotyped for the presence or absence of antigens and cannot be genotyped. Unless a family study has been performed with conclusive results, a genotype is only a probable interpretation of a phenotype. Deduction of the genotype from a family study is illustrated in Fig. 4-9. The Generation I female's phenotype is group B with possible genotypes of *BB* or *BO*, and the male's phenotype is group A with the possible genotypes of *AA* or *AO*. The parental genotypes may be deduced only after phenotyping the offspring. The four offspring's phenotypes are presented in Generation II. To produce a group O offspring, both parents must have passed on the *O* allele. Therefore their genotypes must be *AO* and *BO*.

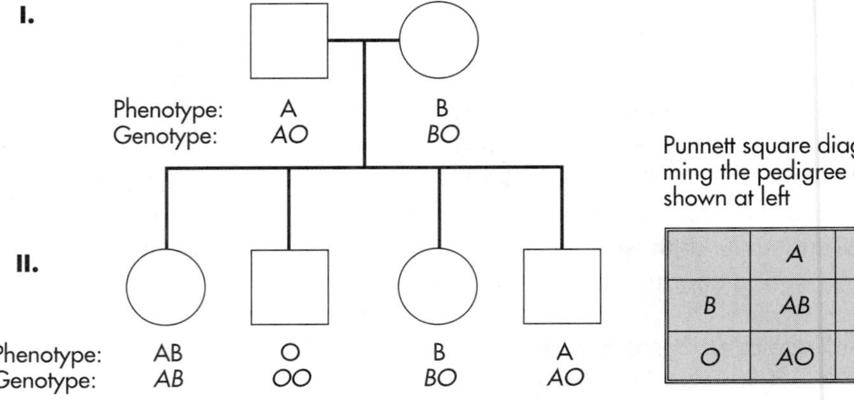

Fig. 4-9 Practical application: ABO inheritance patterns.

ABO SYSTEM ANTIBODIES

As Landsteiner recognized in his early experiments, individuals possess the ABO antibody in their serum directed against the ABO antigen absent from their red blood cells. Landsteiner's rule remains an important consideration in the selection of blood products, since ABO antibodies exist in healthy individuals. These ABO antibodies, present in individuals with no known exposure to blood or blood products, were originally thought to be "naturally occurring." It is currently hypothesized that biochemical structures similar to A and B antigens are present in the environment in bacteria, plants, and pollen. As a result of this environmental exposure to these similar forms of A and B antigens, individuals respond immunologically to these antigens and produce ABO antibodies detectable in plasma and serum.[14] Consequently, the term *naturally occurring* is a misnomer, since an immunologic stimulus is present for antibody development. The term **non–red blood cell stimulated** is more appropriate for describing the ABO antibodies.

Non–red blood cell stimulated: immunologic stimulus for antibody production is unrelated to a red blood cell antigen.
Titers: extent to which an antibody may be diluted before it loses its ability to agglutinate with antigen.

ABO antibodies are not detected in the serum of newborns until 3 to 6 months of age. Maximal ABO **titers** have been reported in children from 5 to 10 years of age. With advancing age the ABO titers tend to decrease and may cause problems in ABO phenotyping. In addition to those in newborn and elderly patients, other situations exist where ABO antibody titers may be weak or not demonstrable in testing.[15] These situations are outlined in Box 4-1. The recognition of these circumstances can assist in resolving ABO phenotyping problems discussed later in this chapter.

BOX 4-1

Reduction in ABO Antibody Titers

AGE-RELATED
Newborn
Elderly

PATHOLOGIC ETIOLOGY
Chronic lymphocytic leukemia
Congenital hypogammaglobulinemia or **acquired hypogammaglobulinemia**
Congenital agammaglobulinemia or **acquired agammaglobulinemia**
Immunosuppressive therapy
Bone marrow transplant
Multiple myeloma

General Characteristics of Human Anti-A and Anti-B

Immunoglobulin Class

The anti-A produced in group B individuals and the anti-B produced in group A individuals contain primarily antibodies of the IgM immunoglobulin class along with small amounts of IgG. In contrast the anti-A and anti-B antibodies found in the serum of group O individuals are composed primarily of IgG class.

Hemolytic Properties and Clinical Significance

Either immunoglobulin class of anti-A and anti-B—IgM or IgG—is capable of the activation and binding of complement and eventual hemolysis of red blood cells in vivo or in vitro. Because of their ability to activate the complement cascade with resultant red blood cell hemolysis, the ABO antibodies are considered of **clinical significance** in transfusion medicine. An antigen-antibody reaction between a recipient's ABO antibody and the ABO phenotype of the transfused red blood cells can cause the activation of complement and the destruction of the transfused donor red blood cells, precipitating the clinical signs and symptoms of an acute hemolytic transfusion reaction. For example, a group A recipient has circulating anti-B antibodies in serum. If this individual is transfused with group B or AB donor red blood cells, the circulating anti-B will recognize the B antigen on the donor red blood cells and combine with the antigens. The complement system is readily activated, causing a decreased survival of transfused red blood cells.

Clinical significance: antibodies that are capable of causing a decreased survival of transfused cells as in a transfusion reaction.
Congenital hypogammaglobulinemia: genetic disease characterized by reduced levels of gamma globulin in the blood.
Acquired hypogammaglobulinemia: less than normal levels of gamma globulin in the blood associated with malignant diseases (chronic leukemias and myeloma) and immunosuppression therapy.
Congenital agammaglobulinemia: genetic disease characterized by the absence of gamma globulin and antibodies in the blood.
Acquired agammaglobulinemia: the absence of gamma globulin and antibodies associated with malignant diseases such as leukemia, myeloma, or lymphoma.

In Vitro Serologic Reactions

ABO antibodies directly agglutinate a suspension of red blood cells in a physiologic saline environment and do not require any additional potentiators. They are optimally reactive in immediate spin phases at room temperature (25° C). The agglutination reactions do not require an incubation period and react without delay upon centrifugation.

Human Anti-A,B from Group O Individuals

Human anti-A,B is detected in the serum of group O individuals and possesses unique activities beyond mixtures of anti-A and anti-B antibodies. Its activity is regarded as a specificity that is cross-reactive with both A and B antigens. A cross-reactive antibody is capable of recognizing a particular molecular structure (antigenic determinant) common to several molecules. This distinguishing characteristic enables the antibody to agglutinate with red blood cells of group A, B, and AB phenotype, since this antibody recognizes a structure shared by both A and B antigens. Human anti-A,B also manifests the property of agglutinating red blood cells of infrequent subgroups of A, particularly A_X. Before the advent of monoclonal reagents, human anti-A,B was widely used to detect these infrequent subgroups in routine ABO typing. Monoclonal antisera has since replaced the use of human anti-A,B in ABO phenotyping.

Anti-A_1

In accordance with Landsteiner's rule for expected ABO antibodies, sera from group O and B individuals contain anti-A antibodies. The anti-A produced by group O and B individuals can be separated by adsorption and elution techniques into two components: anti-A and anti-A_1. Anti-A_1 is specific for the A_1 antigen and does not agglutinate A_2 red blood cells. The optimal reactivity of this antibody is at room temperature or below. Anti-A_1 is not considered clinically significant for transfusion purposes. Anti-A_1 becomes a concern when it causes problems with ABO phenotyping results and **incompatible crossmatches** on immediate spin. Anti-A_2 does not exist, since the A_2 phenotype possesses the same A antigens as the A_1 phenotype but in reduced quantities. Therefore individuals with A_1 phenotype do not respond immunologically on exposure to A_2 red blood cells.

Incompatible crossmatches: occur when agglutination or hemolysis is observed in the crossmatch of donor red blood cells and patient serum, indicating a serologic incompatibility. The donor unit would not be transfused.

ROUTINE ABO PHENOTYPING

A fundamental procedure of immunohematologic testing is the determination of the ABO phenotype. The procedure is straightforward and divided into two components: testing of the red blood cells for the presence of ABO antigens (or forward grouping) and testing of serum or plasma for the expected ABO antibodies (or reverse grouping). According to the *Standards for Blood Banks and Transfusion Services*, donor and recipient red blood cells must be tested using anti-A and anti-B reagents. Donor and recipient serum or plasma must be tested for the expected ABO antibodies using reagent A_1 and B red blood cells.[15] Neither human anti-A,B nor the monoclonal blend anti-A,B is required in ABO typing. Testing of cord blood and samples from infants less than 4 months old require only red blood cell testing in ABO phenotyping, since ABO antibody levels are not detectable. Refer to Chapter 2 for a discussion of the various ABO commercial antisera.

The ABO phenotype is determined when the red blood cells are directly tested for the presence or absence of either A or B antigens. Serum testing provides a control for red blood cell testing, since ABO antibodies would reflect

Landsteiner's rule. Table 4-5 shows the expected reactions observed in ABO phenotyping. An **ABO discrepancy** occurs when red blood cell testing does not agree with the expected serum testing. Any discrepancy in ABO testing should be resolved before transfusion of recipients or labeling of donor units.

ABO discrepancy: occurs when ABO phenotyping of red blood cells does not agree with expected serum testing results for the particular ABO phenotype.

SELECTION OF ABO-COMPATIBLE RED BLOOD CELLS AND PLASMA PRODUCTS FOR TRANSFUSION

In routine transfusion practices donor products (red blood cells and plasma) with identical ABO phenotypes are usually available to the recipient. This transfusion selection is referred to as providing *ABO-identical (ABO group–specific)* blood for the intended recipient. In situations where blood of identical ABO phenotype is not available, *ABO-compatible (ABO group–compatible)* blood may be issued to the recipient. For red blood cell transfusions ABO compatibility between the recipient and the donor is defined as the serologic compatibility between the ABO antibodies present in the recipient's serum and the ABO antigens expressed on the donor's red blood cells. For example, a group A recipient, who concurrently demonstrates anti-B in serum, would be compatible with either group A or O donor red blood cells, since serum anti-B would not react with either the group A or O red blood cells in vivo. However, if this individual receives a transfusion with either group B or AB donor red blood cells, recipient anti-B antibodies will recognize the B antigens present on the red blood cells. Antigen-antibody complexes form, activate the complement cascade, and result in the signs and symptoms of an acute hemolytic transfusion reaction. It is important to note that ABO compatibility applies to red blood cell transfusions but not to those of whole blood. When whole blood is transfused, ABO-identical donor units must be provided, since both plasma and red blood cells are present in the product. The concepts of ABO compatibility for whole blood and red blood cell transfusions are outlined in Table 4-6.

Persons with group O red blood cells are called **universal donors,** since the red blood cell product lacks both A and B antigens and could be transfused to any ABO phenotype. Group O donor red blood cells can be used in times of urgency for emergency release of donor units. Conversely group AB recipients are considered **universal recipients,** since these individuals can receive red blood cells of any ABO phenotype because they lack circulating ABO antibodies.

When plasma products are transfused the selection of an ABO-identical phenotype is the ideal situation. When identical ABO phenotypes are unavailable the rationale for compatible plasma transfusions is the reverse of red blood cell transfusions. In this case the donor's plasma must be compatible with the recipient's red blood cells. This concept translates to the serologic compatibility between the

Universal donors: group O donors for red blood cell transfusions; these red blood cells may be transfused to any ABO phenotype because the cells lack both A and B antigens.

Universal recipients: group AB recipients may receive transfusions of red blood cells from any ABO phenotype; this recipient lacks circulating ABO antibodies in plasma.

Table 4-6 Practical Application: ABO Compatibility for Whole Blood, Red Blood Cells, and Plasma Transfusions

Recipient	Donor		
ABO phenotype	Whole blood	Red blood cells	Plasma
A	A	A, O	A, AB
B	B	B, O	B, AB
AB	AB	AB, A, B, O	AB
O	O	O	O, A, B, AB

Universal donor for red blood cell transfusions is group O; universal donor for plasma transfusions is group AB.

Table 4-5 ABO Phenotyping Reactions

PHENOTYPE	RED BLOOD CELL REACTIONS		SERUM OR PLASMA REACTIONS	
	ANTI-A	ANTI-B	A_1 CELLS	B CELLS
A	+	0	0	+
B	0	+	+	0
O	0	0	+	+
AB	+	+	0	0

+, Agglutination; *0*, no agglutination.

ABO antibodies in the donor unit with and the ABO antigens present on the recipient's red blood cells. For example, group A recipients needing plasma would be compatible with group A and AB plasma products. Because group A plasma contains anti-B, and group AB has no ABO antibodies, these plasma products do not recognize the A antigen on recipient red blood cells. No adverse antigen-antibody reaction would ensue. For the transfusion of plasma group AB is considered the universal donor, and group O is the universal recipient (Table 4-6).

RECOGNITION AND RESOLUTION OF ABO DISCREPANCIES

The recognition and resolution of ABO discrepancies are challenging aspects of problem solving in the blood bank. As defined in a previous section, an ABO discrepancy is an ABO phenotype in which the results of the red blood cell testing do not agree with the results of expected serum testing. Discrepancies may be indicated when the following observations are noted in the results of ABO phenotyping:

- ◆ Agglutination strengths of the typing reactions are weaker than expected. Typically the reactions in ABO red blood cell testing with reagents anti-A and anti-B are 3+ to 4+ agglutination reactions; the results of ABO serum testing with reagent A_1 and B cells are 2+ to 4+
- ◆ Expected reactions in ABO red blood cell testing and serum testing are missing (for example, a group O is missing one or both reactions in the serum testing with reagent A_1 and B cells)
- ◆ Extra reactions are noted in either the ABO red blood cell or serum tests

The source of these discrepancies can be either technical or sample-related problems. The first step in the resolution of an ABO discrepancy is to identify the source of the problem. Is the discrepancy a technical error in testing, or is the discrepancy related to the sample itself?

Technical Considerations in ABO Typing

Several sources of technical errors can transpire in ABO typing and lead to erroneous results. An awareness and recognition of these technical errors can assist in the resolution of an ABO discrepancy. These technical errors can be classified into several categories, including identification and documentation errors, reagent and equipment problems, and standard operating procedure errors. By following the guidelines outlined in Box 4-2, technical sources of error can be pinpointed more readily. A new sample can be obtained to eliminate possible contamination or identification problems. In addition red blood cell suspensions prepared from patient samples can be washed three times before repeated testing. Once a technical error is discovered and corrected, the ABO discrepancy can be quickly resolved upon repeated testing. If the discrepancy still exists after repeated testing, the possibility of a problem related to the sample itself (e.g., related to the patient or donor) should be considered.

Sample-Related ABO Discrepancies

Sample-related problems can be divided into two groups: ABO discrepancies that affect the ABO red blood cell testing and those that affect the ABO serum testing. Is the problem associated with the patient or donor red blood cells, or is it associated with patient or donor antibodies? A logical approach to solving these sample-related problems is to select the side of the ABO test (red blood cell test-

BOX 4-2 Practical Application: Guidelines for Investigating ABO Technical Errors

IDENTIFICATION OR DOCUMENTATION ERRORS
Correct sample identification on all tubes
Results are properly recorded
Interpretations are accurate and properly recorded

REAGENT OR EQUIPMENT ERRORS
Daily quality control on ABO typing reagents is satisfactory
Inspect reagents for contamination and hemolysis
Centrifugation time and calibration are confirmed

STANDARD OPERATING PROCEDURE ERRORS
Procedure follows manufacturer's directions
Correct reagents were used and added to testing
Red blood cell suspensions are at the correct concentration
Cell buttons are completely suspended before grading the reaction

BOX 4-3 Overview of ABO Discrepancies

PROBLEMS WITH RED BLOOD CELL TESTING?
Extra antigens
Acquired B phenotype
B(A) phenotype
Polyagglutination
Rouleaux
Missing or weak antigen
ABO subgroup
Pathologic etiology
Mixed field reactions
Transfusion of group O to A, B, or AB
Bone marrow or stem cell transplants
A_3 phenotype

PROBLEMS WITH SERUM TESTING?
Extra antibodies
A subgroups with anti-A_1
Cold alloantibodies
Cold autoantibodies
Rouleaux
Missing or weak antibodies
Newborn
Elderly population
Pathologic etiology

ing or serum testing) believed to be discrepant and to focus on the problem from this angle. The observed strengths of agglutination reactions in both testing of the red blood cells and serum are keys in determining whether to focus problem solving on a red blood cell or a serum problem. For success with this approach, a working knowledge of the multitude of potential problems relating to ABO red blood cell and serum testing is mandatory (Box 4-3). The most common ABO discrepancies encountered in the immunohematology laboratory are those relating to weak or missing ABO antibodies in serum testing. ABO discrepancies associated with red blood cell testing are examined first before discussion of those associated with serum testing.

ABO Discrepancies Associated with Red Blood Cell Testing

Those ABO discrepancies that affect the testing of red blood cells (forward grouping) can be classified into three categories: extra antigens present, missing antigens, and mixed field reactions.

■ **EXTRA ANTIGENS PRESENT.** ABO red blood cell typing results may demonstrate unexpected positive agglutination reactions with either commercial reagent anti-A or anti-B. Extra reactions are present in red blood cell testing or forward grouping. For the purposes of this book, the scope of the discussion on extra antigens in red blood cell testing is limited to the illustration of the **acquired B phenotype** and the **B(A) phenotype**.

Examples 1 and 2 follow to demonstrate extra antigens present with the acquired B and B(A) phenotype.

Acquired B phenotype: group A_1 individual with diseases of the lower gastrointestinal tract, cancers of the colon and rectum, intestinal obstruction, or gram-negative septicemia who acquires reactivity with anti-B reagents in ABO red blood cell testing and appears as group AB.

B(A) phenotype: group B individual who acquires reactivity with anti-A reagents in ABO red blood cell testing; in these individuals the B gene transfers trace amounts of the immunodominant sugar for the A antigen and the immunodominant sugar for the B antigen.

▼

EXAMPLE 1

Acquired B Phenotype

ABO Typing Results			
Patient RBCs with		Patient Serum with Reagent RBCs	
Anti-A*	Anti-B*	A_1	B
4+	1+	0	4+

RBCs, Red blood cells.
*Monoclonal ABO antisera.

EVALUATION OF ABO RESULTS

1. The agglutination of the patient's red blood cells with anti-A is strong (4+).
2. The agglutination of the patient's red blood cells with anti-B is weaker (1+) than is usually expected (3+ to 4+). These red blood cells react as the phenotype group AB.
3. The results of serum testing reactions are typical of a group A individual.

CONCLUSION

These results are typical of individuals possessing the acquired B phenotype. In acquired B phenotype a group A individual possesses an extra antigen in red blood cell testing (notice the weaker agglutination with anti-B reagents). Anti-B is observed in the serum testing. Serum testing reactions are typical for a group A individual.

BACKGROUND INFORMATION

Usually only group A_1 individuals, with diseases of the lower gastrointestinal tract, cancers of the colon and rectum, intestinal obstruction, or gram-negative septicemia, express the acquired B phenotype. The most common mechanism for this phenotype is usually associated with a bacterial **deacetylating** enzyme that alters the A immunodominant sugar, *N*-acetylgalactosamine, by removing the acetyl group. The resulting sugar, galactosamine, resembles the B immunodominant sugar, D-galactose, and cross-reacts with many anti-B reagents.[16] Recent reports have linked the incidence of the acquired B phenotype with certain monoclonal anti-B blood grouping reagents licensed by the Food and Drug Administration.[17] Red blood cells agglutinated strongly by anti-A, and weakly by anti-B in combination with a serum containing anti-B, suggest the acquired B phenotype. These patients should receive units of group A red blood cells for transfusion purposes.

Deacetylating: removal of the acetyl group (CH_3CO–).

RESOLUTION OF ABO DISCREPANCY

1. Determine the patient's diagnosis and transfusion history. The first step in the resolution of any ABO discrepancy is to obtain more information on the pa-

tient. This information may provide additional clues about the root of the ABO discrepancy.

2. Test the patient's serum against **autologous** red blood cells. Anti-B in the patient's serum does not agglutinate autologous red blood cells with the acquired B antigen.
3. Test red blood cells with additional monoclonal anti-B reagents from other manufacturers that are documented not to react with the acquired B antigen or a source of human polyclonal anti-B.

Autologous: pertaining to self.

EXAMPLE 2

B(A) Phenotype

ABO Typing Results			
Patient RBCs with		Patient Serum with Reagent RBCs	
Anti-A*	Anti-B*	A_1	B
1+	4+	4+	0

RBCs, Red blood cells.
*Monoclonal ABO antisera.

EVALUATION OF ABO RESULTS

1. The agglutination of the patient's red blood cells with anti-A is weak (1+).
2. The agglutination of the patient's red blood cells with anti-B is strong (4+).
3. The results of serum testing are typical of a group B individual.

CONCLUSION

These results are characteristic of a possible B(A) phenotype. In the B(A) phenotype a group B with apparent extra antigen reaction occurring with anti-A in red blood cell testing is observed.

BACKGROUND INFORMATION

The B(A) phenotype has been observed as a result of the increased sensitivity of potent monoclonal reagents for ABO phenotyping.[18] These reagents can detect trace amounts of either A or B antigens that are nonspecifically transferred by the glycosyltransferase enzymes. In the B(A) phenotype the *B* gene transfers trace amounts of the immunodominant sugar for the A antigen (*N*-acetylgalactosamine) and the immunodominant sugar for the B antigen (D-galactose) to the H antigen acceptor molecules. The trace amounts of A antigens are detected with certain clones from the monoclonal reagents. A similar mechanism can cause an A(B) phenotype analogous to the acquired B phenotype.

RESOLUTION OF ABO DISCREPANCY

1. Determine the patient's diagnosis and transfusion history.
2. Test red blood cells with additional monoclonal anti-A reagents from other manufacturers or a source of human polyclonal anti-A.

Other potential explanations for extra antigens in ABO red blood cell testing include the following:

- **Polyagglutination** of red blood cells by most human sera as a result of the exposure of a hidden T antigen on the red blood cell membrane because of a bacterial infection

Polyagglutination: agglutination of red blood cells by most human sera regardless of blood type.

Wharton's jelly: gelatinous tissue contaminant in cord blood samples that may interfere in immunohematologic tests.

- Nonspecific aggregation of serum-suspended red blood cells because of abnormal concentrations of serum proteins or **Wharton's jelly** in cord blood samples (false agglutination)

■ **MISSING OR WEAKLY EXPRESSED ANTIGENS.** In this category of ABO discrepancies, patient or donor red blood cells demonstrate weaker than usual reactions with reagent anti-A and anti-B or may fail to demonstrate any reactivity. Phenomena associated with this category include:

- ABO subgroups
- Weakened A and B antigen expression in patients with leukemia or Hodgkin's disease

Example 3, illustrating missing or weakly expressed antigens in a subgroup of A, follows.

EXAMPLE 3

Subgroup of A

ABO Typing Results			
Patient RBCs with		Patient Serum with Reagent RBCs	
Anti-A*	Anti-B*	A_1	B
0	0	0	3+

RBCs, Red blood cells.
*Monoclonal ABO antisera.

EVALUATION OF ABO RESULTS

1. No agglutination of the patient's red blood cells with both anti-A and anti-B is observed. The individual appears to be a group O phenotype.
2. The results of serum testing are typical of a group A individual. Agglutination of anti-B with reagent B cells is strong (3+).

CONCLUSION

These results are characteristic of a missing antigen in the red blood cell testing. The serum testing results are those expected in a group A individual. Anti-A, found in group O individuals, is absent in the serum testing.

BACKGROUND INFORMATION

As previously discussed in this chapter, weak or missing reactions with anti-A and anti-B correlate with subgroups of A and B. Subgroups of A represent less than 1% of the group A population, and the subgroups of B are even rarer. The inheritance of an alternative allele at the *ABO* locus results in a quantitative reduction of antigen sites per red blood cell and in weakened or missing reactions with anti-A and anti-B.

RESOLUTION OF ABO DISCREPANCY

1. Determine the patient's diagnosis and transfusion history.
2. Repeat the red blood cell testing with extended incubation times and include human polyclonal anti-A,B or monoclonal blend anti-A,B. The extended incubation time may enhance the antigen-antibody reaction.

Additional Testing Results	
	Anti-A,B
Patient Red Blood Cell	1+

Conclusion: Probable subgroup of A (A_x).

Additional Testing Results	
	Anti-A,B
Patient Red Blood Cell	0

Next Step: Perform adsorption and elution studies with anti-A. These studies assist in determining the presence of A antigens on the patient's red blood cells.

■ **MIXED FIELD REACTIONS.** Mixed field reactions can occur in red blood cell testing with either anti-A or anti-B reagents. As noted earlier a mixed field reaction contains agglutinates with a mass of unagglutinated red blood cells. Usually a mixed field reaction is due to the presence of two distinct cell populations. For example, testing red blood cells from a patient recently transfused with non–ABO-identical red blood cells (group O donor red blood cells to a group AB recipient) can yield mixed field observations. In addition to the transfusion of group O red blood cells to group A, B, or AB individuals, recipients of recent **bone marrow transplant** and **stem cell transplant,** individuals with the A_3 phenotype, and patients with **Tn-polyagglutinable red blood cells** can demonstrate mixed field reactions. Example 4, showing mixed field reactions, follows.

Bone marrow transplant: procedure that transplants bone marrow from healthy donors to stimulate the production of blood cells.

Stem cell transplant: procedure that uses peripheral blood stem cells in lieu of bone marrow to stimulate the production of blood cells.

Tn-polyagglutinable red blood cells: type of polyagglutination that results from a mutation in the hematopoietic tissue, characterized by mixed field reactions in agglutination testing.

EXAMPLE 4

Group B Transfused with Group O Red Blood Cells			
ABO Typing Results			
Patient RBCs with		Patient Serum with Reagent RBCs	
Anti-A*	Anti-B*	A_1	B
0	2+mf	3+	0

RBCs, Red blood cells; *mf*, mixed field.
*Monoclonal ABO antisera.

EVALUATION OF ABO RESULTS

1. The strength of the agglutination reaction with anti-B is weaker than expected for group B individuals.
2. The anti-B mixed field grading of reactivity is a 2+ reaction with a sufficient number of unagglutinated cells.
3. The results of serum testing are typical of a group B individual.

CONCLUSION

These results demonstrate a group B individual possibly transfused with group O red blood cells.

BACKGROUND INFORMATION

In certain situations ABO-identical red blood cell products may not be available for transfusion, and group O red blood cells are transfused. If many group O donor red blood cell units are transfused in respect to the recipient's total body mass, mixed field reactions may appear in the ABO red blood cell testing.

RESOLUTION OF ABO DISCREPANCY

1. Determine the patient's diagnosis and recent transfusion history.
2. Determine if the patient is a recent bone marrow or stem cell recipient.
3. Investigate pretransfusion ABO phenotype history, if possible.

ABO Discrepancies Associated with Serum Testing

ABO discrepancies that affect the serum testing (reverse grouping) include the presence of additional antibodies other than anti-A and anti-B or the absence of expected ABO antibody reactions. The most commonly encountered ABO discrepancies involve the absence of expected ABO antibody reactions.

ADDITIONAL ANTIBODIES IN SERUM TESTING. This section of ABO discrepancies addresses the detection of anti-A_1, **cold alloantibodies, cold autoantibodies,** and rouleaux in ABO typing. Examples 5 through 7 illustrate additional antibodies in serum testing.

Cold alloantibodies: red blood cell antibodies specific for other human red blood cell antigens that typically react at or below room temperature.
Cold autoantibodies: red blood cell antibodies specific for autologous antigens that typically react at or below room temperature.

EXAMPLE 5

Group A_2 with Anti-A_1

ABO Typing Results			
Patient RBCs with		Patient Serum with Reagent RBCs	
Anti-A*	Anti-B*	A_1	B
4+	0	2+	4+

RBCs, Red blood cells.
*Monoclonal ABO antisera.

EVALUATION OF ABO RESULTS

1. The agglutination pattern with anti-A and anti-B reagents is typical of a group A individual.
2. The results of serum testing with reagent A_1 and B cells indicate a group O individual.

CONCLUSION

These results demonstrate an extra reaction in the serum testing with the reagent A_1 red blood cells (2+). Possible explanations for these results include an anti-A_1, a cold alloantibody, a cold autoantibody, or rouleaux.

RESOLUTION OF ABO DISCREPANCY

1. Determine the patient's diagnosis and transfusion history.
2. Test the patient's red blood cells with anti-A_1 lectin to ascertain if a subgroup of A is present.

Additional Testing Results	
Patient Red Blood Cells with Anti-A_1 Lectin	Conclusion
0	Subgroup of A; suspect anti-A_1 antibody

3. Test the patient's serum with three examples of A_1 and A_2 cells to confirm the presence of anti-A_1 antibody.

Additional Testing Results					
Patient Serum Testing with					
A_1 Cells	A_1 Cells	A_1 Cells	A_2 Cells	A_2 Cells	A_2 Cells
2+	2+	2+	0	0	0

CONCLUSION

Agglutination is observed with A_1 red blood cells providing the evidence for anti-A_1. The serum does not agglutinate with A_2 red blood cells. Remember that anti-A_1 may be present in 1% to 8% of the group A_2 phenotype.

EXAMPLE 6

Cold Autoantibody and Cold Alloantibody			
ABO Typing Results			
Patient RBCs with		Patient Serum with Reagent RBCs	
Anti-A*	Anti-B*	A_1	B
4+	4+	0	1+

RBCs, Red blood cells.
*Monoclonal ABO antisera.

EVALUATION OF ABO RESULTS

1. Strong agglutination reactions are observed in the red blood cell testing and are consistent with a group AB individual.
2. The results of serum testing with reagent B cells demonstrate a weaker extra reaction. This serum testing appears to be consistent with a group A individual.

CONCLUSION

These results indicate a possible extra reaction in the serum testing with the reagent B red blood cells. Possible considerations include a cold alloantibody or a cold autoantibody.

BACKGROUND INFORMATION

Donors and patients may possess antibodies to other blood group system red blood cell antigens in addition to those of the ABO system. These *alloantibodies* may appear as additional serum antibodies in ABO typing as one of the following specificities: anti-P_1, anti-M, anti-N, anti-Le^a, and anti-Le^b. Because they react at or below room temperature, these antibodies are sometimes referred to as *cold*. Reagent A_1 and B red blood cells used in ABO serum testing may possess these antigens in addition to the A and B antigens. Screening cells, group O reagent red blood cells, are used to detect an alloantibody because they lack A and B antigens. Any serum reactivity caused by an existing ABO antibody would be eliminated in the reaction with group O cells. It is logical to conclude that screening cells are valuable in distinguishing between ABO antibodies and alloantibodies.

Patients and donors may also possess serum antibodies directed toward their own red blood cell antigens. These antibodies are classified as autoantibodies. If autoantibodies are reactive at or below room temperature, they are also called *cold*. Cold autoantibodies usually possess the specificity of anti-I or anti-IH and react against all adult red blood cells, including screening cells, A_1 and B cells,

Autocontrol: testing a person's serum with his or her own red blood cells to determine if an autoantibody is present.

and autologous cells. An **autocontrol** (autologous control) is tested to differentiate a cold autoantibody from a cold alloantibody. If the autocontrol is positive, the reactions observed with the A_1 and B cells and screening cells are probably the result of autoantibodies. Refer to Chapter 7 for more information on cold autoantibody test methods and techniques useful in negating their reactivity in ABO typing tests.

RESOLUTION OF ABO DISCREPANCY

1. Determine the patient's diagnosis and transfusion history.
2. Test the patient's serum with screening cells and an autocontrol at room temperature. This strategy helps distinguish if a cold alloantibody or cold autoantibody is present.

Interpretation of Testing Results

	Screening Cells	Autologous Cells	Conclusion
Patient Serum	Pos*	Neg	Cold alloantibody
Patient Serum	Pos	Pos	Cold autoantibody

*Positive reaction if the corresponding antigen is present on the screening cell.

3. If an alloantibody is detected, antibody identification techniques can be performed (see Chapter 7).
4. If an autoantibody is detected, special techniques to identify the antibody (a minicold panel) and remove antibody reactivity (prewarming techniques) can be used (see Chapter 7).

EXAMPLE 7

Rouleaux

ABO Typing Results

Patient RBCs with		Patient Serum with Reagent RBCs	
Anti-A*	Anti-B*	A_1	B
4+	4+	2+	2+

RBCs, Red blood cells.
*Monoclonal ABO antisera.

EVALUATION OF ABO RESULTS

1. Strong agglutination reactions are observed in the red blood cell testing and are consistent with the expected results of a group AB individual.
2. The serum testing results are consistent with those of a group O individual.

CONCLUSION

Consider the possibility of extra reactions in the serum testing with the reagent red blood cells because of an alloantibody, an autoantibody, or rouleaux. The phenomenon of rouleaux is demonstrated in this example.

BACKGROUND INFORMATION

Rouleaux can produce false positive agglutination in testing. The red blood cells resemble stacked coins under microscopic examination. Increased concentrations of serum proteins can affect this spontaneous agglutination of red blood cells. Diseases associated with rouleaux include **multiple myeloma** and **Waldenström's macroglobulinemia**. In addition to creating problems with the serum testing in ABO phenotyping, rouleaux can create extra reactions in the ABO red blood cell typing if unwashed red blood cell suspensions are used.

Multiple myeloma: malignant neoplasm of the bone marrow characterized by abnormal proteins in the plasma and urine.

Waldenström's macroglobulinemia: overproduction of IgM by the clones of a plasma B cell in response to an antigenic signal; increased viscosity of blood is observed.

RESOLUTION OF ABO DISCREPANCY

1. Determine the patient's diagnosis and transfusion history.
2. Wash a red blood cell suspension and repeat the phenotyping.
3. Perform the **saline replacement technique** to help distinguish true agglutination from rouleaux (Fig. 4-10).

Saline replacement technique: test to distinguish rouleaux and true agglutination.

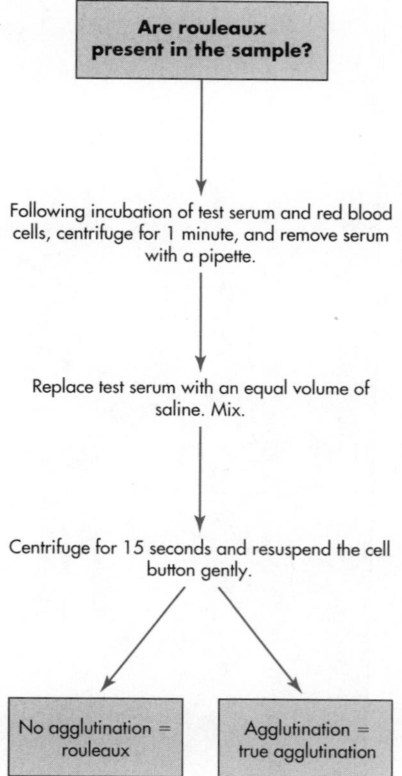

Fig. 4-10 Saline replacement technique.

Modified from Mallory D: *Immunohematology methods and procedures*, Rockville, Md, 1993, American Red Cross.

ABO Discrepancies Associated with Serum Testing

MISSING OR WEAK ANTIBODIES IN SERUM TESTING. ABO antibodies may be missing or weakened in certain patient-related situations and may result in an ABO discrepancy. Example 8 illustrates this discrepancy.

EXAMPLE 8

ABO Typing Results			
Patient RBCs with		Patient Serum with Reagent RBCs	
Anti-A*	Anti-B*	A_1	B
0	0	0	0

RBCs, Red blood cells.
*Monoclonal ABO antisera.

EVALUATION OF ABO RESULTS

1. The agglutination pattern with anti-A and anti-B is typical of a group O individual.
2. The results of serum testing with reagent A_1 and B cells indicate a group AB individual.

CONCLUSION

Consider approaching this problem from the angle of missing serum reactions with reagent A_1 or B cells.

BACKGROUND INFORMATION

An investigation of the patient's history, including age, diagnosis, and immunoglobulin levels, provides clues to explaining the missing reactions in the serum testing. The patient's age is an important factor, since the concentrations of ABO antibodies are reduced in the newborn and the elderly population. Knowledge of the patient's diagnosis is essential, since reduced immunoglobulin levels are also associated with several pathologic states (see Box 4-1). In conjunction with the patient's diagnosis, the immunoglobulin levels and serum protein electrophoretic patterns are helpful data in the resolution of, and in finding the cause of, this ABO discrepancy.

RESOLUTION OF ABO DISCREPANCY

1. Determine the patient's diagnosis, age, and immunoglobulin levels if available.
2. Incubate serum testing for 15 minutes at room temperature, and then centrifuge and examine for agglutination. This simple incubation often solves the

problem. If the results are still negative, place the serum testing at 4° C for 5 minutes with an autologous control. The control validates the test by ensuring that positive reactions are not attributable to a cold autoantibody.

Interpretation of Additional Testing Results				
4° C	A_1 Cells	B Cells	Autologous Cells	Conclusion
Patient Serum	Pos	Pos	Neg	Group O
Patient Serum	Pos	Pos	Pos	Cold autoantibody

SPECIAL TOPICS RELATED TO ABO AND H BLOOD GROUP SYSTEMS

Classic Bombay Phenotype

The classic Bombay phenotype is an unusual genetic occurrence associated with the ABO and H blood group systems. A 1952 report describing a family living in Bombay, India, is the source of the descriptive term for the phenotype.[1] This family's red blood cells were unusual because they lacked H antigens and subsequently any ABO antigen expression. Interestingly, both red blood cells and secretions were deficient in H and ABO antigen expression. The red blood cell reactions were characteristic of the group O phenotype in routine ABO testing. Serum testing demonstrated reactions similar to those of group O individuals. Another related antibody, anti-H, was detected in the family's serum in addition to the ABO antibodies of anti-A, anti-B, and anti-A,B. The anti-H in the Bombay phenotype is of clinical significance, since this antibody is capable of high thermal activity at 37° C and complement activation with resulting hemolysis.

Today more than 130 Bombay phenotypes have been reported with a relatively greater incidence in India.[19] Genetic family studies have identified the genotype required for this phenomenon. An individual who is homozygous for the *h* allele (*hh*) expresses the Bombay phenotype (the *H* and *h* genes of the *H* locus were previously described in this chapter). The *hh* genotype does not produce the L-fucosyltransferase necessary to transfer the immunodominant sugar, L-fucose, to the acceptor oligosaccharide chain to form the H antigen. As a result, the H antigen is not assembled on the red blood cells. Since H antigen is the building block for the development of the A and B antigens, neither A nor B glycosyltransferases can act on their substrate to produce the corresponding antigen structures, even though the ABO alleles are inherited. The resulting phenotype lacks expression of both H and ABO antigens. Transfusion for these individuals presents an especially difficult problem, since they are compatible only with the Bombay phenotype. If transfusion is necessary, stored autologous units, siblings, and rare donor files are potential options.

Secretor Status

The interrelationship of the secretor locus with the expression of ABO antigens in body fluids has been mentioned several times throughout this chapter. There are two allelic genes at this locus: *Se* and *se.* The *Se* allele's gene product is an L-fucosyltransferase that preferentially adds L-fucose to type 1 oligosaccharide chain structures. The *H* gene preferentially adds fucose to type 2 chains. The *Se* gene is directly responsible for the expression of H antigen on the glycoprotein structures located in body secretions such as saliva. An individual who inherits the *Se* allele

Example 1

Genes inherited				Antigen expression RBC	Saliva
AB	*HH*	*SeSe*	⟶	A, B, H	A, B, H
AB	*HH*	*sese*	⟶	A, B, H	None

Example 2

Genes inherited				Antigen expression RBC	Saliva
OO	*HH*	*Sese*	⟶	H	H
OO	*HH*	*sese*	⟶	H	None

Fig. 4-11 Practical application: interaction of ABO, H, and secretor genes in the expression of soluble antigens in saliva. *RBC*, Red blood cell.

in either a homozygous (*SeSe*) or a heterozygous (*Sese*) manner is classified as a **secretor**. About 80% of the random population inherit the *Se* allele and are classified as secretors. These individuals express soluble forms of H antigens in secretions that can be converted to A or B antigens by the A and B glycosyltransferases. These soluble antigens are found in saliva, urine, tears, bile, amniotic fluid, breast milk, exudate, and digestive fluids. An individual with the genotype (*sese*) is classified as a **nonsecretor**. Approximately 20% of the random population can be considered nonsecretors. The *se* allele is an amorph. A homozygote does not convert glycoprotein antigen precursors to H antigen and has neither soluble H antigens nor soluble A or B antigens present in body fluids. Fig. 4-11 illustrates the genetic interaction of the *ABO*, *H*, and *Se* loci.

Secretor: individual who inherits *Se* allele and expresses soluble forms of H antigens in secretions.

Nonsecretor: individual who inherits the genotype *sese* and does not express soluble forms of H antigen in secretions.

CHAPTER SUMMARY

The major concepts of ABO antigens and ABO antibodies presented in this chapter are summarized below.

IMPORTANT FACTS: ABO AND H SYSTEM ANTIGENS

Widespread antigen distribution	Blood cells, tissues, body fluids, secretions
Biochemical composition	Glycolipid/glycoprotein
Common structures	Type 1 and type 2 oligosaccharide chains
Gene products	Glycosyltransferases
Immunodominant sugars	H Antigen: L-fucose
	A Antigen: *N*-acetylgalactosamine
	B Antigen: D-galactose
Antigen expression	Cord blood cells: weak
Genetic loci	ABO system: chromosome 9
	H system: chromosome 19
Major alleles	A^1, A^2, *B*, *O*
	H, *h*
Bombay phenotype	Genotype *hh;* no H or ABO antigens
Secretor status	*Se* allele; soluble H and ABO antigens

IMPORTANT FACTS: ABO AND H SYSTEM ANTIBODIES

Landsteiner's rule	ABO antibody directed toward the A or B antigen that is absent from red blood cells
Antibody production	Not detectable in first few months of life; decreases in elderly population
Immunoglobulin class	IgM and IgG
In vitro reactions	At or below room temperature
Complement binding	Yes; some hemolytic
Clinical significance	Yes

◊ CRITICAL THINKING EXERCISES

◆ ***EXERCISE 4-1*** Case Study

RT, a 37-year-old woman, is a first-time donor at your blood center. She is a healthy donor with an unremarkable medical history and is not taking any medications. Initial ABO results indicate an ABO discrepancy.

ABO Typing Results

Donor RBCs with		Donor Serum with Reagent RBCs	
Anti-A*	Anti-B*	A_1	B
0	4+	3+	1+

RBCs, Red blood cells.
*Monoclonal ABO antisera.

1. Evaluate the ABO phenotyping results. Is the discrepancy associated with the red blood cell testing or the serum testing? State the reasons for this selection.
2. How would you classify the category of ABO discrepancy shown in this problem?
3. What are the potential causes of an ABO discrepancy in this category?

◆ ***Additional Testing***

No technical errors were found. The donor's red blood cells were washed and the ABO phenotyping was repeated. Red blood cell testing results were identical to the first set. In addition to A_1 and B cells, screening cells and an autologous control were tested with the donor's serum. The results of the testing are depicted in the following table.

Additional Testing Results

Donor's Serum Testing with			
A_1 Cells	B Cells	Screening Cells	Autologous Cells
3+	1+	1+	0

4. What conclusions can be drawn from the results of additional serum testing?
5. What additional steps are required to resolve this ABO discrepancy?

◆ ***EXERCISE 4-2***

What are the possible ABO phenotypes of offspring with parents of the genotypes A^1A^2 and BO?

◆ ***EXERCISE 4-3***

Why is group O considered a universal donor for the transfusion of red blood cells and a universal recipient for plasma transfusions?

◆ ***EXERCISE 4-4***

Create a diagram to illustrate the genetic pathways for ABO antigen production and the Bombay phenotype.

◆ ***EXERCISE 4-5***

For a Bombay phenotype encountered in the immunohematology laboratory:

1. Predict the agglutination reactions of patient's red blood cells with the following reagents: anti-A, anti-B, anti-A,B, and *Ulex europaeus*.
2. Predict the agglutination reactions of the patient's serum sample with the following reagent red blood cells: A_1, B, and O.

◆ ***EXERCISE 4-6***

Why does an individual with the genotyping of *AB, HH,* and *sese* possess A, B, and H antigens on red blood cells but not have any soluble forms of these antigens in the saliva?

STUDY QUESTIONS

1. Given the following ABO typing results, what conclusion can be drawn from these results?

ABO Typing Results			
Patient RBCs with		Patient Serum with Reagent RBCs	
Anti-A*	Anti-B*	A_1	B
4+	4+	1+	0

RBCs, Red blood cells.
*Monoclonal ABO antisera.

   a. expected results for a group O individual
   b. expected results for a group AB individual
   c. discrepant results; patient has A antigen on red blood cells with anti-A in serum
   d. discrepant results; patient has B antigen on red blood cells with no anti-B in serum

2. What are the gene products of the *A* and *B* genes?
   a. glycolipids
   b. glycoproteins
   c. oligosaccharides
   d. transferase enzymes

For questions 3 through 5, use the following ABO typing results.

ABO Typing Results			
Patient RBCs with		Patient Serum with Reagent RBCs	
Anti-A*	Anti-B*	A_1	B
0	0	4+	4+

RBCs, Red blood cells.
*Monoclonal ABO antisera.

3. What is the ABO interpretation?
   a. group O
   b. group A
   c. group B
   d. group AB

4. What ABO phenotypes would be compatible if the patient in question 3 required a transfusion of red blood cells?
   a. group AB, O, A, or B
   b. group O or B
   c. group AB or O
   d. only group O

5. What ABO phenotypes would be compatible if the patient in question 3 required a transfusion of fresh frozen plasma?
   a. group AB, O, A, or B
   b. group O or B
   c. group AB or O
   d. only group O

6. Using known sources of reagent antisera (known antibodies) to detect ABO antigens on a patient's red blood cells is known as:
   a. Rh typing
   b. reverse grouping
   c. direct antiglobulin test
   d. forward grouping

7. Which of the following results is discrepant if the red blood cell typing shown in the following chart is correct?

ABO Typing Results

Patient RBCs with		Patient Serum with Reagent RBCs	
Anti-A*	Anti-B*	A_1	B
0	4+	0	0

RBCs, Red blood cells.
*Monoclonal ABO antisera.

   a. negative reaction with B cells
   b. positive reaction with anti-B
   c. negative reaction with A_1 cells
   d. no discrepancies in these results

8. What ABO antibody is expected in this patient's serum based on the following information?

Patient Red Blood Cells with	
Anti-A*	Anti-B*
0	4+

*Monoclonal ABO antisera.

   a. anti-B
   b. anti-A
   c. anti-A and anti-B
   d. none

9. According to Landsteiner's rule, if a patient has no ABO antibodies after serum testing, what ABO antigens are present on the patient's red blood cells?
   a. A
   b. B
   c. both A and B
   d. none

10. Select the ABO phenotypes, in order from most frequent to least frequent, that occur in the White population:
   a. A, B, O, AB
   b. O, A, B, AB
   c. B, A, AB, O
   d. AB, O, B, A

11. Which of the following statements is true about ABO antibody production?
    a. ABO antibodies are present in newborns
    b. ABO titers remain at constant levels throughout life
    c. ABO antibodies are stimulated by bacteria and other environmental factors
    d. all of these statements are true

12. What immunoglobulin class is primarily associated with ABO antibodies?
    a. IgA
    b. IgG
    c. IgE
    d. IgM

13. What immunodominant sugar confers B blood group specificity?
    a. D-galactose
    b. L-fucose
    c. *N*-acetylgalactosamine
    d. L-glucose

14. An individual has the genotype of *AO, hh*. What antigens would be present on the red blood cells of this individual?
    a. A only
    b. A and H
    c. A and O
    d. none of the above

15. What gene controls the presence of soluble H antigens in saliva?
    a. *H*
    b. *A*
    c. *Se*
    d. *B*

16. Which lectin agglutinates A_1 red blood cells?
    a. *Dolichos biflorus*
    b. *Ulex europaeus*
    c. *Dolichos europaeus*
    d. *Ulex biflorus*

17. What immunodominant sugar builds H antigens?
    a. D-galactose
    b. L-fucose
    c. *N*-acetylgalactosamine
    d. L-glucose

18. Which of the following situations may produce ABO discrepancies in the serum testing?
    a. newborn
    b. patient with hypogammaglobulinemia
    c. cold alloantibody
    d. all of the above

19. What soluble antigen forms are detectable in saliva based on the following genotype: *AB, HH, SeSe*?
    a. none (nonsecretor)
    b. only H
    c. A, B, and H
    d. A and B

20. Which ABO discrepancy is the best explanation for the results shown in the following chart?

ABO Typing Results			
Patient RBCs with		Patient Serum with Reagent RBCs	
Anti-A*	Anti-B*	A_1	B
4+	0	2+	4+

RBCs, Red blood cells.
*Monoclonal ABO antisera.

a. an elderly patient
b. subgroup of A
c. deterioration of reagents
d. hypogammaglobulinemia

REFERENCES

1. Issitt PD, Anstee DJ: *Applied blood group serology*, ed 4, Durham, NC, 1998, Montgomery Scientific Publications.
2. Lewis M, Anstee DJ, Bird GWG, et al: *Blood group terminology 1990*, from the ISBT working party on terminology for red cell surface antigens, *Vox Sang* 58:152, 1990.
3. Lewis M, Anstee DJ, Bird GWG, et al: ISBT Working party on terminology for red cell surface antigens: Los Angeles report, *Vox Sang* 61:158, 1991.
4. Landsteiner K: Zur Kenntnis der antifermentativen, lytischen und agglutinierenden Wirkungen des Blutserums und der Lymphe, *Zbl Bakt* 27:357, 1900.
5. von Decastello A, Sturli A: Über die Isoagglutinine im Serum gesunder und kranker Menschen, *Munchen Med Wochenschr* 95:1090, 1902.
6. Reid ME, Lomas-Francis C: *The blood group antigen facts book*, San Diego, 1997, Academic Press.
7. Economidou J, Hughes-Jones N, Gardner B: Quantitative measurements concerning A and B antigen sites, *Vox Sang* 12:321, 1967.
8. Mourant AE, Kopeâc AC, Domaniewska-Sobczak K: *The distribution of the human blood groups and other biochemical polymorphisms*, ed 2, London, 1976, Oxford University Press.
9. Vengelen-Tyler V, editor: *Technical manual*, ed 12, Bethesda, Md, 1996, American Association of Blood Banks.
10. Pittiglio DH: Genetics and biochemistry of A, B, H and Lewis antigens. In Wallace ME, Gibbs FL, editors: *Blood group systems: ABH and Lewis*, Arlington, Va, 1986, American Association of Blood Banks.
11. Yamamoto F, Clausen H, White T, et al: Molecular genetic basis of the histo-blood group ABO system, *Nature* 345:229, 1990.
12. Fukuda MN, Hakamori S: Structures of branched blood group A–active glycosphingolipids in human erythrocytes and polymorphism of A- and H-glycolipids in A_1 and A_2 subgroups, *J Biol Chem* 257:446, 1982.
13. Lopez M, Benali J, Bony V, Salmon C: Activity of IgG and IgM ABO antibodies against some weak A (A_3, A_x, A_{end}) and weak B (B_3, B_x) red cells, *Vox Sang* 37:281, 1979.
14. Nance ST: Serology of the ABH and Lewis blood group systems. In Wallace ME, Gibbs FL, editors: *Blood group systems: ABH and Lewis*, Arlington, Va, 1986, American Association of Blood Banks.
15. Menitove JE, editor: *Standards for blood banks and transfusion services*, ed 18, Bethesda, Md, 1997, American Association of Blood Banks.
16. Gerbal A, Maslet C, Salmon C: Immunological aspects of the acquired B antigen, *Vox Sang* 28:398, 1975.
17. Beck ML, Kowalski MA, Kirkegaard JR, et al: Unexpected activity with monoclonal anti-B reagents, *Immunohematology* 8:22, 1992.
18. Beck ML, Yates AD, Hardman J, Kowalski MA: Identification of a subset of group B donors reactive with monoclonal anti-A reagent, *Am J Clin Pathol* 92:625, 1989.
19. Bhatia HM: Serologic reactions of ABO and Oh (Bombay) phenotypes due to variations in H antigens. In Mohn JF, Plunkett RW, Cunningham RK, Lambert RM, editors: *Human blood groups: proceedings of the fifth international convocation on immunology*, Basel, 1977, Karger.

SUGGESTED READINGS

Harmening D: *Modern blood banking and transfusion practices*, ed 4, Philadelphia, 1999, FA Davis.

Wallace ME, Gibbs FL, editors: *Blood group systems: ABH and Lewis*, Arlington, Va, 1986, American Association of Blood Banks.

Rh BLOOD GROUP SYSTEM 5

Kathy D. Blaney

CHAPTER OUTLINE

Historical Overview of the Discovery of the D Antigen
Genetics and Biochemistry
Rh Terminology
Fisher-Race: CDE Terminology
Wiener: Rh-Hr Terminology
Rosenfield: Numeric Terminology
International Society of Blood Transfusion: Standardized Numeric Terminology
Determining the Genotype from the Phenotype
Antigens of the Rh System
D Antigen
Other Rh System Antigens
Unusual Phenotypes
Rh Antibodies
General Characteristics
Clinical Considerations
LW Blood Group System
Relationship to the Rh System

LEARNING OBJECTIVES

Upon completion of this chapter, the reader should be able to:

1. Explain how the D antigen was named *Rh*.
2. Describe the current genetic theory of the inheritance of Rh system antigens.
3. Discuss the biochemistry of the Rh system, including the gene products and antigen structures.
4. Compare and contrast the genetic theories behind the Fisher-Race and Wiener terminology and be able to translate from one to the other.
5. Compare the Rosenfield and International Society of Blood Transfusion terminology with the Fisher-Race and Wiener terminology and discuss their use.
6. Predict the Rh genotype given a phenotype.
7. Define *weak D* and list the genetic circumstances that cause this phenotype.
8. Explain the test for the weak D antigen and the importance of an appropriate control.
9. Discuss the significance of testing for weak D.
10. Define *cis product antigens* and give two examples of this phenotype.
11. Describe the inheritance and significance of the G antigen.
12. Explain the significance of Rh_{null}, Rh_{mod}, and deletion phenotypes.
13. Describe the characteristics of the Rh system antibodies and their clinical significance with regard to transfusion and hemolytic disease of the newborn.
14. Compare and contrast the LW blood group system to the Rh system.
15. Describe anti-LW in terms of recognition and clinical significance.

The Rh blood group system is highly complex, polymorphic, and the second most important blood group system after the ABO system. Since the initial discovery of the D antigen in 1939, more than 50 related antigens have been added to the system. This chapter focuses on the five principal antigens, including D, C, E, c, and e, and their corresponding antibodies that account for most clinical transfusion issues. Readers are encouraged to review the suggested reading list for more details regarding theoretical considerations, rare phenotypes, and unusual antibodies.

HISTORICAL OVERVIEW OF THE DISCOVERY OF THE D ANTIGEN

The terms *Rh positive* and *Rh negative* refer to the presence or absence of the D red blood cell antigen. Unlike in the ABO system, the absence of Rh antigens on red blood cells does not typically correspond with the presence of the antibody in the plasma. The production of Rh antibodies requires immune red blood cell stimulation from red blood cells positive for the antigen in individuals lacking the antigen. This exposure may occur during transfusion or pregnancy.

The discovery of the Rh system, as with many other blood group systems, followed the investigation of an adverse transfusion reaction or hemolytic disease of the newborn (HDN). In 1940 the cause of HDN was linked to the Rh system by Levine and Stetson.[1] *Rh* was the name given to the system because of the similarity of this antibody to one made from stimulating guinea pigs and rabbits with rhesus monkey cells.[2] This Rh antibody, described by Landsteiner and Wiener, agglutinated 85% of human red blood cells tested and was nonreactive with 15%. This characterized the population as Rh positive or Rh negative. Later experiments demonstrated that the Rh antibody made from the guinea pigs and rabbits was similar, but not identical, in reactivity to the anti-Rh produced by humans. The rhesus antibody specificity was actually directed toward another red blood cell antigen named *LW* in honor of Landsteiner and Wiener. The name of the Rh system had been established by then and was not changed.

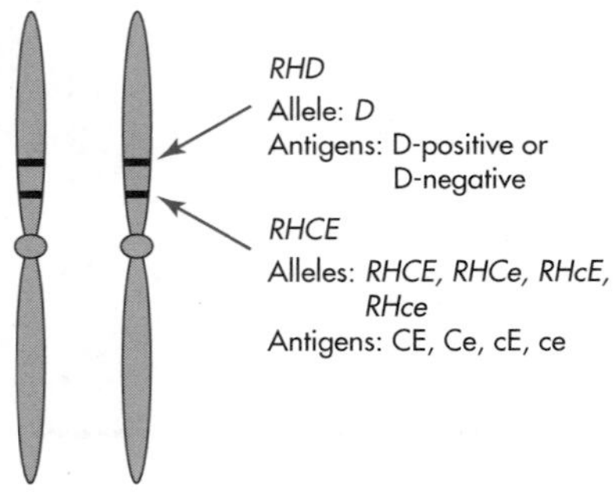

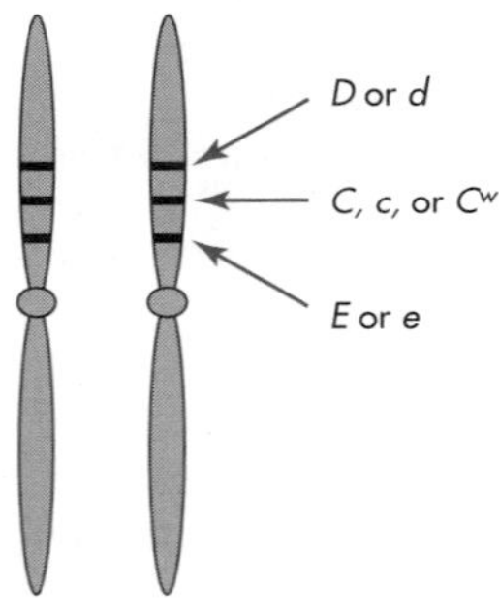

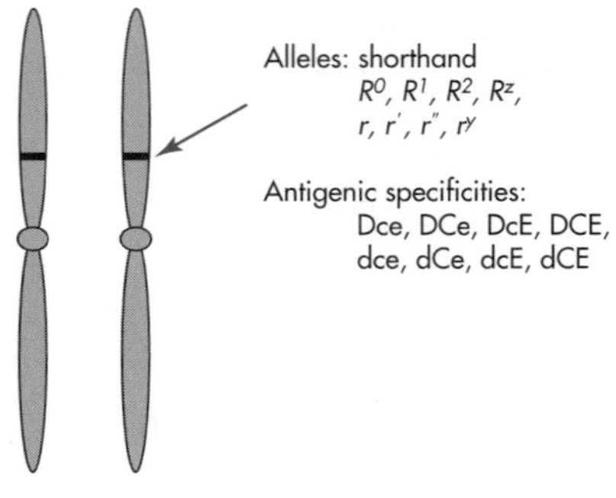

Fig. 5-1 Comparison of Rh genetic theories. Comparison of three Rh genetic theories that have influenced the nomenclature of the Rh system.

GENETICS AND BIOCHEMISTRY

Current theory explaining genetic control of Rh antigen expression has been enhanced with the ability to characterize the amino acid sequences produced by genes that code for proteins on the red blood cell membrane. A theory, originally postulated by Tippett,[3] describes two closely linked genes—*RHD* and *RHCE*—on chromosome 1. *RHD* determines the D antigen expression on the surface of red blood cells. D-negative individuals have no genetic material at this site.[4] An antithetical *d* allele does not exist. Adjacent to the *RHD* locus, the gene *RHCE* determines the C, c, E, and e antigens. The alleles at this locus are *RHCE, RHCe, RHcE,* and *RHce* (Fig. 5-1).[5] These genes encode the red blood cell antigens CE, Ce, cE, and ce. The *RHCE* gene codes for two similar polypeptides; only one critical amino acid distinguishes C,c and E,e,[6] as illustrated in Fig. 5-2. The assortment of other antigens in the Rh system occurs as a result of variations of these polypeptides embedded in the cell membrane bilayer in unique configurations. The more commonly encountered Rh antigens are listed in Table 5-1.

The products of both the *RHD* and *RHCE* genes are proteins of 416 amino acids that traverse the membrane 12 times and display short loops of amino acids on the exterior (Fig. 5-2).[7] The Rh system polypeptides, unlike most blood

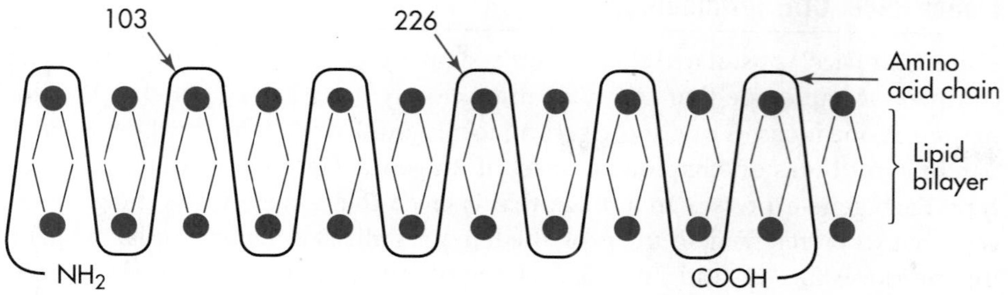

Antigen	Amino acid	Number
C	Serine	103
c	Proline	103
E	Proline	226
e	Alanine	226

Fig. 5-2 Model of the Rh Polypeptide. A model of the differences in the amino acid sequence for the antigens produced by the *RHCE* gene. An identical basic structure differs in the amino acid at the residue number indicated.

Table 5-1 Common Antigens in the Rh System: Equivalent Notations

NUMERIC	FISHER-RACE	WIENER	OTHER NAMES	ISBT NO.
Rh1	D	Rh_0	Rh+	004001
Rh2	C	rh′		004002
Rh3	E	rh″		004003
Rh4	c	hr′		004004
Rh5	e	hr″		004005
Rh6	ce	hr	*cis*-ce or f	004006
Rh7	Ce	rh_i	*cis*-Ce	004007
Rh8	C^w	rh^{w1}		004008
Rh9	C^x	rh^x		004009
Rh10	ce^s	hr^v	V	004010
Rh12	G	rh^G		004012

ISBT, International Society of Blood Transfusion.

group–associated proteins, carry no carbohydrate residues. Rh antigens have been detected only on red blood cell membranes, and the proteins are not recognized by antibodies once the proteins separate from the membrane.[8] The functions of the Rh antigens on the red blood cells may be cation transport and membrane integrity.[9] The lack of Rh system antigens, called *Rh null,* causes a membrane abnormality that shortens red blood cell survival. Further discussion of Rh_{null} appears later in this chapter.

Rh TERMINOLOGY

Two systems of nomenclature were developed before recent advances in molecular genetics. These systems reflect serologic observations and inheritance theories based on family studies. Since these systems are used interchangeably in the transfusion setting, it is necessary to understand these theories well enough to "translate" from one to another. Two additional systems were developed because of a need for a universal language compatible with computers. Table 5-1 lists the equivalent notations for the more common Rh antigens.

Fisher-Race: CDE Terminology

Fisher and Race[10] postulated that the Rh system antigens were inherited as a gene complex or haplotype that codes for three closely linked sets of alleles. D is inherited at one locus, C or c at the second locus, and E or e at the third locus. Each parent contributes one haplotype or set of Rh genes. Fig. 5-1 illustrates this concept. Each gene expresses an antigen that is given the same letter as the gene except that when referring to the gene the letter is italicized. For example, the gene that produces the "C" antigen is *C*. Each red blood cell antigen can be recognized by testing with a specific antibody. The original theory assumed the *d* allele was present when the *D* allele was absent. The "d" is still sometimes written to denote the absence of the D antigen. The order of the genes on the chromosome, according to the Fisher-Race theory, is *DCE*; however, it is often written alphabetically as *CDE*.

Wiener: Rh-Hr Terminology

In contrast to the Fisher-Race theory, Alexander Wiener[11] postulated that alleles at *one* gene locus were responsible for the expression of the Rh system antigens on the red blood cells. Each parent contributes one Rh gene. The inherited form of the gene may be identical (homozygous) to or different (heterozygous) from each parent. According to Wiener, eight alleles exist at the Rh gene locus: R^0, R^1, R^2, R^z, *r*, *r′*, *r″*, and r^y (written in shorthand). The gene encodes a structure on the red blood cell called an **agglutinogen**, which can be identified by its parts or factors. These factors are identified with the same antisera that agglutinates the D, C, c, E, and e antigens mentioned earlier in the Fisher-Race nomenclature. The difference between the Wiener and Fisher-Race theories is the inheritance of the Rh system on a *single* gene locus rather than *three* separate genes. The antigen complex or agglutinogen is made up of factors that are identifiable as separate antigens (Table 5-2). For example, in Wiener terminology, the R^1 gene codes for the Rh_1 agglutinogen, which is made up of factors Rh_0, rh′ and hr″ that correspond to D, C, and e, respectively. The *r* gene codes for the rh agglutinogen, made up of factors hr′ and hr″ that correspond to c and e, respectively. The longhand factor notations of Rh_0, rh′, hr′, rh″, and hr″ that correspond to D, C, c, E, and e, respectively, are outdated and rarely used.

Agglutinogen: group of antigens or factors.

Wiener terminology can be easily translated to Fisher-Race terminology when the following points are kept in mind: R is the same as D; r indicates no D antigen; the number 1 and the character ′ denote C; and the number 2 and the character ″ are the same as E (Table 5-3). For example, in Wiener nomenclature, having the c, D, and E factors or antigens would be written as R_2. Although most workers prefer the Fisher-Race terminology to Wiener's, it is often easier to describe a phenotype as R_2R_2 than as D+, C−, c+, E+, e−.

Table 5-2 Wiener Theory: Genes and the Factors or Antigens They Encode

Gene	Antigens (Fisher-Race)	Gene	Antigens (Fisher-Race)
R^0	cDe	*r*	ce
R^1	CDe	*r′*	Ce
R^2	cDE	*r″*	cE
R^z	CDE	r^y	CE

Factors in Wiener terminology: D = Rh_0; C = rh′; E = rh″; c = hr′; e = hr″.

Table 5-3 Converting Fisher-Race Terminology to Wiener Terminology

Fisher-Race Antigen	R (D+)	r (D−)
C	1	′
E	2	″
CE	Z	y
ce	0	

Upper-case R indicates the D antigen is present; lower-case r indicates the D antigen is absent; 1, ′, 2, ″, 0, Z, and ^{y} refer to the presence or absence of the C, E, c, and e antigens.

Rosenfield: Numeric Terminology

Both the Wiener and Fisher-Race terminologies are based on genetic concepts. The Rosenfield system was developed to communicate phenotypic information more suited for computerized data entry; it does not address genetic information.[12] In this system, each antigen is given a number that corresponds to the order of its assignment in the Rh system. The phenotype of a cell is expressed by the system *Rh* followed by a colon and then the numbers corresponding to the tested antigens. If a red blood cell sample is negative for the antigen tested, a minus sign is written before the number. For example, a red blood cell sample that tested D+, C+, E−, c+, e+ would be written as Rh:1,2,-3,4,5. Table 5-1 compares Fisher-Race, Wiener, and Rosenfield terminology.

International Society of Blood Transfusion: Standardized Numeric Terminology

The International Society of Blood Transfusion (ISBT), in an effort to standardize blood group system nomenclature, assigned a six-digit number to each blood group specificity.[13] The first three numbers represent the system, and the remaining three represent the antigen specificity. The Rh system's assigned number is 004, and the remaining three numbers correspond to the Rosenfield system. For example, the C antigen's ISBT number is 004002. An ISBT "symbol" or alphanumeric designation similar to the Rosenfield terminology is used to refer to a specific antigen. The term *Rh* is written in upper-case letters, and the antigen number immediately follows the system designation. The ISBT symbol for C is RH2. A partial list of Rh antigens that includes the ISBT numerical designation appears in Table 5-1.

DETERMINING THE GENOTYPE FROM THE PHENOTYPE

The term *phenotype* refers to the test results obtained with specific antisera, and the term *genotype* refers to the genetic makeup of an individual. The genotype cannot be absolutely determined without family studies but can be inferred from the phenotype based on the frequency of genes in a population. Five antisera used to determine the Rh system phenotypes include anti-D, anti-C, anti-c, anti-E, and anti-e.

Once the phenotype is known, the most probable genotype can be determined by knowing the most common Rh system genes for the race of the person being tested (Table 5-4). In the White population the four most common genes encountered, in order of frequency from highest to lowest, are *CDe* (R^1), *cde* (*r*), *cDE* (R^2), and *cDe* (R^0). In the Black population the order of gene frequency from highest to lowest is *cDe* (R^0), *cde* (*r*), *CDe* (R^1), and *cDE* (R^2). The genes *Cde* (*r′*), *cdE* (*r″*), *CDE* (R^z), and *CdE* (r^y) are not commonly found in either race. If a red blood cell specimen is typed as D+, C+, E−, c+, e+, the phenotype would be CcDe. When the genotype is inferred in the White population, the combination *CDe/cde* or R^1r would be the most probable genotype. In the Black population, however, the most probable genotype would be *CDe/cDe* or R^1R^0 because R^0 is more common than *r*. Table 5-5 lists phenotypes determined by reactions with specific antisera and the most probable genotype based on gene frequency in the population.

Table 5-4 Order of Frequency of the Common Rh System Haplotypes

	Rh GENE FREQUENCY	
	Whites	Blacks
Highest	*CDe* (R^1)	*cDe* (R^0)
↓	*cde* (*r*)	*cde* (*r*)
↓	*cDE* (R^2)	*CDe* (R^1)
Lowest	*cDe* (R^0)	*cDE* (R^2)

Cde (*r′*) is 2% or less; *cdE* (*r″*), *CDE* (R^Z), *CdE* (R^y) are less than 1%.

Pedigree diagrams illustrate inheritance patterns. In Fig. 5-3 the inheritance of the Rh system is diagrammed to illustrate the concept that the Rh system is inherited as a haplotype. Since the *RHD* and *RHCE* loci are close on chromosome 1, it is easy to follow the inheritance of the gene complex using Wiener terminology. A Punnett square, which can predict phenotypes and genotypes, can also be used to illustrate the probability of being Rh positive or Rh negative (Fig. 5-4).

ANTIGENS OF THE Rh SYSTEM

D Antigen

The D antigen is the most immunogenetic antigen in the Rh system. **Immunogenicity** refers to the ability of an antigen to elicit an immune response. More

Immunogenicity: ability to stimulate an immune response.

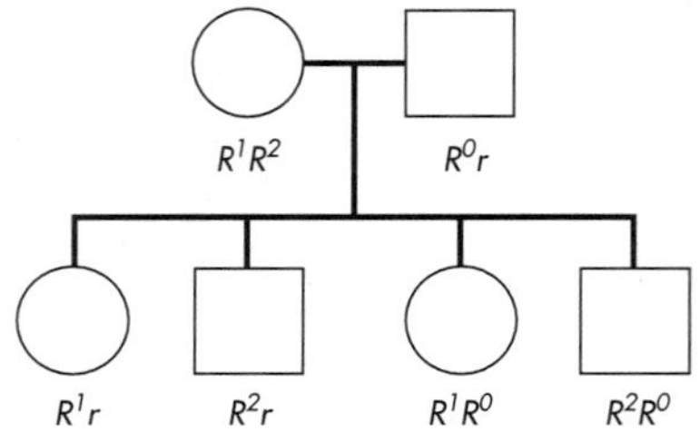

	R^1	R^2
R^0	R^1R^0	R^2R^0
r	R^1r	R^2r

Fig. 5-3 Inheritance of Rh haplotypes. Rh antigens are inherited as haplotype, which is illustrated in a pedigree chart and in a Punnett square.

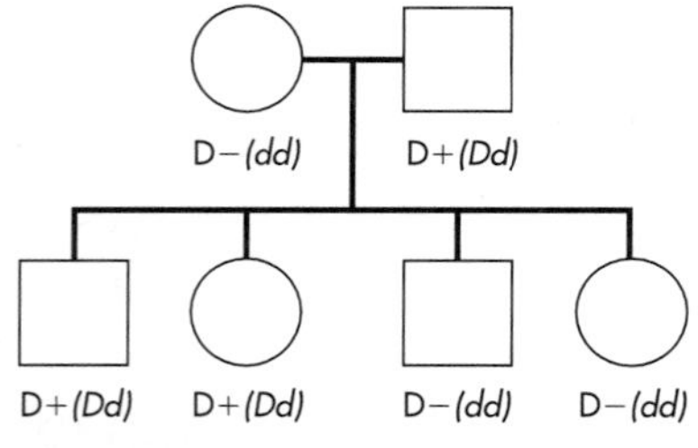

	D	d
d	Dd	dd
d	Dd	dd

Fig. 5-4 Inheritance of the D antigen. Predicting the probability of D-positive offspring from a D-negative mother and a heterozygous (Dd) father. The *d* gene does not exist and is being used only for illustrative purposes. Fifty percent of the children are D positive.

Table 5-5 Rh Phenotypes and Genotypes

RESULTS WITH ANTISERA Anti-D	-C	-E	-c	-e	PHENOTYPE	GENOTYPE CDE	Rh-hr	GENOTYPE FREQUENCY White	Black
+	+	−	+	+	CcDe	***CDe/ce***	$\mathbf{R^1r}$	**31**	9
						CDe/cDe	$\mathbf{R^1R^0}$	3	**15**
						Ce/cDe	$r'R^0$	<1	2
+	+	−	−	+	CDe	***CDe/CDe***	$\mathbf{R^1R^1}$	**18**	3
						CDe/Ce	R^1r'	2	<1
+	−	+	+	+	cDEe	***cDE/ce***	$\mathbf{R^2r}$	**10**	6
						cDE/cDe	$\mathbf{R^2R^0}$	1	**10**
+	−	+	+	−	cDE	*cDE/cDE*	R^2R^2	2	1
						cDE/cE	R^2r''	<1	<1
+	+	+	+	+	CcDEe	***CDe/cDE***	$\mathbf{R^1R^2}$	**12**	4
						CDe/cE	R^1r''	1	<1
						Ce/cDE	$r'R^2$	1	<1
+	−	−	+	+	cDe	***cDe/ce***	$\mathbf{R^0r}$	3	**23**
						cDe/cDe	$\mathbf{R^0R^0}$	<1	**19**
−	−	−	+	+	ce	*ce/ce*	rr	15	7
−	+	−	+	+	Cce	*Ce/ce*	$r'r$	<1	<1
−	−	+	+	+	cEe	*cE/ce*	$r''r$	<1	<1
−	+	+	+	+	CcEe	*Ce/cE*	$r'r''$	<1	<1

The more common genotypes and genotype frequencies are shown in bold.

-D- > R_2R_2 > R_1R_1 > R_1r or R_0r > R_1r' or R_0r'

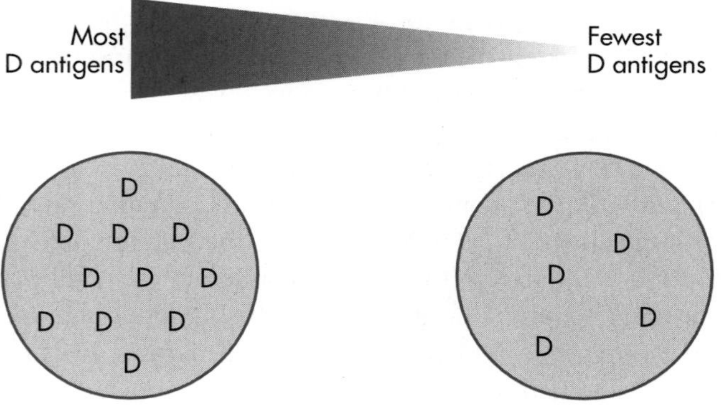

Fig. 5-5 D-antigen concentration. The D-antigen concentration varies depending on the antigens inherited at the *RHCE* gene. The D deletion phenotype has the most D-antigen sites. The *C* gene weakens the D expression if inherited on the opposite chromosome. R^2R^2 cells show stronger D expression than R^1R^1 cells.

than 80% of D-negative people receiving a D-positive red blood cell transfusion produce an antibody with anti-D specificity.[14] For that reason a D-negative patient should receive D-negative red blood cells. Fig. 5-5 illustrates the variation of the D antigen concentration in different phenotypes.

Weak D (D^u)

Most red blood cells can be typed for the D antigen directly with anti-D reagents. Although the antibody to D is typically IgG, reagent manufacturers have developed anti-D antisera that can be used concurrently with anti-A and anti-B testing. When the D antigen is weakly expressed on the red blood cell, its detection requires the indirect antiglobulin test (IAT). Red blood cells that are positive for D only by the IAT are referred to as **weak D.** Table 5-6 shows the interpretation of this test, which must always include a control. If the control is positive, additional serologic techniques may be required, which are discussed in Chapter 7.

Older terminology classified weak D antigens as D^u. The IAT used to determine whether a weak form of D is present is still sometimes referred to as the D^u test. Newer monoclonal typing reagents for Rh system antigens have enhanced the ability to detect the weaker D antigens without additional testing. Refer to Chapter 3 for a discussion of reagents and controls.

Weaker D expression can result from several different genetic circumstances that are outlined briefly in the following section. Note that only the first type of weak D requires the detection of the D antigen by the antiglobulin test.

Table 5-6 Weak D Test (D^u) Interpretation (with Control Results)

Anti-D	Rh control	Interpretation
+	0	Weak D positive
0	0	D negative
+	+	Unable to interpret

Weak D: weak form of the D antigen that requires the IAT for its detection.

Weak D: Genetic

Some *RHD* genes code for a weaker expression of the D antigen. This quantitative variation in the *RHD* gene is more common in Blacks and is often part of the *cDe* (R_0) haplotype. An IAT using anti-D is usually required to detect this form of D.

Partial D: D antigen that is missing part of its typical antigenic structure.

Weak D: Position Effect

Weaker expression of the D antigen can be found when the C antigen is inherited in *trans* to the D antigen (Fig. 5-6). The *Cde* (*r′*) gene paired with a *CDe* (R^1) or *cDe* (R^0) gene weakens the expression of D. This type of D antigen is usually detected without additional testing by the IAT using anti-D because of the increased sensitivity of monoclonal reagents. The occurrence of the *Cde* (*r′*) gene in the White population is less than 2%.

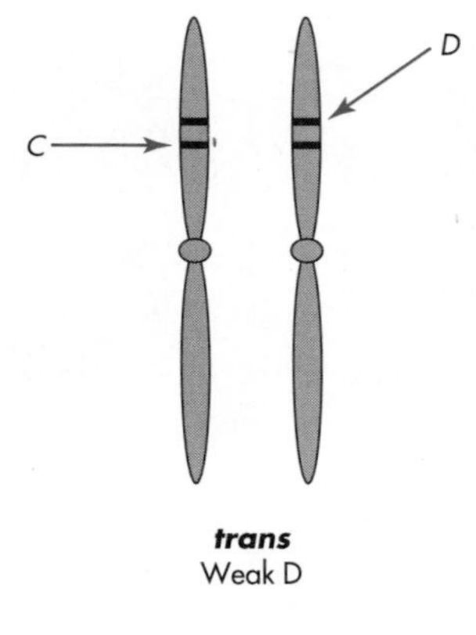

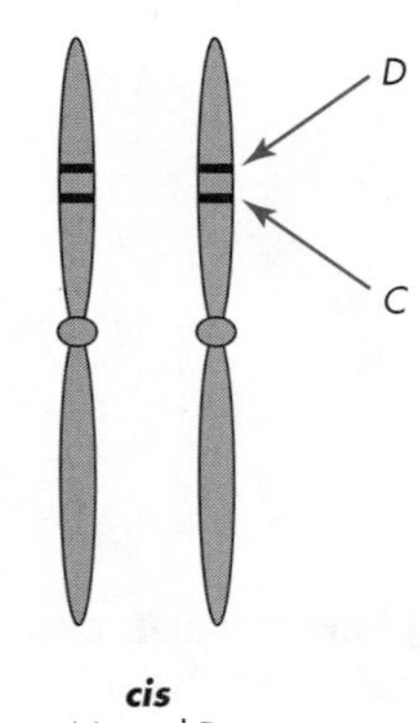

Fig. 5-6 Weak D caused by C inherited in *trans.* The D-antigen expression will be weaker when the *D* and *C* genes are inherited on the opposite chromosome.

Weak D: Partial D

Although rare, some individuals who are positive for the D antigen can make an alloantibody that appears to be anti-D after exposure to D-positive red blood cells. Investigation of this phenomenon revealed that some D-positive cells could be missing parts of the D antigen complex. When these individuals are exposed to the "whole D" antigen, they can make an antibody to the part they are missing. In the past the **partial D** phenotype was termed *D variant* or *D mosaic.* Lomas, McColl, and Tippett[15] have established as many as nine partial D phenotypes, which are classified by their parts or epitopes.

Red blood cells of most partial D phenotypes react as strongly with monoclonal anti-D reagents as red blood cells made up of the complete D antigen. For this reason partial D phenotypes are infrequently detected. A partial D phenotype should be suspected if a D-positive individual makes anti-D that is nonreactive with his or her own cells.[14] In addition the partial D phenotype should be suspected if two different manufacturers' monoclonal anti-D reagents are used and the interpretation as D positive or D negative does not agree. In this circumstance the clone used to manufacture the antisera may vary in the ability to detect all the epitopes or parts of the D antigen.

Significance of Testing for Weak D

The American Association of Blood Banks[16] requires testing for weak D on all donor red blood cells that do not directly agglutinate with anti-D reagents. Weak D-positive units are labeled D positive and should be transfused only to

D-positive recipients. A D control or an autocontrol is an important part of the weak D test, because it verifies that a positive result is not due to red blood cells already coated with antibodies. If red blood cells are coated with IgG antibodies before testing with anti-D at the antiglobulin phase, the test is invalid and additional procedures are required to determine the D status of the donor.

A D control is a reagent made by some manufacturers that consists of all additives except the D antibody. It is used to determine whether agglutination by anti-D at immediate spin is false positive, which could be due to the reagent additives, such as albumin. A D control tested at the antiglobulin phase then determines whether patient cells are already coated with autoantibodies. Reagent manufacturers specify the use of controls in their package inserts, and it is important to become familiar with these guidelines. Chapter 2 discusses Rh reagents in detail.

Testing for weak D on recipient samples is not required. Many facilities perform only the direct test for the D antigen and do not complete the antiglobulin procedure if the reaction is negative. This policy may be most cost effective in terms of time and reagents, since the majority of D-negative individuals do not test positive for the weak D antigen. The patients are classified as D negative in this case and transfused with D-negative blood.

Some facilities test for weak D on recipient samples. If a weak D is detected, D-negative blood is provided. Although unlikely, a patient with a weak D because of the partial-D phenotype can, theoretically, make anti-D. Partial-D phenotype is rare and, with current monoclonal reagents, usually does not require the antiglobulin test for detection. Some workers consider the practice of providing D-negative blood to weak D–positive recipients a waste of D-negative blood, since it is extremely rare that an antibody is formed.

Another acceptable policy is to test for weak D and, if positive, provide D-positive blood. Although unlikely, an individual may be a partial D and make an antibody to the epitope he or she is missing.

Some debate about these policies exists; however, the important element in weak D testing by the IAT is that the interpretation be made with proper controls to detect cells already coated with IgG antibodies.

Other Rh System Antigens

Antigens in the Rh system other than D, C, E, c, and e are alternate forms or variations produced by the *RHD* and *RHCE* genes. These antigens and corresponding antibodies, along with their clinical relevance, are outlined in the following section. Table 5-7 provides a summary of less common antigens and antibody characteristics. Refer to the suggested reading list for a more thorough discussion of these rare phenotypes, which lies beyond the scope of this text.

Compound Antigens

Compound antigens: distinct antigens produced when two other antigens are encoded by the same gene.
***cis*-Product antigens:** compound antigens produced when two genes are inherited on the same chromosome.

Examples of **compound antigens** or ***cis*-product antigens** in the Rh system include Rh6 (*cis* ce or f), Rh7 (*cis* Ce or rh_i), Rh27 (*cis* cE), and Rh22 (*cis* CE). A *cis*-product antigen is the additional antigen product formed when two genes are inherited on the same chromosome (Fig. 5-7). For example, when c and e are inherited as a haplotype (*cde* or *cDe*) in addition to the c and e antigens, another determinant, or epitope, called "f" is inherited. This epitope can also elicit its own immune response. The f antigen would not be present on the red blood cell if the person's genotype was *CDe*/*cDE*, even though the red blood cells would type pos-

Table 5-7 Summary of Less Common Rh System Antigens and Antibodies

ANTIGEN	ANTIGEN CHARACTERISTICS	ANTIBODY CHARACTERISTICS
f or ce	*cis*-Product antigen; present when c and e are inherited as a haplotype	Rare antibody; can cause HTR and HDN; c– or e– blood is f–
Ce or rh_i	*cis*-Product antigen; present when C and e are inherited as a haplotype	Anti-Ce is often made by D+ patients who make anti-C
C^w	Low-frequency antigen, found in 2% of Whites and rarely in Blacks; most C^w+ are also C+	Can be naturally occurring; immune examples can cause HDN and HTR
C^x	Low (<0.01%) occurrence; C^x+ is C+	Rare, can cause mild HTR and HDN
V or Ce^s	Found in 30% of Blacks and less than 1% of Whites	Often found with other antibodies; can cause HTR but not HDN
G or rh^G	Present on most D+ and all C+ cells	Antibody appears to be anti-D and anti-C; can cause HDN and HTR
Rh29 or total Rh	Present on all red blood cells except Rh_{null} cells	Antitotal Rh is made by Rh_{null} individuals (amorph and regulator)
RH:17 or Hr_0	Present on all red blood cells except -D- cells (D deletion)	Antibody made by individuals who are -D-
hr^s, hr^B	e-Like antigens (e variants) produced by all Rh genes that make e; antigen hr^s or hr^b is associated with weak e-antigen typing	Antibodies found when an e+ person makes an apparent anti-e

HTR, Hemolytic transfusion reaction; *HDN*, hemolytic disease of the newborn.

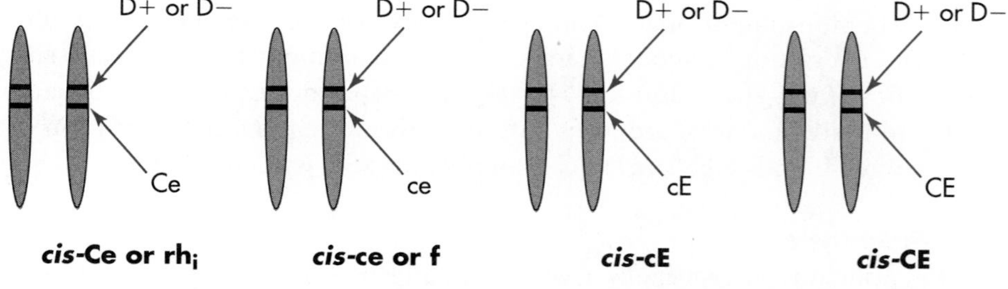

Fig. 5-7 ***cis*-Product antigens.** A *cis*-product antigen is the product of two alleles inherited on the same gene.

itive for both the c and e antigens. In this case the *c* and *e* alleles were inherited on opposite chromosomes and f would not be formed.

Antibodies to compound antigens are infrequently encountered. If they are identified, locating antigen-negative units would require the use of common Rh antisera, such as anti-E, anti-C, anti-c, and anti-e. For example, if anti-f were identified, red blood cell units that are c negative or e negative would also be negative for the f antigen. When red blood cells are required, units that are negative for one of the antigens creating the compound antigen can be safely transfused.

G Antigens

Almost all genes that code for C or D antigens also code for a G antigen. Additionally, cells that are negative for C and D are negative for the G antigen. Anti-G mimics anti-D and anti-C. D-negative persons immunized by C+, D- red blood cells sometimes appear to produce an anti-C as well as anti-D when they have actually made anti-G. A D-positive person who is negative for C can also make an antibody that appears to be anti-D and anti-C. Distinguishing anti-G, anti-D, and anti-C antibodies requires adsorption and elution procedures.[17] Extensive testing to identify anti-G is not usually necessary. Individuals making anti-G (or what appears to be anti-D or anti-C) should receive red blood cells that are negative for *both* D and C antigens. Rare cells do exist that are negative for D and positive for G (r^G). G is not a compound antigen; G is present when D *or* C is inherited.

Unusual Phenotypes

Null phenotypes: absences of a particular blood group system from the red blood cell membrane.

Unusual phenotypes in the Rh system are rarely encountered in routine blood bank testing. Unusual phenotypes include cells that have diminished or undetectable Rh system antigen expression. Understanding the inheritance patterns and cell characteristics of unusual phenotypes provides insight into the genetics and biochemistry of the system. **Null phenotypes** are found in many blood group systems and have led to an understanding of the role of the antigen on the red blood cell. Serologically, null phenotypes have provided the mechanism to categorize blood group systems.

D-Deletion Phenotype

Rare Rh phenotypes demonstrate no reactions when the red blood cells are tested with anti-E, anti-e, anti-C, or anti-c. Genetic material has been deleted or rendered nonfunctional at the RHCE site. Red blood cells that lack C/c or E/e antigens may demonstrate stronger D antigen activity (see Fig. 5-4). Individuals who are of the "D-deletion" phenotype may produce an antibody that reacts as a single specificity (anti-Hr_0 or anti-Rh17) or separable specificities such as anti-e and anti-C. An individual who produces anti-Rh17 would require the transfusion of D-deleted red blood cells. The D-deletion phenotype is written as -D- or D--.

Rh_{null} Phenotype

The Rh_{null} phenotype appears to have no Rh antigens and can be produced from two distinct genetic mechanisms. Cells that type as Rh_{null} demonstrate membrane abnormalities that shorten their survival and cause hemolytic anemia of varying severity.[18] Other blood group antigens, such as S, s, U, and LW, are affected, since Rh_{null} cells are negative for these antigens as well. Antibodies produced by immunized individuals who lack all Rh antigens may be directed to "total-Rh" (Rh29) or to an individual Rh-antigen specificity. If an anti-Rh29 is detected, Rh_{null} cells are needed for transfusion. Siblings, autologous donations, and the rare donor registry could be potential sources of compatible red blood cell units.

Regulator gene: gene inherited at another locus or chromosome that affects the expression of another gene.

The inheritance of the Rh_{null} phenotype can result from a **regulator** (X^0r) **gene** or an amorph ($\overline{\overline{r}}$) gene. A normal regulator gene (X^1r) is inherited separately from the Rh genes and allows normal Rh antigen expression. When homozygous X^0r genes are inherited instead, no Rh antigens are expressed. In the regulator type Rh_{null}, the Rh genes are inherited but not expressed. The amorph $\overline{\overline{r}}$ Rh_{null} phenotype is less well understood. The *RHD* gene is absent, and there is a lack of expression of the *RHCE* gene.[19]

Rh_{mod} Phenotype

The Rh_{mod} phenotype is similar to the regulator Rh_{null}. In this phenotype red blood cells lack most of their Rh antigen expression as a result of the inheritance of an X^Qr gene. Hemolytic anemia is also a characteristic of this phenotype.

Rh ANTIBODIES

General Characteristics

Rh system antibodies are usually made by exposure to Rh antigens through transfusion or pregnancy. Antibodies to Rh system antigens show similar serologic characteristics. Most antibodies are IgG (IgG_1) and bind at 37° C; agglutination is observed by the IAT. Enhancement with high-protein, low–ionic strength solution (LISS), proteolytic enzymes, and polyethylene glycol (PEG) **potentiators** is useful in identification procedures. Some Rh antibodies may be IgM (anti-E) or found in individuals never transfused or pregnant (anti-C^W). Stronger reactivity with homozygous antigen expression (dosage) is characteristic of antibodies to C, c, E, and e, although this is not typical of anti-D. Anti-D is typically stronger with *cDE/cDE* (R_2R_2), since these cells have more D antigen sites. Rh antibodies are not associated with complement activation, which would be detected by hemolysis in tube testing or the use of polyspecific antihuman globulin reagent.

Potentiators: reagents added to the serum-cell mixture to enhance antibody uptake during the incubation phase of the IAT.

When an R^1R^1 individual makes an anti-E, anti-c often may be present, although weak or undetectable. Because of this association some workers provide c-negative and E-negative blood when anti-E is identified. It is recommended that more sensitive methods to detect anti-c be used when anti-E is present.

Clinical Considerations

Transfusion Reactions

Antibodies to Rh system antigens can cause hemolytic transfusion reactions. Although antibodies often remain detectable for many years, their reactivity in agglutination procedures can fall below detectable levels. Reexposure to the antigen once the antibody has formed produces a rapid secondary immune response. Antigen-negative red blood cells should be transfused if antibodies to Rh system antigens are identified or have been previously noted in the patient's history. It is important to check previous records of patients who may be transfused for a history of red blood cell antibodies that may have developed from previous transfusions or pregnancies. A more detailed discussion of antibody detection appears in Chapter 7.

Hemolytic Disease of the Newborn

HDN was initially observed in babies from D-negative women with D-positive mates. Initial pregnancies were not usually affected. Infants from subsequent pregnancies were often stillborn or severely anemic and jaundiced. The initial pregnancy stimulated the mother to produce anti-D from the exposure to D-positive cells that occurs during birth when the baby's and mother's circulations mix. Since anti-D can cross the placenta, fetal cells in subsequent pregnancies were hemolyzed by the mother's antibody. **Rh immune globulin** (RhIG) protects D-negative mothers against the production of anti-D following delivery. Anti-C, anti-c, anti-E, and anti-e are not protected by RhIG and can cause HDN. An important aspect of prevention of HDN is antibody screening early in pregnancy and the determination of the D status of mothers to ascertain RhIG candidacy. Refer to Chapter 13 for a discussion of HDN and RhIG.

Rh immune globulin: immune serum globulin consisting of anti-D that is given to prevent the formation of anti-D by Rh-negative individuals.

LW BLOOD GROUP SYSTEM

Relationship to the Rh System

The LW blood group system is presented in this chapter because of the phenotypic relationship to the Rh system. The antigens and antibodies are similar in

Table 5-8 LW Blood Group System

GENOTYPE	PHENOTYPE	CHARACTERISTICS
LW^aLW^a *or* LW^aLW	LW(a+b−)	Most common (97%) LW phenotype
LW^aLW^b	LW(a+b+)	3%
LW^bLW^b *or* LW^bLW	LW(a−b+)	Rare
LWLW	LW(a−b−)	Rare; can make anti-LW, which reacts more strongly with D+ cells

serologic properties but are not genetically related. As discussed earlier the LW antibody made by guinea pigs and rabbits that were immunized with red blood cells from rhesus monkeys in early experiments is similar to the anti-D antibody. Anti-LW reacts strongly with D-positive cells and weakly with D-negative cells. Rh_{null} cells are negative for LW antigens as well. The theory suggesting a precursor relationship between the Rh system and LW antigens has been discounted, although the membrane biochemistry is still being studied.[20] A summary of LW system antigens and antibodies appears in Table 5-8.

The LW locus is on chromosome 19. The LW system alleles are LW^a, LW^b, and *LW*. LW(a+b−) is the most common phenotype in the population, since the LW^a gene is of high frequency. The *LW* gene is an amorph, and inheriting two *LW* genes produces the rare LW(a−b−) phenotype. Antibodies to the LW system are clinically significant and rare.

CHAPTER SUMMARY

The major concepts of the Rh system regarding inheritance theories, nomenclature, antigens, and antibodies are summarized below.

SUMMARY OF Rh SYSTEM ANTIGENS

Biochemical composition	Polypeptides with no carbohydrate residues
Gene products	416 amino acids that traverse the membrane 12 times
Current genetic theory	Two genes: RHD and RHCE; alleles include *RHCE, RHCe, RHcE, RHce*
Fisher-Race theory	Three genes; alleles include *D/d, C/c, E/e*
Wiener theory	One gene; alleles include R^0, R^1, R^2, R^z, *r*, *r′*, *r″*, r^y
Rosenfield terminology	Numeric: D=Rh1, C=Rh2, E=Rh3, c=Rh4, e=Rh5
International Society of Blood Transfusion: Standard numeric	Rh system is 004; each antigen has a number as shown in the Rosenfield system
Genetic loci	Chromosome 1
Weak D (D^u)	D antigen that can be detected only by the indirect antiglobulin test
Compound antigens	f(*cis*-ce), rh_i(*cis*-Ce), *cis*-CE, and *cis*-cE
G antigen	Present whenever the D or C antigen is on the red blood cell

SUMMARY OF Rh SYSTEM ANTIGENS—CONT'D

Rh_{null} phenotype	Results from the *r* amorph gene or the X^0r regulator gene; no Rh antigens; abnormal red blood cell membrane

SUMMARY OF Rh SYSTEM ANTIBODIES

Antibody production	Red blood cell stimulation through transfusion or pregnancy
Immunoglobulin class	IgG; usually IgG1 and IgG3
In vitro reactions	Binds at 37° C, agglutination seen using the indirect antiglobulin test
Enhancement	Proteolytic enzymes, albumin, and polyethylene glycol
Complement binding	No
Clinical significance	Yes; can cause delayed transfusion reactions and hemolytic disease of the newborn
Dosage	Yes; stronger reactions with homozygous expression

CRITICAL THINKING EXERCISES

◆ *EXERCISE 5-1*

A request was received for 4 units of R_2R_2 from an outside facility. From this request, determine the following:

1. Which antigens are requested to be negative?
2. Is it an easy request to fill?
3. How many units need to be screened to satisfy the request?
4. What corresponding antibody does the patient receiving these units have?
5. How would the requested units in Fisher-Race and Rosenfield terminology be written?

◆ *EXERCISE 5-2*

The following reactions were obtained by testing red blood cells from a donor unit with antisera:

Anti-D:	+
Anti-C:	+
Anti-E:	0
Anti-c:	0
Anti-e:	+

1. What Rh antigens does the donor possess?
2. What is the phenotype?
3. Determine the most probable genotype if the donor is White.
4. Is the genotype different in this case if the donor is Black?
5. What antibodies could this donor make if he were to be transfused?
6. Is this phenotype rare or common?

◆ ***EXERCISE 5-3***

The following results were obtained from a 65-year-old patient with cancer:

Anti-A	Anti-B	Anti-D	Rh Control	A_1 Cells	B Cells	Interpretation
4+	4+	1+	1+	0	0	AB positive

1. Is the interpretation of the patient's blood type correct?
2. What test should be performed next to determine the problem?
3. Should a weak-D test be performed if the patient has a positive DAT?
4. If the patient needed a transfusion before the resolution of the discrepancy, what blood type should this patient receive?

◆ ***EXERCISE 5-4***

The following results were obtained from a first-time blood donor:

Anti-A	Anti-B	Anti-D	Weak D (D^u)	Rh Control	A_1 Cells	B Cells	Interpretation
4+	0	0	2+	0	0	4+	

1. What is the correct ABO/Rh interpretation for this donor?
2. Is the testing valid?
3. Why is it unnecessary to perform an Rh control with the immediate-spin anti-D test?
4. Would the interpretation of this individual's blood type be the same if he were to receive red blood cells?

◆ ***EXERCISE 5-5***

A 25-year-old man received 5 units of O-negative red blood cells in the emergency room following a serious car accident. His blood type, which was determined from a specimen collected before he received the red blood cell units, was O negative. Two weeks following the accident a sample was resubmitted for a type and screen before orthopedic surgery. The screen was positive, and the antibodies identified were anti-D and anti-C.

1. What are possible explanations for the antibodies identified?
2. What additional testing should be performed to explain the problem?
3. If it is determined that the blood type of the units he received was correct, what is the Rh phenotype of the units that he received?
4. What antigen(s) should be negative if he needs red blood cell transfusions in the future?
5. Will it be difficult to obtain these units?

STUDY QUESTIONS

1. The Rh genotype *CDE/cDE* is written in Wiener notation as:
   a. R^0R^1
   b. R^yR^2
   c. R^2R^1
   d. R^zR^2

2. In Rosenfield notation the phenotype of a donor may be written as Rh:1,-2,-3,4,5. What is the correct phenotype in Fisher-Race (CDE) notation?
   a. cDe
   b. CcDe
   c. CcDE
   d. CDEe

3. Anti-f was identified in a patient. Since commercial antisera are not available, what is the best course of action to locate compatible red blood cell units?
   a. crossmatch E-negative units
   b. contact the rare donor registry
   c. release O-negative units
   d. crossmatch c-negative units

4. A patient's Rh phenotype was determined to be D+, c+, e+, C-, E-. The race of this donor is most likely:
   a. Black
   b. White
   c. Asian
   d. Native American

5. The test for the weak D antigen involves:
   a. the indirect antiglobulin test
   b. the direct antiglobulin test
   c. anti-D^u typing sera
   d. anti-D antisera with an LISS potentiator

6. The anti-G antibody would be negative with which red blood cell?
   a. R_0r
   b. rr
   c. R_2r
   d. r'r

7. Results of a weak-D test on a patient with a positive DAT would be:
   a. accurate as long as the check cells were positive
   b. unreliable because of immunoglobulins already on the cell
   c. reliable if a high-albumin anti-D was used
   d. false negative because of antibody neutralization

8. The Rh_{null} phenotype is associated with:
   a. elevated D antigen expression
   b. increased LW antigen expression
   c. the Bombay phenotype
   d. red blood cell membrane abnormalities

9. The blood group system that was originally identified as the Rh system is now called:
   a. Kell
   b. Lutheran
   c. Lewis
   d. LW

10. A donor tested Rh negative using commercial anti-D reagent. The antiglobulin or weak-D test was positive. How should the red blood cell unit be labeled?
   a. Rh positive
   b. Rh negative
   c. D variant
   d. will vary with blood bank policy

11. Which offspring is **NOT** possible from a mother who is R_2r and a father who is R_1r?
   a. *DcE/DcE*
   b. *DCe/DcE*
   c. *DcE/ce*
   d. *ce/ce*

12. How are antibodies to the Rh system antigens usually characterized?
   a. naturally occurring IgM
   b. immune IgG
   c. immune IgM
   d. naturally occurring IgG and IgM

13. Which of the following genotypes is heterozygous for the C antigen?
   a. R^1r
   b. R^2R^2
   c. R^1R^1
   d. $r'r'$

14. What is the likelihood that two heterozygous D-positive parents will have a D-negative child?
   a. less than 1%
   b. not possible
   c. 25%
   d. 75%

15. Which of the following genotypes could make anti-rh$_i$ (anti-Ce)?
   a. R^2R^2
   b. R^1R^0
   c. R^1R^2
   d. $r'r$

REFERENCES

1. Levine P, Stetson RE: An unusual case of intragroup agglutination, *JAMA* 113:126, 1939.
2. Landsteiner K, Wiener AS: An agglutinable factor in human blood recognized by immune sera for rhesus blood, *Proc Soc Exp Biol NY* 43:223, 1940.
3. Tippett P: A speculative model for the Rh blood groups, *Ann Human Genet* 50:241, 1986.
4. Colin Y, Cherif-Zahar B, Le Van Kim C, et al: Genetic basis of the RhD-positive and RhD-negative blood group polymorphism as determined by Southern analysis, *Blood* 78:2747, 1991.
5. Mouro I, Colin Y, Cherif-Zahar B, et al: Molecular genetic basis of the human Rhesus blood group system, *Nat Genet* 5:62, 1993.
6. Arge P, Cartron JP: Molecular biology of the Rh antigens, *Blood* 78:551, 1991.
7. Cartron JP: Defining the Rh blood group antigens: biochemistry and molecular genetics, *Blood* 8:199, 1994 (review).
8. Cherif-Zahar B, Bloy C, Le Van Kim C, et al: Molecular cloning and protein structure of a human blood group Rh polypeptide, *Proc Natl Acad Sci USA* 87:6243, 1990.
9. Daniels G, Lomas-Francis C, Wallace M, Tippett P: Epitopes of Rh D: serology and molecular genetics. In Silberstein LE, editor: *Molecular and functional aspects of blood group antigens*, Bethesda, Md, 1995, American Association of Blood Banks.
10. Race RR: The Rh genotypes and Fisher's theory, *Blood* 2:27, 1948.
11. Wiener AS: Genetic theory of the Rh blood types, *Proc Soc Exp Biol Med* 54:316, 1943.
12. Rosenfield RE, Allen FH Jr, Swisher SN, Kochwa S: A review of Rh serology and presentation of a new terminology, *Transfusion* 2:287, 1962.
13. Lewis M, Anstee DJ, Bird GWG, et al: Blood group terminology 1990: the ISBT working party on terminology for red cell surface antigens, *Vox Sang* 58:152, 1990.
14. Vengelen-Tyler V, editor: *Technical manual,* ed 12, Bethesda, Md, 1996, American Association of Blood Banks.
15. Lomas C, McColl K, Tippett P: Further complexities of the Rh antigen D disclosed by testing category D^{II} cells with monoclonal anti-D, *Transfus Med* 3:67, 1993.
16. Klein HG, editor: *Standards for blood banks and transfusion services,* ed 17, Bethesda, Md, 1996, American Association of Blood Banks.
17. Issitt PD: *Applied blood group serology,* ed 3, Miami, 1985, Montgomery Scientific Publications.
18. Schmidt PJ: Hereditary hemolytic anemias and the null blood types, *Arch Intern Med* 139:570, 1979.
19. Cherif-Zahar B, Raynal V, Le Van Kim C, et al: Structure and expression of the RH locus in the Rh-deficiency syndrome, *Blood* 82:656, 1993.
20. Bloy C, Hermand P, Cherif-Zahar B, et al: Comparative analysis by two-dimensional iodopeptide mapping of the RhD protein and LW glycoprotein, *Blood* 75:2245, 1990.

SUGGESTED READINGS

Harmening D: *Modern blood banking and transfusion practices*, ed 4, Philadelphia, 1999, FA Davis.

Issitt PD, Anstee, DJ: *Applied blood group serology*, ed 4, Durham, NC, 1998, Montgomery Scientific Publications.

Reid ME, Lomas-Francis C: *The blood group antigen facts book*, San Diego, 1997, Academic Press.

Vengelen-Tyler V, Pierce SR, editors: *Blood group systems: Rh*, Arlington, Va, 1987, American Association of Blood Banks.

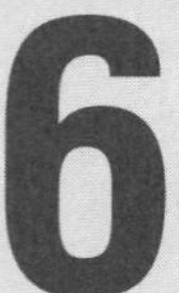

6 OTHER BLOOD GROUP SYSTEMS

Kathy D. Blaney
Paula R. Howard

CHAPTER OUTLINE

LEARNING OBJECTIVES

Upon completion of this chapter, the reader should be able to:

1. Identify the major antigens classified within the other blood group systems.
2. List the frequencies of the observed phenotypes and the association of phenotypes with ethnic group diversity.
3. Describe the biochemical characteristics of antigens within each blood group system.
4. Describe the genetic mechanisms for antigen inheritance in each blood group system.
5. Discuss the serologic characteristics and clinical relevance of the antibodies associated with each blood group system.
6. Discuss unique characteristics of selected blood group systems regarding disease association and biologic functions.

WHY STUDY OTHER BLOOD GROUP SYSTEMS?

In addition to the antigens of the ABO and Rh blood group systems, more than 200 unique antigens have been documented on red blood cells. The International Society for Blood Transfusion (ISBT) has currently defined 23 blood group systems. As previously discussed, the antigens of the ABO and Rh systems are of primary importance in transfusion. The antibodies to ABO and Rh system antigens are capable of effecting a decreased survival of transfused red blood cells and playing a role in the pathogenesis of hemolytic disease of the newborn (HDN). Antigens assigned to other blood group systems may also elicit immune responses in transfusion or pregnancy. Some of these antibodies produced are considered clinically relevant in transfusion medicine. Knowledge of the blood group systems provides the foundation for solving complex antibody problems in a logical and efficient manner.

In traditional terms the blood group antigen has been considered the target of a red blood cell alloantibody or autoantibody. The antigen-antibody complex may then trigger a process leading to the immune-mediated destruction of red blood cells. The primary effort in the blood bank has revolved around problem resolution relating to this pathophysiologic role.

In addition to these pathophysiologic roles, the molecular cloning of blood group genes has provided insight into the primary functional roles of these blood group antigens. Recent studies have linked blood group systems with unique roles in the following physiologic functions related to red blood cell membranes[1]:

- Molecules that function in transporting water-soluble molecules across the lipid bilayer for intake of nutrients and excretion of waste products
- Molecules that function in the complement pathway
- Molecules that play a role in the ability of cells to adhere to other cells
- Molecules that function as structural proteins to maintain red blood cell shape and mechanical deformability
- Molecules with suggested enzymatic activities

In addition to serving these physiologic functions, red blood cell antigens can function as microbial receptors for the infection by microorganisms (bacteria, viruses, or protozoan parasites). For example, the Duffy antigens, Fy^a and Fy^b, serve as the attachment sites for certain malarial parasites. An overview of the relationships of the blood group systems and their unique functional roles is presented in Box 6-1.[1]

BOX 6-1

Functional Roles of the Blood Group Systems

GLYCOSYLTRANSFERASES

ABO, P, Lewis, and H blood group systems

STRUCTURAL RELATIONSHIP TO RED BLOOD CELL

MNS, Diego, and Gerbich blood group systems

TRANSPORT PROTEINS

Rh, Kidd, Diego, Colton, and Kx blood group systems

COMPLEMENT PATHWAY MOLECULES

Chido/Rodgers, Cromer, and Knops blood group systems

ADHESION MOLECULES

Lutheran, Xg, Landsteiner-Wiener, and Indian blood group systems

MICROBIAL RECEPTORS

MNS, Duffy, P, Lewis, and Cromer blood group systems

BIOLOGIC RECEPTORS

Duffy, Knops, and Indian blood group systems

Many of these functional relationships have been predicted based on molecular cloning studies and remain under investigation.

ORGANIZATION OF THE CHAPTER

This chapter highlights the major facts relating to the antigens and antibodies of the other blood group systems. Each blood group system section begins with a box that outlines the major features of each system. The following information is featured:

- ISBT blood group system symbol
- ISBT blood group system number
- Clinical significance of the blood group system antibodies
  - **YES** = Antibodies are of clinical significance; reports of decreased red blood cell survival in vivo (e.g., transfusion reactions and HDN) are associated with the presence of these antibodies
  - **NO** = Antibodies are not of clinical significance; there is no association of decreased red blood cell survival in vivo (e.g., transfusion reactions and HDN) with the presence of the antibodies
- Immunoglobulin class of most antibodies produced: *IgM or IgG immunoglobulin class*

- **Optimal in vitro reaction temperature**

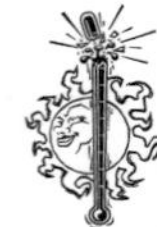
= Agglutination is observed at 37° C

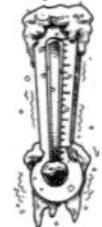
= Agglutination is observed at or below room temperature

- Optimal in vitro reaction phases
  IS = Agglutination reactions are observed on immediate spin
  4C = Agglutination reactions are enhanced on incubation at 4° C
  RT = Agglutination reactions are observed after incubation at room temperature
  37C = Agglutination reactions are enhanced on incubation at 37° C
  AHG = Agglutination reactions are enhanced in indirect antiglobulin tests (IATs)
- Antibody reactivity with enzyme-treated reagent red blood cells (ficin or papain)

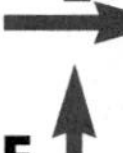
E → = No significant changes in the strength of agglutination reactions are observed with enzyme-treated reagent red blood cells

E ↑ = Agglutination reactions with enzyme-treated reagent red blood cells are increased in strength (e.g., enhanced)

= No agglutination is observed with enzyme-treated reagent red blood cells; the agglutination reactions disappear with enzyme-treated reagent red blood cells

VAR = Variable agglutination reactions are observed with enzyme-treated reagent red blood cells

KELL BLOOD GROUP SYSTEM

ISBT SYSTEM SYMBOL	ISBT SYSTEM NUMBER	CLINICAL SIGNIFICANCE	ANTIBODY CLASS	OPTIMAL TEMPERATURE	REACTIVE PHASES	ENZYME PHASES
KEL	006	YES	IgG		AHG	E → NO EFFECT

Characteristics and Biochemistry of the Kell Antigens

Antigen Nomenclature

In 1946 Coombs and associates[2] reported the detection of a new blood group antibody after using their antiglobulin test. This antibody was associated with a case of HDN, a disease characterized by the decreased survival of fetal red blood cells because of their sensitization with maternal IgG antibodies. This antibody, designated as anti-Kell, defined a red blood cell antigen called the Kell antigen. Therefore the Kell blood group system was established. Since its discovery 50 years ago, the Kell blood group system has grown into a complex polymorphism of 22 red blood cell antigens.[3] Numerical and alphabetical terminologies similar to those of the Rh system have evolved for the Kell blood group system. Currently the preferred terminology for the original antigen is K or K1 rather than Kell. The correct terminology for the originally described antibody is anti-K or anti-K1 rather than anti-Kell. Any references to the blood group system as an entity are called *Kell*, whereas appropriate references to the antigens within the system are made through the numerical or alphabetical notations. The original names of the Kell antigens are appropriately used only in an historical context.

Population studies have determined that the K (K1) antigen has about a 9% frequency in the White population. Its antithetical antigen, k or K2 (originally designated as Cellano), possesses a 99.8% frequency in Whites and was first reported in 1949.[4] Additional pairs of high- and low-frequency antithetical antigens intrinsic to the Kell blood group system were discovered over the next several years. These antigens were designated as Kp^a or K3 (originally designated as Penney) and Kp^b or K4 (originally designated as Rautenberg).[5,6] The Kp^b (K4) antigen possesses a high frequency (99.9%), whereas the Kp^a (K3) antigen is rarely expressed in the White population (2%). The Js^a or K6 antigen (originally designated as Sutter) and the Js^b or K7 antigen (originally known as Matthews) were added to the Kell blood group system as a pair of high- and low-frequency antithetical antigens.[7,8] The Js^a antigen has a 20% frequency in the Black population and a 0.1% frequency in Whites. Presently 22 red blood cell antigens numbered K1 to K25 have been assigned to this system (three antigens have been removed from the system). Box 6-2 summarizes the Kell blood group system antigens. Similarities to the Rh system include the confinement of Kell antigens to red blood cells and the presence of detectable antigens on fetal red blood cells. As a result of this early antigen development, Kell antibodies have been implicated in HDN cases.

BOX 6-2

Summary of Antigens: Kell Blood Group System

ANTITHETICAL ANTIGENS: HIGH AND LOW FREQUENCY

- K (K1) and k (K2)
- Kp^a (K3), Kp^b (K4), and Kp^c (K21)
- Js^a (K6) and Js^b (K7)
- Cote (K11) and Wk^a (K17)
- K14 and K24 (suspected relationship)

HIGH-FREQUENCY ANTIGENS

- Ku (K5)
- K12
- K13
- K16
- K18
- K19
- K20
- K22

LOW-FREQUENCY ANTIGENS

- Ul^a (K10)
- K23
- K25 (VLAN)

K8 and K9 are obsolete; K15 (Kx) is no longer included in the Kell system.
From Oyen R, Halverson GR, Reid ME: Review: conditions of causing weak expression of Kell system antigens, *Immunohematology* 13:75, 1997.

Antigen Biochemistry

In biochemical terms, the Kell blood group system antigens are located on a glycoprotein that is integral to the red blood cell membrane.[9] With the exception of K24, all Kell antigens have been shown to reside on this glycoprotein.[7] Special studies of the Kell glycoprotein have revealed that 4,000 to 18,000 Kell antigen sites exist per red blood cell.[10]

The Kell antigens are characteristically sensitive to treatment with **sulfhydryl reagents,** such as 2-mercaptoethanol (2-ME), dithiothreitol (DTT), or 2-aminoethylisothiouronium bromide (AET). These reagents reduce the disulfide bonds, which results in a disruption of multiple disulfide bonds in the protein. Antigens with three-dimensional highly folded protein structures are susceptible to any agent that interferes with its tertiary structure. Molecular cloning studies have shown that the Kell glycoprotein possesses an extensively folded disulfide-bonded region. This factor explains Kell antigen sensitivity to disulfide-reducing agents.[11] Treatment of red blood cells with these sulfhydryl reagents creates red blood cells that lack Kell antigens.

Sulfhydryl reagents: reagents that disrupt the disulfide bonds between cysteine amino acid residues in proteins; dithiothreitol, 2-mercaptoethanol, and 2-aminoethylisothiouronium bromide function as sulfhydryl reagents.

Immunogenicity of Kell Antigens

The K (K1) antigen is strongly immunogenic. Its immunogenicity ranks second to the D antigen in terms of eliciting an immune response in transfusions. Studies have reported that one in ten individuals negative for K antigen (K:-1) who are transfused with donor red blood cells positive for K antigen (K:1) develop anti-K in response to transfusion. Other antigens within the Kell blood group system are less immunogenic. Antibodies to these antigens are not commonly observed because of a combination of two factors: antigen frequency and immunogenicity of structure.

K_o or $Kell_{null}$ Phenotype

A red blood cell phenotype lacking the expression of the Kell glycoprotein, and consequently the Kell antigens, was identified by Chown and associates[12] in 1957. This null phenotype is designated as K_o or $Kell_{null}$ phenotype. The inheritance of two recessive K_o genes in a homozygote (K_oK_o) results in the null phenotype. These individuals lack all Kell system antigens but express another related antigen, Kx antigen. This antigen is discussed later in this chapter.

The alloantibody stimulated immunologically in K_o individuals, who have received transfusions, has been called *anti-Ku* or *anti-K5* and is clinically significant for transfusion purposes. Anti-Ku is produced because the Ku antigen is present on all red blood cells except K_o cells. Immunized K_o individuals require transfusion with rare K_o donor units. Rare donor units can be obtained by contacting the American Rare Donor Program sponsored by the American Association of Blood Banks and the American Red Cross.

Genetics of the Kell Blood Group System

The *Kell* blood group system locus is located on chromosome 7. The *Kell* locus is the site of the different *Kell* genes that produce the antigens of the Kell blood group system. Four sets of alleles that produce the Kell system's antithetical antigens exist within the *Kell* locus. These alleles include the following:

- *K* and *k*
- Kp^a and Kp^b
- Js^a and Js^b
- *KEL11* and *KEL17* (Wk^a)

The existence of a fifth set of alleles with an antithetical relationship, *KEL14* and *KEL24*, is suspected but not yet proven.[13] The high-incidence genes include *k*, Kp^b, Js^b, and *KEL11*. This haplotype is common in all populations. Low-incidence genes include *K*, Kp^a, Js^a, and *KEL17*. The incidence of low-frequency alleles varies in different ethnic groups. The *K*, Kp^a, and *K17* alleles are more common in the White population, whereas the Js^a allele is more common in the Black population. Table 6-1 summarizes the common phenotypes and their frequency distribution of the Kell blood group system.

Other unrelated genetic loci may affect the expression of Kell antigens on red blood cells. The Kell antigens may be modified by regulator genes on the X chromosome in relation to the Xk blood group system. This is discussed later in this chapter.

Table 6-1 Common Phenotypes and Frequencies in the Kell System

	PHENOTYPE FREQUENCY (%)	
Phenotype	**White**	**Black**
K−k+	91	98
K+k−	0.2	rare
K+k+	8.8	2
Kp(a+b−)	rare	0
Kp(a−b+)	97.7	100
Kp(a+b+)	2.3	rare
Js(a+b−)	0	1
Js(a−b+)	100	80
Js(a+b+)	rare	19

From Reid ME, Lomas-Francis C: *The blood group antigen facts book*, San Diego, 1997, Academic Press.

Characteristics of the Kell Antibodies

Most Kell system antibodies possess the following characteristics:

- Immunoglobulin class is IgG
- Antibodies are produced in response to antigen exposure through transfusion or pregnancy
- Antibodies agglutinate optimally in the IAT
- Antibodies usually do not bind complement
- Antibodies have been associated with transfusion reactions and HDN
- Enzyme phases show no enhancement or depression of antibody reactivity
- Depressed reactivity of anti-K is observed in some low–ionic strength solution (LISS) reagents

Anti-K (K1) is the most commonly observed antibody of the Kell blood group system in the transfusion service. Most examples of anti-K are IgG and react well in IATs. Despite its low frequency (9%), the K antigen's high degree of immunogenicity is responsible for the antibody's occurrence in a patient population.

Antibodies to k, Kp^b, and Js^b are not commonly detected, since individuals who lack these high-incidence antigens are scarce. An antibody to one of these antigens should be considered when patient serum reacts with the majority of or all of the panel cells in antibody identification studies. Anti-k and anti-Kp[b] production is associated with the White population, whereas anti-Js[b] is associated with the Black population. Sources of compatible donor red blood cell units are difficult to obtain when dealing with an antibody to a high-frequency antigen. Often suitable donors may be obtained from the patient's siblings or the American Rare Donor Program.

Antibody production to the Kp[a] and Js[a] antigens is also infrequent in a patient population, since both antigens possess low frequencies. Donor units possessing these antigens are uncommon; therefore exposure to these antigens by transfusion recipients is minimal.

Xk BLOOD GROUP SYSTEM

ISBT SYSTEM SYMBOL: **XK**
ISBT SYSTEM NUMBER: **019**

Kx Antigen and Its Relationship to the Kell Blood Group System

As previously discussed in the genetics section, the autosomal gene responsible for the production of the Kell glycoprotein is located on chromosome 7. Another gene, assigned to the X chromosome and designated as *XK1*, encodes a protein that carries the Kx antigen. Kx has been assigned to the Xk blood group system. A discussion of this blood group system is included here, since the absence of Kx antigen in the McLeod phenotype (discussed in the next section) weakens the expression of Kell antigens.

Although the Kx antigen is genetically independent of the Kell antigens, it possesses a phenotypic relationship to the Kell blood group system. Red blood cells with normal Kell phenotypes carry trace amounts of Kx antigen. Red blood cells from K_o individuals possess elevated levels of Kx antigen.

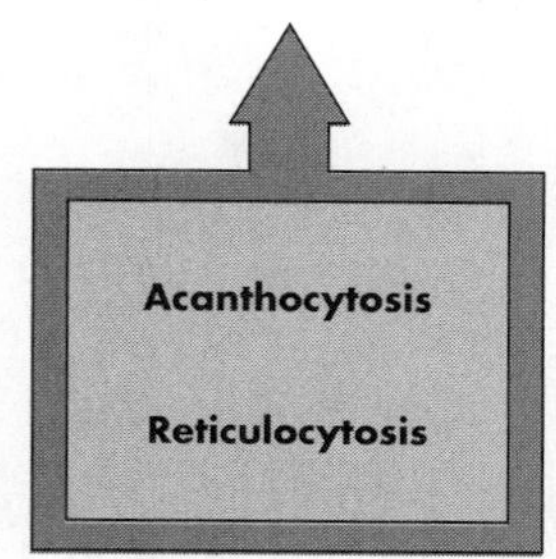

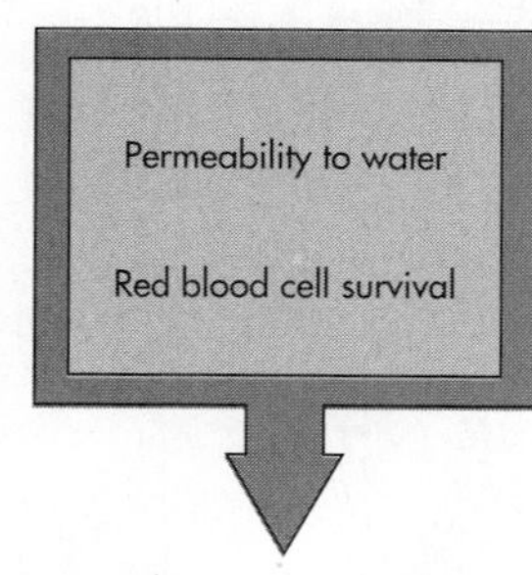

Fig. 6-1 McLeod phenotype: morphologic and functional red blood cell abnormalities.

McLeod Phenotype

When the *XK1* gene is not inherited, Kx antigen is not expressed on the red blood cells. The absence of Kx antigen from red blood cells and a concurrent reduced expression of the Kell blood group system antigens are characteristically associated with a red blood cell abnormality known as the McLeod phenotype. Individuals with the McLeod phenotype have red blood cell morphologic and functional abnormalities characterized by decreased red blood cell survival (Fig. 6-1). The McLeod phenotype is rare and is seen almost exclusively in the White male population as a result of the X chromosome–borne gene. Only about 60 individuals with the phenotype are known.[12] Table 6-2 summarizes the Kx antigen, the McLeod phenotype, and the K_o phenotype.

McLeod Syndrome

The McLeod phenotype is just one phenomenon attributed to the McLeod syndrome. Individuals with the McLeod syndrome, in addition to having red blood cell abnormalities, may possess associated defects of muscular and neurologic origins. Elevated levels of creatine kinase accompany the syndrome. The correlation of depressed Kell antigens and these defects currently remains undetermined. The X-linked disorder of **chronic granulomatous disease** is occasionally associated with the McLeod syndrome. In this disorder the normal functional

Acanthocytosis: presence of abnormal red blood cells with spurlike projections in the circulating blood.

Reticulocytosis: increase in the number of reticulocytes in the circulating blood.

Chronic granulomatous disease: inherited disorder where the phagocytic white blood cells are able to engulf but not kill certain microorganisms.

Table 6-2 Summary of Kell Phenotypes

PHENOTYPE	ANTIGEN EXPRESSION KELL	Kx	POSSIBLE SERUM ANTIBODIES?	NORMAL RED BLOOD CELL MORPHOLOGY?
Common	Normal	Weak	Kell alloantibodies	✓
K_o	None	↑↑↑	Anti-Ku	✓
McLeod	↓↓↓	None	Anti-KL (anti-Kx and anti-Km)	Acanthocytes
DTT-treated	None	↑	N/A	N/A

✓, Yes; ↑↑↑, marked increase; ↓↓↓, marked reduction; ↑, slight increase; *N/A*, not applicable.
Modified from Reid ME, Lomas-Francis C: *The blood group antigen facts book*, San Diego, 1997, Academic Press.

properties of phagocytic white blood cells are impaired. The phagocytes are able to engulf but not kill microorganisms. Because of this functional defect, patients possess an increased susceptibility to infections. A genetic deletion of chromosomal material encompassing both genetic loci on the X chromosome accounts for the association of the McLeod phenotype and chronic granulomatous disease.

DUFFY BLOOD GROUP SYSTEM

ISBT SYSTEM SYMBOL	ISBT SYSTEM NUMBER	CLINICAL SIGNIFICANCE	ANTIBODY CLASS	OPTIMAL TEMPERATURE	REACTIVE PHASES	ENZYME PHASES
FY	008	YES	IgG		AHG	E

Characteristics and Biochemistry of the Duffy Antigens

Duffy Antigen General Facts

The Duffy blood group system was first described in 1950 when a previously unrecognized antibody was discovered in the serum of a multiple-transfused hemophiliac, Mr. Duffy.[14] The antigen that defined this antibody was called Fy^a. Its antithetical antigen, Fy^b, was described the following year.[15] When phenotypic studies of the Fy^a and Fy^b antigens were performed, investigators observed that the White population commonly phenotyped as Fy(a+b+), Fy(a−b+), or Fy(a+b−). Sanger and associates[16] reported in 1955 that the majority of Blacks lacked both Fy^a and Fy^b antigens and phenotyped as Fy(a−b−).[16] This phenotype is rare among the White population. Common phenotypes and frequencies of the Duffy antigens are presented in Table 6-3, which shows that phenotype frequencies differ significantly between Whites and Blacks. A White Australian woman with the rare Fy(a−b−) phenotype was the first to produce anti-Fy3, which reacted with all Fy(a+) and Fy(b+) red blood cells.[17] This Duffy antigen was called Fy3. Several additional antigens (Fy4, Fy5, and Fy6) have been assigned to the system that now includes six antigens. Antigens are well developed at birth and detectable on fetal red blood cells. As with the Kell blood group system antigens, the Duffy antigens have not been identified on granulocytes, lymphocytes, monocytes, or platelets. The Fy^a and Fy^b antigens are considered of

Table 6-3 Common Phenotypes and Frequencies in the Duffy System

PHENOTYPE			PHENOTYPE FREQUENCY (%)	
REACTIONS WITH ANTI-Fy[a]	ANTI-Fy[b]	INTERPRETATION	WHITE	BLACK
+	0	Fy(a+b−)	17	9
0	+	Fy(a−b+)	34	22
+	+	Fy(a+b+)	49*	1
0	0	Fy(a−b−)	rare	68†

*Most common phenotype in the White population.
†Most common phenotype in the Black population.
From Reid ME, Lomas-Francis C: *The blood group antigen facts book*, San Diego, 1997, Academic Press.

Table 6-4 Summary of Antigens and Their Characteristics in the Duffy Blood Group System

Fy[a] and Fy[b]	◆ Antithetical antigens ◆ Expressed on cord blood cells ◆ Sensitive to ficin/papain treatment ◆ Receptors for *Plasmodium vivax* and *Plasmodium knowlesi*
Fy3	◆ Expressed on cord blood cells ◆ Resistant to ficin/papain treatment ◆ Red blood cells that are Fy(a−b−) are also Fy:-3
Fy4	◆ Expressed on cord blood cells ◆ Resistant to ficin/papain treatment
Fy5	◆ Expressed on cord blood cells ◆ Resistant to ficin/papain treatment ◆ Common in Whites ◆ Altered expression in Rh_{null} phenotype ◆ Possible antigen interaction between the Duffy and Rh proteins
Fy6	◆ Expressed on cord blood cells ◆ Red blood cells that are Fy(a-b-) are also Fy:-6 ◆ Sensitive to ficin/papain treatment ◆ Antigen has been defined by murine monoclonal antibodies; no human anti-Fy6 has been described

greatest importance for transfusion purposes. A summary of the antigens in this blood group system is presented in Table 6-4.

Biochemistry of the Duffy Antigens

The Duffy antigens have been mapped to a glycoprotein of the red blood cell membrane.[18] Molecular studies of the Duffy glycoprotein have determined that the glycoprotein spans the lipid bilayer of the membrane multiple times. The Fy[a], Fy[b], and Fy6 antigens are susceptible to proteolytic degradation by the enzymes papain and ficin. When red blood cells are treated with papain or ficin, these antigens are destroyed.

In 1993 Horuk and associates[19] identified the Duffy glycoprotein as an erythrocyte receptor for a number of proinflammatory **chemokines**. These chemokines are involved in the activation of white blood cells. In this functional role the Duffy glycoprotein is capable of binding molecules responsible

Chemokines: group of cytokines involved in the activation of white blood cells during migration across the endothelium.

for cell-to-cell communication. Research suggests that the Duffy glycoprotein functions as a biologic sponge for these excess chemokines.

Genetics of the Duffy Blood Group System

Syntenic: genetic term referring to genes closely situated on the same chromosome without being linked.

In 1968 Donahue and associates[20] demonstrated that the *Fy* locus was located on chromosome 1. Their report marked the first assignment of a human gene to a specific chromosome. The *Fy* locus is **syntenic** with the *Rh* locus and consists of these alleles:

- Fy^a and Fy^b, which are codominant alleles that produce Fy^a and Fy^b antigens, respectively
- Fy^x allele, which encodes a weakened Fy^b antigen
- *Fy* allele, which encodes no identifiable Duffy antigen

The genetic mechanisms for the remaining Duffy blood group system antigens are not completely understood at this time.

Characteristics of the Duffy Antibodies

For the scope of this book the discussion of Duffy antibodies is limited to anti-Fy^a and anti-Fy^b.

Common characteristics of anti-Fy^a and anti-Fy^b include the following:

- The antibodies are stimulated by antigen exposure through transfusion or pregnancy
- Agglutination reactions are best observed in IATs
- Immunoglobulin class is IgG
- The antibodies usually do not bind complement
- The antibodies possess clinical significance in transfusion and are an uncommon cause of HDN
- The antibodies are nonreactive in enzyme test phases; since the antigens are degraded by these enzymes, anti-Fy^a and anti-Fy^b do not agglutinate with enzyme-treated red blood cells
- Weaker examples of Duffy antibodies demonstrate stronger agglutination reactions with the homozygous expression of antigen [Fy(a−b+) or Fy(a+b−)] versus the heterozygous expression of antigen [Fy(a+b+)]; antibodies are detecting dosage of antigen expression
- Anti-Fy^a is more commonly observed than anti-Fy^b

Duffy System and Malaria

The majority of African and American Blacks are resistant to infection from certain forms of malarial parasites. Miller and associates[21] first made the connection between malaria and the Duffy blood group system in 1975. Their studies demonstrated that Fy(a−b−) red blood cells were not invaded by *Plasmodium knowlesi* parasites. Later observations confirmed that *P. knowlesi* and *P. vivax* invaded Fy(a+) or Fy(b+) red blood cells, but Fy(a−b−) red blood cells were resistant to infection. The Duffy antigens serve as biologic receptor molecules to assist the attachment of the merozoite to the red blood cell. The high incidence of the Fy(a−b−) phenotype in the West African population supports the hypothesis that this phenotype offered a selective evolutionary advantage for resistance to *P. vivax* infection. However, resistance to *P. falciparum* is not a characteristic of the Fy(a−b−) phenotype.

KIDD BLOOD GROUP SYSTEM

ISBT SYSTEM SYMBOL	ISBT SYSTEM NUMBER	CLINICAL SIGNIFICANCE	ANTIBODY CLASS	OPTIMAL TEMPERATURE	REACTIVE PHASES	ENZYME PHASES
JK	009	YES	IgG		AHG	E ↑

Characteristics and Biochemistry of the Kidd Antigens

In contrast to the polymorphism of the Rh and Kell blood group systems, the Kidd blood group system is relatively uncomplicated at both the serologic and genetic levels. The unique characteristic of the Kidd blood group system arises from the challenge for the transfusion service personnel to detect Kidd alloantibodies in vitro. The Kidd antibodies are often linked to extravascular hemolysis in delayed hemolytic transfusion reactions, where the removal of antibody-sensitized red blood cells is facilitated by the reticuloendothelial system.

Three antigens—Jk^a, Jk^b, and Jk3—define the Kidd blood group system. The original reports of the antibodies to Jk^a and Jk^b appeared in the early 1950s,[22,23] followed by the discovery of the Jk(a−b−) phenotype, or the Kidd null phenotype.[24] Individuals with this null phenotype are usually from the Far East and Pacific Island areas and may produce an antibody, anti-Jk3, that is reactive serologically as an inseparable combination of anti-Jk^a and anti-Jk^b. This unique antibody defined an antigen specified as Jk3. The Jk3 antigen is present whenever Jk^a or Jk^b antigens are also produced. This antigen is analogous to Fy3 antigen in that Fy3 antigen is present on Fy(a+) and Fy(b+) red blood cells. Kidd antigens develop early in fetal life and are detectable on fetal red blood cells. In general the Kidd antigens do not rank high in terms of red blood cell immunogenicity. The Kidd antigens are not denatured after exposure to routine proteolytic enzyme reagents. The common phenotypes and frequencies of the Kidd antigens are presented in Table 6-5.

Heaton and McLoughlin[25] reported the first evidence in clarifying the biochemical structure of the Kidd antigens in 1982. These investigators demonstrated that Jk(a−b−) red blood cells were more resistant to lysis in the

Table 6-5 Common Phenotypes and Frequencies in the Kidd System

PHENOTYPE			PHENOTYPE FREQUENCY (%)	
REACTIONS WITH ANTI-Jk^a	ANTI-Jk^b	INTERPRETATION	WHITES	BLACKS
+	0	Jk(a+b−)	26.3	51.1*
0	+	Jk(a−b+)	23.4	8.1
+	+	Jk(a+b+)	50.3†	40.8
0	0	Jk(a−b−)	rare	rare

*Most common phenotype in the Black population.
†Most common phenotype in the White population.
From Reid ME, Lomas-Francis C: *The blood group antigen facts book,* San Diego, 1997, Academic Press.

presence of 2M urea than red blood cells possessing either the Jk^a or Jk^b antigens. Red blood cells of normal Kidd phenotypes swell and lyse rapidly on exposure to 2M urea. From these observations they suggested that the molecule expressing the Kidd antigens was a urea transporter, since the absence of the Kidd antigens resulted in a defect in urea transport. It was recently reported that the Kidd blood group and urea transport function of human erythrocytes were carried by the same protein.[26] From a practical perspective screening methods based on the property of resistance to 2M urea can be used to identify rare Jk(a−b−) donor units.

Genetics of the Kidd Blood Group System

The Kidd blood group system has been assigned to a genetic locus located on chromosome 18. Characteristics of the alleles within the locus include the following:

- Jk^a allele encodes the Jk^a and Jk3 antigens and is codominant with the Jk^b allele
- Jk^b allele encodes the Jk^b and Jk3 antigens and is codominant with the Jk^a allele
- *Jk* allele is a silent allele that produces neither Jk^a nor Jk^b antigens; it is a common allele in Polynesian, Filipino, and Chinese populations; the *JkJk* genotype results in a Jk(a−b−) phenotype
- Jk(a−b−) phenotype can also be derived by the action of a dominant suppressor gene, *In(Jk)*

Characteristics of the Kidd Antibodies

As previously mentioned the alloantibodies produced in response to Kidd antigen exposure are of clinical significance for transfusion recipients. Their importance lies in their characteristic weak reactivity in vitro combined with the capacity to effect severe red blood cell destruction in vivo. After immune stimulation antibody titers rise and quickly plummet to undetectable levels. Delayed hemolytic transfusion reactions and extravascular hemolysis are commonly associated with the antibodies of this blood group system. In addition, rare examples of Kidd antibodies capable of the activation and binding of complement proteins may cause intravascular red blood cell destruction in a transfusion reaction. The consultation of a patient's previous records before the selection of donor units is important in reducing the incidence of these transfusion reactions.

Common serologic characteristics of anti-Jk^a and anti-Jk^b include the following:

- The immunoglobulin class is IgG
- Agglutination reactions are best observed by the IAT
- The antibodies detect dosage of Kidd antigens on red blood cells; weak examples of antibodies demonstrate stronger agglutination reactions with the homozygous expression of antigen [Jk(a−b+) or Jk(a+b−)] versus the heterozygous expression of antigen [Jk(a+b+)]
- The antibodies bind complement molecules
- The antibodies are produced in response to antigen exposure through transfusion or pregnancy
- The antibodies usually appear in combination with multiple antibodies in the sera of individuals who have formed other red blood cell antibodies
- Antibody detection is aided with enzyme reagents, LISS, and polyethylene glycol (PEG)
- The antibodies do not store well; antibody concentration quickly declines in vivo

Table 6-6 Characteristics of Antibodies in the Kell, Duffy, and Kidd Blood Group Systems

CHARACTERISTIC	KELL SYSTEM	DUFFY SYSTEM	KIDD SYSTEM
◆ RBC stimulated	Yes	Yes	Yes; weak antibody
◆ IgG	Yes	Yes	Yes
◆ IAT phase	Yes	Yes	Yes
◆ Enzyme phase	No effect	No reactivity	Enhanced
◆ Clinical significance	Yes	Yes	Yes
◆ Unique features	Anti-K most common Anti-Js^b more common in Blacks Anti-Kp^b more common in Whites		Bind complement Common cause of delayed hemolytic transfusion reactions

RBC, Red blood cell; *IAT,* indirect antiglobulin test.

Since antibodies to the Kell, Duffy, and Kidd blood group antigens are of great clinical significance, their recognition in antibody identification testing is vital to ensure that patients receive antigen-negative donor red blood cell units when necessary. Each of these blood group systems shares similar antibody characteristics. A comparison of the important characteristics of these system antibodies is provided in Table 6-6.

LUTHERAN BLOOD GROUP SYSTEM

ISBT SYSTEM SYMBOL	ISBT SYSTEM NUMBER	CLINICAL SIGNIFICANCE	ANTIBODY CLASS	OPTIMAL TEMPERATURE	REACTIVE PHASES	ENZYME PHASES
LU	005	YES Lu^b	IgG/IgM		RT AHG	E →

Characteristics and Biochemistry of the Lutheran Antigens

Lutheran Phenotypes

The Lutheran blood group system comprises 18 antigens, numbered from LU1 to LU20 (LU10 and LU15 are obsolete). The Auberger antigens Au^a and Au^b, first reported in 1961 and 1989, respectively, were recently added to the Lutheran system and assigned to LU19 and LU20.[27] Lutheran antigens have not been found on lymphocytes, granulocytes, monocytes, or platelets. In addition, Lutheran antigens are weakly expressed on cord blood cells. Most of the 18 Lutheran antigens are of high incidence; therefore corresponding red blood cell alloantibodies are infrequently encountered in the transfusion service. The two primary antigens of this system include the antithetical antigens, Lu^a (LU1) and Lu^b (LU2). Antibodies to these antigens are occasionally observed in patient samples. Lu^a (LU1) and Lu^b (LU2) antigens are resistant to ficin and papain treatment of red blood cells. Individuals in most populations have the Lu(a−b+) phenotype (Table 6-7).

The Lu$_{null}$ phenotype, Lu(a−b−), rarely occurs and may manifest itself in any of the following three unique genetic mechanisms:

- Recessive: only true Lu_{null} phenotype; homozygosity for a rare recessive amorph, *Lu*, at the *LU* locus
- Dominant inhibitor or In(Lu) phenotype: heterozygosity for a rare dominant inhibitor gene, *In(Lu)*, that is not located at the *LU* locus
- X-linked suppressor gene: inherited in a recessive manner

Lutheran Antigen Biochemistry

In biochemical studies using monoclonal antibodies, the Lutheran antigens were located on a membrane glycoprotein.[28] The biologic importance of the Lutheran glycoproteins remains unresolved.

Genetics of the Lutheran Blood Group System

The *LU* locus has been assigned to chromosome 19 and is linked to the *Se* (secretor) locus. The *H*, *Le*, and *LW* genetic loci are also located on chromosome 19. The Lu^a and Lu^b codominant alleles genetically encode the production of the low-frequency antigen, Lu^a, and the high-frequency antigen, Lu^b.

Characteristics of the Lutheran Antibodies

Important serologic characteristics of the Lutheran antibodies are outlined below.

*Anti-Lu^a^*

- Anti-Lu^a may be present without immune red blood cell stimulation
- Immunoglobulin class: IgM and IgG
- Optimal in vitro agglutination reactions are observed at room temperature
- Anti-Lu^a has characteristic mixed-field pattern of agglutination; small agglutinates are surrounded by unagglutinated free red blood cells
- No clinical significance in transfusion; mild cases of hemolytic disease of the newborn reported

*Anti-Lu^b^*

- Anti-Lu^b is a rare antibody because of antigen's high incidence
- Immunoglobulin class: IgG
- Most examples of anti-Lu^b agglutinate within antiglobulin phases
- Some examples of anti-Lu^b demonstrate a mixed-field agglutination pattern

Table 6-7 Common Phenotypes and Frequencies in the Lutheran Blood Group System

PHENOTYPE			PHENOTYPE FREQUENCY (%)
REACTIONS WITH ANTI-Lu^a	ANTI-Lu^b	INTERPRETATION	MOST POPULATIONS
+	0	Lu(a+b−)	0.2
0	+	Lu(a−b+)	92.4
+	+	Lu(a+b+)	7.4
0	0	Lu(a−b−)	rare

From Reid ME, Lomas-Francis C: *The blood group antigen facts book*, San Diego, 1997, Academic Press.

◆ Anti-Lu^b has been associated with transfusion reactions and mild cases of HDN

LEWIS BLOOD GROUP SYSTEM

ISBT SYSTEM SYMBOL	ISBT SYSTEM NUMBER	CLINICAL SIGNIFICANCE	ANTIBODY CLASS	OPTIMAL TEMPERATURE	REACTIVE PHASES	ENZYME PHASES
LE	007	NO	IgM		IS 37C AHG	E ↑

Characteristics of the Lewis Antigens

The Lewis antigens, unlike other blood group antigens, are manufactured by tissue cells and secreted into body fluids.[29] Lewis antigens are found primarily in secretions and plasma and are adsorbed onto the red blood cell membrane. In contrast to the antigens of the Kell, Duffy, and Kidd blood group systems, the Lewis antigens are not integral to the red blood cell membrane. The development of the Lewis antigen structure begins in the first week after birth and may continue its development for up to 6 years. The Lewis system is similar to the ABO system in that the antigen development depends on three sets of independently inherited genes. Lewis genes encode a glycosyltransferase that adds a sugar to an antigen precursor structure. The Lewis antigen system is not particularly relevant from a clinical standpoint, since Lewis antibodies do not usually cause in vivo red blood cell destruction. The antibodies are common, however, and an understanding of antigen genetics and biochemistry is helpful in the discernment of the serologic characteristics. Frequency distributions of the Lewis antigens appear in Table 6-8.

Biochemistry of the Lewis Antigens

The product of the Lewis gene is L-fucosyltransferase, which adds L-fucose to the number 4 carbon of *N*-acetylglucosamine of type 1 precursor structures. The structure acquires Le^a antigen specificity and is adsorbed onto the red blood cell membrane, thus creating the Le(a+) phenotype. If type 1 H structures are also present in the secretions, the Lewis transferase adds L-fucose to this structure. This resulting product, Le^b, is adsorbed preferentially over the Le^a glycoprotein onto

Table 6-8 Lewis System Phenotypes and Frequencies

PHENOTYPE			PHENOTYPE FREQUENCY (%)	
REACTIONS WITH ANTI-Le^a	ANTI-Le^b	INTERPRETATION	WHITES	BLACKS
+	0	Le(a+b−)	22	23
0	+	Le(a−b+)	72	55
0	0	Le(a−b−)	6	22
+	+	Le(a+b+)	rare	rare

From Vengelen-Tyler V: *Technical manual*, ed 12, Bethesda, Md, 1996, American Association of Blood Banks.

the red blood cell membrane. As discussed in Chapter 4, the difference between type 1 and type 2 structures is the linkage between the carbons of the D-galactose and *N*-acetylglucosamine on the H precursor chain. In type 2 H chains the number 4 carbon is not available for fucose attachment. Therefore type 2 chains never express Lewis antigen activity.

Newborn red blood cells possess the Le(a−b−) phenotype. As the Lewis antigens begin development, the cells may type as Le(a+b+) until the transition to Le(a−b+) is complete. Reliable Lewis phenotyping may not be possible until about 6 years of age.

Inheritance of the Lewis System Antigens

As previously mentioned the Lewis system depends on three genes to produce the Lewis antigen structures: *Hh*, secretor (*Se*), and Lewis (*Le*). The *H*, *Se*, and *Le* gene products are glycosyltransferases. The secretor gene encodes the H transferase available in the secretions. The *le*, *h*, and *se* genes are amorphs and produce no detectable products. If an *Le* gene is inherited, Le^a antigens are found in the secretions and are adsorbed onto the red blood cells, regardless of the secretor status. If the *Se* gene is inherited in addition to the *Le* gene, the Lewis transferase converts the available H structure to an Le^b antigen, and the red blood cells adsorbs Le^b instead of Le^a. This concept is illustrated in Fig. 6-2. If the gene inherited from both parents is *le*, no antigen structure is present on the red blood cells.

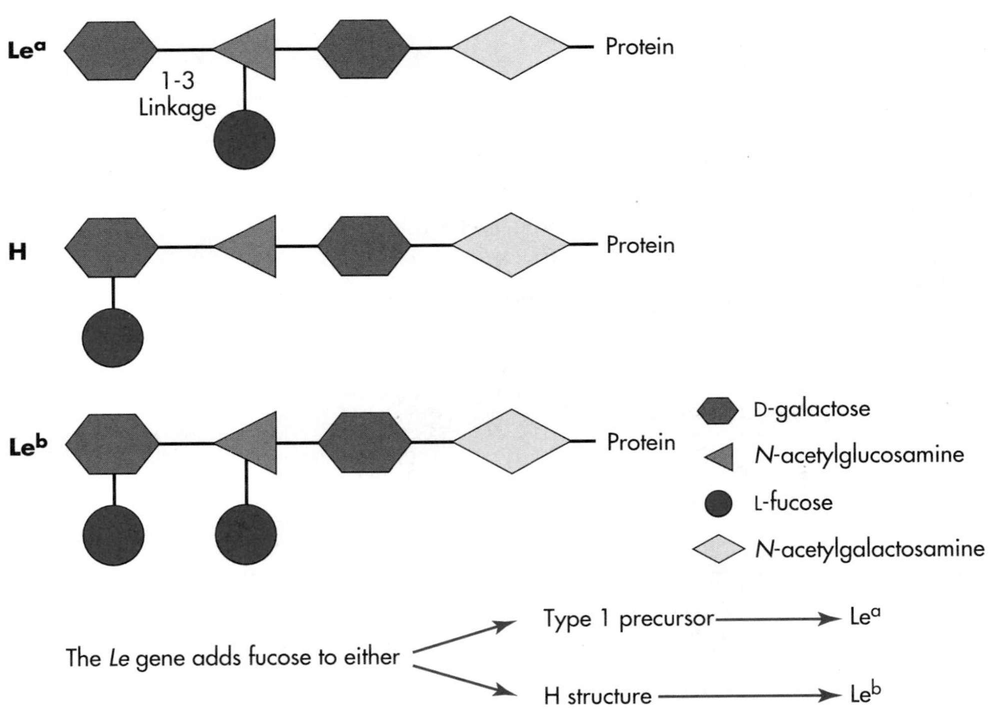

Fig. 6-2 Formation of the Lewis antigens.

A summary of Lewis inheritance and biochemistry concepts is listed in Box 6-3, and a summary of the genes, plasma products, and red blood cell phenotypes that arise from the *Le*, *Se*, and *H* genes can be found in Table 6-9.

Characteristics of the Lewis Antibodies

Lewis antibodies occur almost exclusively in the serum of Le(a−b−) individuals, usually without known red blood cell stimulus.[30] Le(a−b+) individuals do not produce anti-Le^a, and it is rare to find anti-Le^b in an Le(a+b−) individual. Anti-Le^a or anti-Le^b can be found in an Le(a−b−) person. Lewis antibodies are IgM and have no clinical significance. If a donor unit of Lewis antigen–positive blood was transfused to a patient with a Lewis antibody, the Le^a or Le^b antigens in the donor plasma would readily neutralize Lewis antibodies. For this reason it is exceedingly rare that Lewis antibodies cause decreased survival of transfused Le(a+) or Le(b+) cells. Phenotyping donor blood for the presence of Lewis antigens when a recipient has an anti-Lewis antibody is unnecessary. Crossmatching for compatibility using anti-IgG antihuman globulin, with or without prewarming, provides a good indication of transfusion safety.[31] Avoiding room temperature reactions in the antibody screen or antibody identification panel also avoids anti-Lewis antibody reactivity. Lewis antibodies have not been implicated in HDN, because the antibodies do not cross the placenta and the antigens are not well developed at birth. Anti-Le^a and anti-Le^b are found during and immediately following pregnancy more often than would be expected.

BOX 6-3

Summary of Lewis Inheritance and Biochemistry Concepts

- Le^a and Le^b are *not* alleles
- The Le(b+) red blood cell phenotype arises from the inheritance of an *Le*, *Se*, and *H* gene
- Individuals who type as Le(a+b−) are not secretors
- A Bombay phenotype *(hh)* cannot express the Le^b antigen
- A person can be a nonsecretor *(sese)* and still secrete Le^a into body fluids
- Lewis antigens found in the secretions are glycoproteins
- Lewis antigens found in plasma are glycolipids
- Red blood cells only adsorb glycolipids, not glycoproteins, onto the membrane
- Adult red blood cells that type as Le(a+b+) are very rare

Serologic Characteristics

Lewis system antibodies can be challenging to identify, because the reactions can have a wide temperature range. Some of the challenges include the following:

- Agglutination observed at immediate spin, 37° C, and the antiglobulin phase
- Agglutination is often fragile and easily dispersed
- Enzymes enhance anti-Le^b antibody reactivity
- Hemolysis is sometimes seen in vitro, especially if fresh serum is used, because anti-Le^a efficiently binds complement
- Neutralization techniques using commercially prepared Lewis substance may be helpful to confirm the presence of a Lewis antibody or eliminate the reactions to identify other antibodies mixed in the serum

Table 6-9 Lewis Genes and Red Blood Cell Phenotypes

GENES PRESENT	ANTIGENS IN SECRETIONS	RED BLOOD CELL PHENOTYPE
Le sese H	Le^a	Le(a+b−)
Le Se H	Le^a Le^b H	Le(a−b+)
lele sese H	None	Le(a−b−)
lele Se H	H	Le(a−b−)
Le sese hh	Le^a	Le(a+b−)
Le Se hh	Le^a	Le(a+b−)
lele sese hh	None	Le(a−b−)
lele Se hh	None	Le(a−b−)

Ii BLOOD GROUP COLLECTION

ISBT SYSTEM SYMBOL	ISBT SYSTEM NUMBER	CLINICAL SIGNIFICANCE	ANTIBODY CLASS	OPTIMAL TEMPERATURE	REACTIVE PHASES	ENZYME PHASES
I	207	NO	IgM		IS 4C RT	E ↑

The I blood group collection is composed of two antigens: I and i. The antigens are formed from the sequential action of multiple gene products encoding glycosyltransferases. I and i are not antithetical antigens.[3] The i antigen is expressed on newborn and cord blood cells, whereas the I antigen is expressed on adult cells. Anti-I is a commonly encountered autoantibody with optimal reactivity at colder temperatures. The antibody has no clinical significance, since it does not elicit red blood cell destruction during transfusion or pregnancy. This antibody, however, often causes a great deal of confusion in serologic testing.

Biochemistry of the I and i Structures

The I and i antigens exist on the precursor A, B, and H oligosaccharide chains at a position closer to the red blood cell membrane. The I antigen is associated with branched chains, and the i antigen is associated with linear chains (Fig. 6-3). The I and i antigens are present on both glycolipid and glycoprotein structures on the red blood cell membrane. They also can be found as soluble glycoprotein antigens in plasma and in body secretions such as human milk and amniotic fluid.

The I antigen is not well developed at birth, since linear chains of the oligosaccharide precursor chain are predominantly found in newborns. As the straight chains develop into branched chains, the i antigen converts to the I-antigen structure over a 2-year period.

Serologic Characteristics of Autoanti-I

Clinically insignificant: antibody that does not cause red blood cell destruction or clearance.

Anti-I is usually found as a cold-reacting, **clinically insignificant,** IgM autoantibody. Most individuals possess an autoanti-I detectable at 4° C. Anti-I is often de-

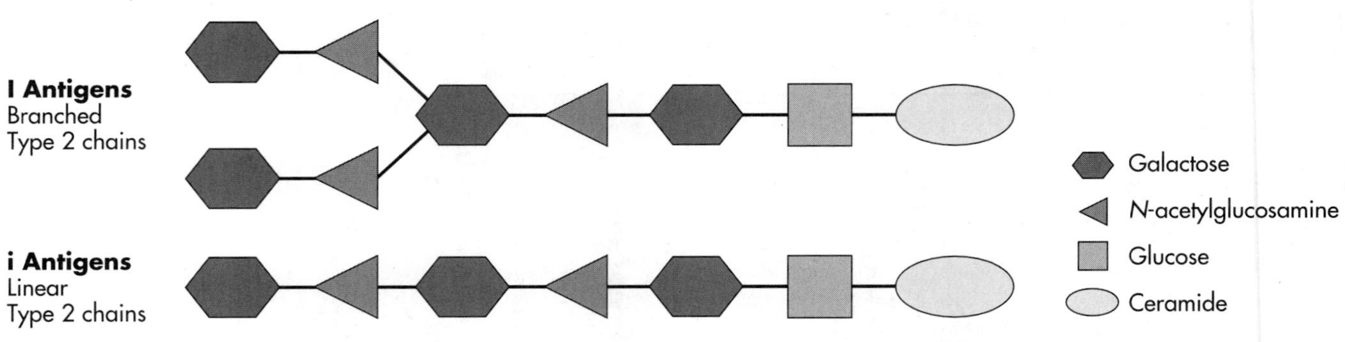

Fig. 6-3 I and i antigen structures.

tected when samples are tested at room temperature. Anti-I varies in its reactivity with different adult red blood cells because the branching oligosaccharide chain structures vary.[30] Since anti-I binds complement, polyspecific antiglobulin reagents may detect the C3 component attached to the red blood cell. Once anti-I is detected, efforts to avoid its reactivity are often accomplished with **prewarming techniques.** This procedure is discussed further in Chapter 7. The use of enzyme reagents in antibody detection enhances anti-I reactivity.

Prewarming techniques: techniques in which patient serum and test cells are prewarmed separately before combining to prevent reactions of cold antibodies binding at room temperature and activating complement.

Anti-I also reacts as a compound antibody. It is often found as an anti-IH and demonstrates stronger agglutination with red blood cells having greater numbers of H antigens, such as group O and group A_2 cells. This antibody is also clinically insignificant. When crossmatching a group A individual this specificity is noted if agglutination reactions are stronger with panel and screening reagent red blood cells than with group A donor units.

Disease Association

Strong autoanti-I is associated with *Mycoplasma pneumoniae* infections and **cold hemagglutinin disease.** Anti-i is associated with infectious mononucleosis, lymphoproliferative disease, and occasionally cold hemagglutinin disease. In these situations, if transfusion becomes necessary, finding serologically compatible blood may be more difficult. I- or i-negative donor units are not required. Serologic techniques to evaluate these antibodies are further discussed in Chapter 7. The frequency of alloanti-I is rare.

Cold hemagglutinin disease: autoimmune hemolytic anemia produced by an autoantibody that reacts best in colder temperatures (less than 37° C).

P BLOOD GROUP SYSTEM

ISBT SYSTEM SYMBOL	ISBT SYSTEM NUMBER	CLINICAL SIGNIFICANCE	ANTIBODY CLASS	OPTIMAL TEMPERAURE	REACTIVE PHASES	ENZYME PHASES
P1	003	NO	IgM		IS 4C RT	E ↑

The antigens associated with this system are located in two systems: P1 (ISBT 003) and the GLOB collection (ISBT 209). The antigen in the P1 system is P_1, and the antigens assigned to the "globoside collection" include P, P^k, and Luke (LKE).[32] The antigens from both systems are reviewed in this section and are collectively referred to as the P system.

Antigens of the P System

The P blood group antigens are structurally related to the ABH antigens and exist as glycoproteins and glycolipids. The antigens are formed by the action of glycosyltransferases, and the P_1 antigen is present in soluble form in some secretions. The phenotypes and corresponding antigens in the P system are shown in Table 6-10. A summary of the antigen and antibody characteristics appears in Table 6-11.

The most common phenotypes in the P blood group system are P_1 and P_2, analogous to the A_1 and A_2 phenotypes in the ABH system. Individuals with the P_1 phenotype have both P and P_1 antigens on their red blood cells. Individuals with the P_2 phenotype express only P antigen on their red blood cells and may produce an anti-P_1. The P_1 antigen is poorly developed at birth and is variably

Table 6-10 P System Phenotypes, Antigens, and Frequencies

PHENOTYPE	ANTIGENS	PHENOTYPE FREQUENCIES (%) BLACKS	PHENOTYPE FREQUENCIES (%) WHITES
P_1	P_1 P P^k	94	79
P_2	P P^k	6	21
P_1^k	P_1 P^k	Very rare in both races	
P_2^k	P^k	Very rare in both races	
p	—	Very rare in both races	

Table 6-11 P System Antigen and Antibody Characteristics

ANTIGEN	ANTIGEN CHARACTERISTICS	POSSIBLE ANTIBODIES	ALLOANTIBODY CHARACTERISTICS
P_1	Red blood cells express P, P_1, and P^k antigens; P_1 is not well developed at birth; most common phenotype	None	Not applicable
P_2	Lacks P_1 antigen but expresses P and P^k antigens; second-most common phenotype	Anti-P_1	IgM; room temperature; variable reactions with adult cells; not clinically significant
P_1^k	Red blood cells express P_1 and P^k antigens; very rare phenotype	Anti-P	Clinically significant; associated with spontaneous abortions (rare)
P_2^k	Red blood cells express only P^k antigens; very rare phenotype	Anti-P and anti-P_1	Anti-P and anti-P_1 characteristics
p	Null phenotype of the P system; negative for P, P_1, and P^k antigens; very rare phenotype	Anti-PP_1P^k (Tj^a)	Hemolytic; clinically significant; can be separated into three specificities

expressed on adult cells. The antigen expression decreases upon storage of the red blood cells. The P_1 antigen exists in a soluble form and can be detected in plasma and **hydatid cyst fluid**.

Hydatid cyst fluid: fluid obtained from a cyst of the dog tapeworm.

P, P^k, and LKE antigens are high-frequency antigens. Their relevance in routine testing is uncommon, because antibodies are not usually discovered with these specificities. The P^k antigen was thought to be expressed only by the P^k phenotype until the discovery that all red blood cells except p cells express P^k.[3] LKE-negative cells have a stronger expression of the P^k antigen.

Genetics and Biochemistry

Expression of the P system antigens originates from two independently inherited genes.[3] Alleles at one locus include P^{1k}, P^k, and *p*. Alleles at the second locus include P^2 and $P^{2.0}$. The interaction of the transferase produced by these two genes creates the antigens of the P system. Fig. 6-4 illustrates the antigen structures, and Fig. 6-5 shows the genes and their resulting products. Note that the P_1 antigen is formed from the same paragloboside precursor as the H antigen. Lactosylceramide is the precursor structure for antigens of the globoside collection.

A

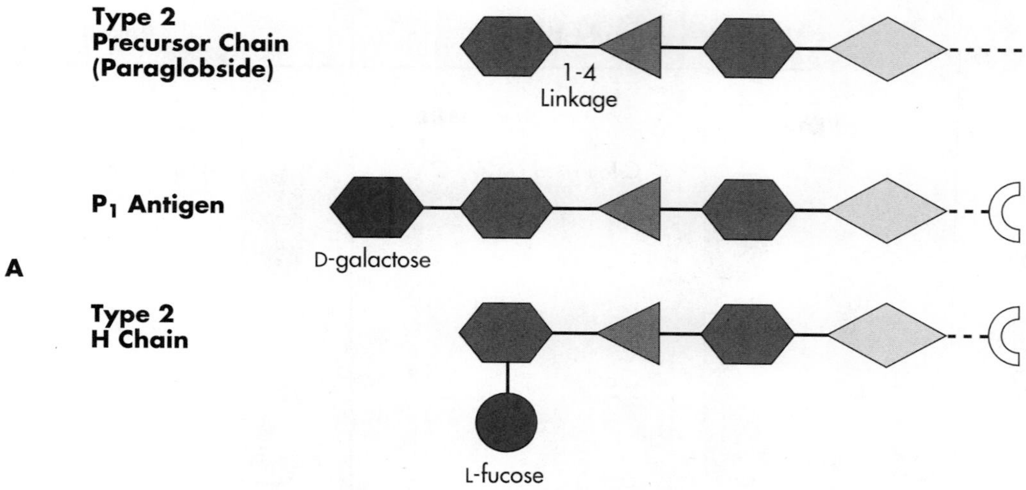

The type 2 precursor chain is the substrate for the P_1 antigen as well as the H antigen.

B

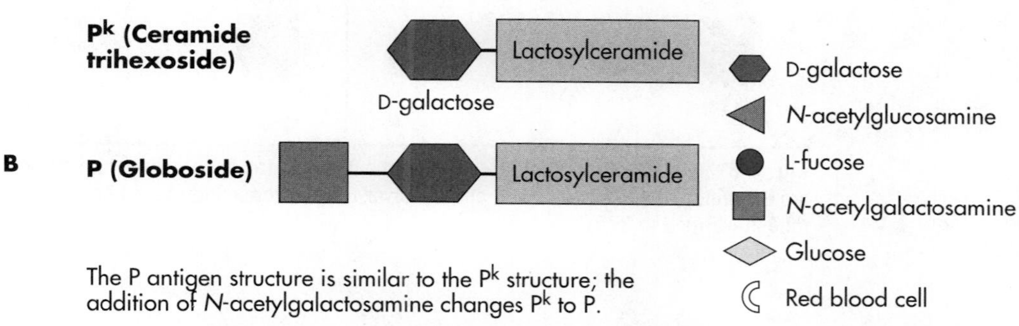

The P antigen structure is similar to the P^k structure; the addition of *N*-acetylgalactosamine changes P^k to P.

Fig. 6-4 P system antigen structures. *A,* P_1 antigen; *B,* P^k and P antigen structure.

P System Antibodies

Anti-P_1

Anti-P_1 is frequently encountered in the serum of P_2 individuals and does not require red blood cell immune stimulation. This antibody is an IgM cold-reactive agglutinin enhanced with enzymes. Commercially available P_1 substance can be used to neutralize the antibody to confirm the antibody presence or eliminate the reactions.

Anti-P_1 rarely decreases red blood cell survival. Providing P_1 positive red blood cells is acceptable if compatible at 37° C and at the antiglobulin phase.[33] If reactions are interfering with the crossmatch, avoiding the immediate spin reading usually eliminates the antibody reactions.

Other alloantibodies in the P system are rarely encountered and are summarized in Table 6-10.

Autoanti-P

Autoanti-P is associated with an immune hemolytic anemia called **paroxysmal cold hemoglobinuria** (PCH). Autoanti-P is an IgG antibody known as the Donath-Landsteiner antibody. This **biphasic hemolysin** binds to P-positive (P_1 or P_2) red blood cells at lower temperatures in the extremities. Complement

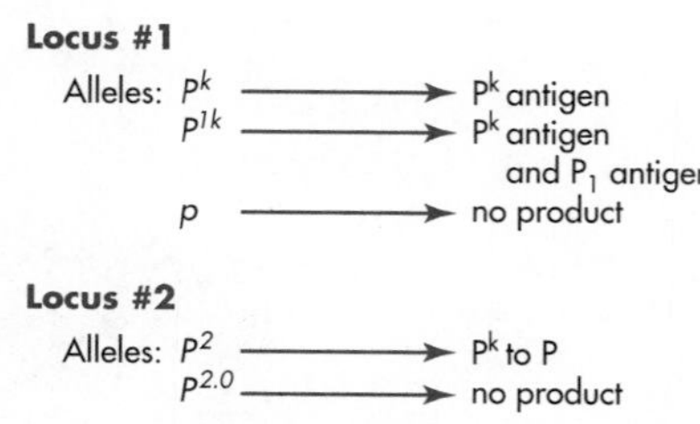

Fig. 6-5 Relationship of the P system genes and their antigen products.

Paroxysmal cold hemoglobinuria: rare autoimmune disorder characterized by hemolysis and hematuria associated with exposure to cold.

Biphasic hemolysin: antibody, such as the Donath-Landsteiner antibody, that requires a period of cold and warm incubations to bind complement with resulting hemolysis.

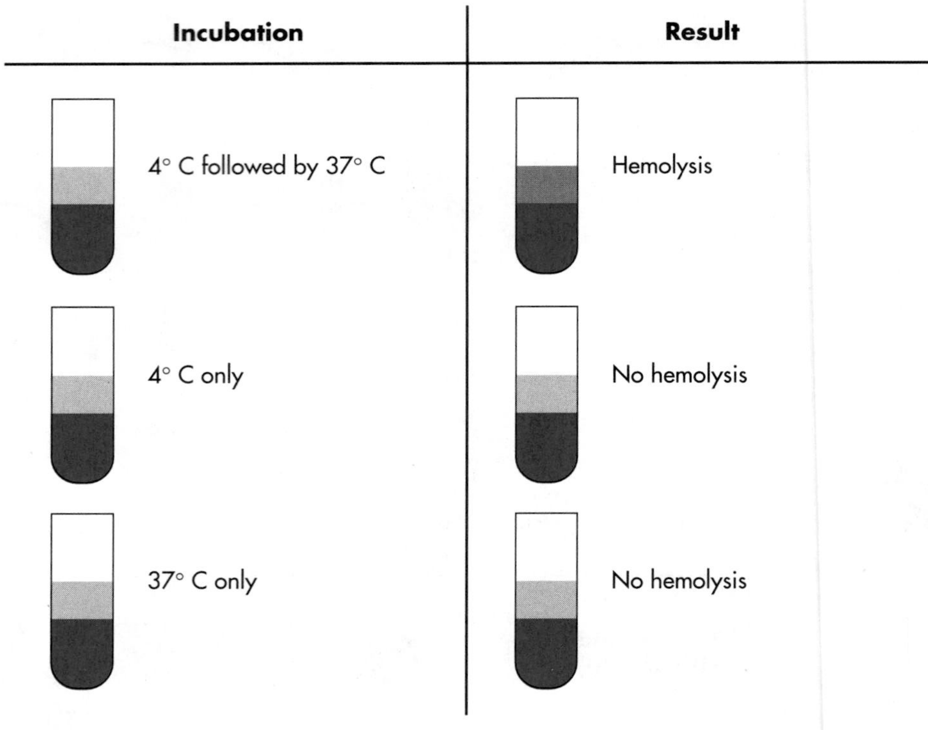

Fig. 6-6 Donath-Landsteiner test. After the patient's freshly drawn serum and red blood cells are incubated, complement binds only at lower temperatures and causes hemolysis when the tube is warmed to 37° C.

is attached, which effects hemolysis when the red blood cells are subsequently warmed to 37° C. This rare autoantibody may appear transiently in children following viral infections and in adults with tertiary syphilis. The autoantibody reacts weakly or not at all in routine in vitro test methods and requires the Donath-Landsteiner test for confirmation. A summary of this test appears in Fig. 6-6. Another autoantibody that has been implicated in PCH is anti-Pr.

Patients with an autoanti-P have a weak positive direct antiglobulin test only because of complement coating. An eluate prepared from their red blood cells is nonreactive with reagent red blood cells. If transfusion becomes necessary, P-negative blood is not required. However, the red blood cell unit may be administered through a **blood warmer**.[34] Patients should be kept warm at all times.

Blood warmer: medical device that prewarms donor blood to 37° C before transfusion.

Anti-PP$_1$P^k

Individuals homozygous for the "*p*" gene (P null) can make an antibody with an anti-PP$_1$P^k specificity. This antibody was originally referred to as anti-Tj^a before it became associated with the P system. It can be separated into three antibodies and often demonstrates hemolysis in vitro. Anti-PP$_1$P^k is a clinically significant antibody, and red blood cells from donors who are also "p" are required if transfusion becomes necessary.[35]

MNS BLOOD GROUP SYSTEM

M and N Antigens

ISBT SYSTEM SYMBOL	ISBT SYSTEM NUMBER	CLINICAL SIGNIFICANCE	ANTIBODY CLASS	OPTIMAL TEMPERATURE	REACTIVE PHASES	ENZYME PHASES
MNS	002	NO	IgM		IS 37C AHG	

S and s Antigens

ISBT SYSTEM SYMBOL	ISBT SYSTEM NUMBER	CLINICAL SIGNIFICANCE	ANTIBODY CLASS	OPTIMAL TEMPERATURE	REACTIVE PHASES	ENZYME PHASES
MNS	002	YES	IgG		AHG	VAR

The MNS system includes 40 antigens that are expressed primarily on red blood cells.[3] Molecular genetics have provided insight into the genetic nature of the various MNS system antigens, many of which result from crossing over, gene recombination, and substitutions. This section limits the discussion of the MNS antigens and antibodies to M, N, S, s, and U.

Genetics and Biochemistry

The two genes that encode the MNS system antigens are located on chromosome 4. Because of their proximity, they are usually inherited as a haplotype. One gene codes for M or N, and the other codes for S or s. The most frequently inherited haplotype is Ns, followed by Ms, MS, and NS.

The genes *GYPA* and *GYPB* code for **glycophorin** A (GPA) and glycophorin B (GPB), respectively. GPA codes for the M and N antigens, and GPB codes for S and s antigens.

Glycophorin: glycoprotein that projects through the red blood cell membrane and carries many blood group antigens.

The structures that carry the MNS blood group system antigens are glycoproteins; since the majority of the sugars carry **sialic acid** structures, the membrane structures are called sialoglycoproteins.[36] The MN sialoglycoprotein (GPA) and the Ss sialoglycoprotein (GPB) structures are similar but distinct. The amino acid sequence makes each a unique structure, and Fig. 6-7 compares the antigen structures.

Sialic acid: constituents of the sugars attached to proteins on red blood cells that lend a negative charge to the red blood cell membrane.

GPA: M and N Antigens

Characteristics of M and N antigens include the following:

- GPA consists of 131 amino acids with 72 outside of the cell membrane
- M and N antigens differ at positions 1 and 5; the first and fifth amino acid residues for the M antigen structure are serine and glycine, respectively, whereas the N antigen structure has leucine and glutamic acid at positions one and five, respectively.
- Inheriting M or N in the homozygous state [(M+N−) or (M−N+)] greatly enhances the strength of the antigen expression.

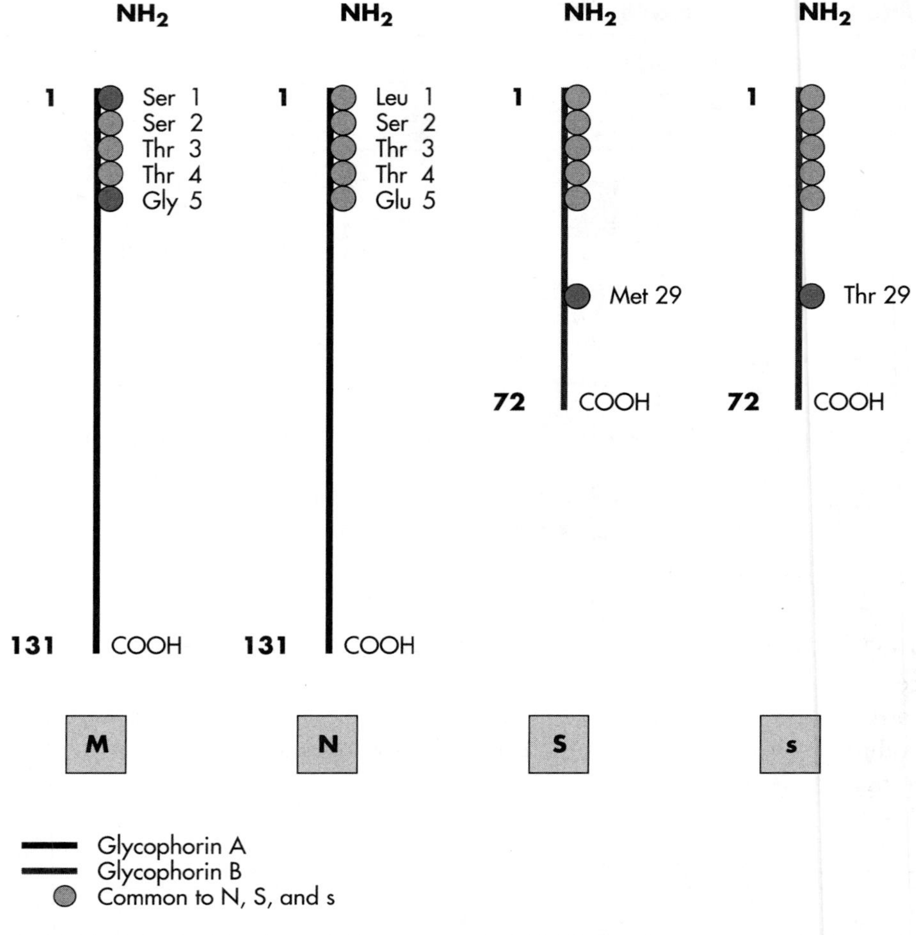

Fig. 6-7 MN and Ss sialoglycoprotein structural comparison. *NH_2,* Amino terminal; *1,* amino acid 1; *131,* amino acid 131; *Ser,* serine; *Thr,* threonine; *Gly,* glycine; *Leu,* leucine; *Glu,* glutamic acid; *Met,* methionine; *COOH,* carboxy terminal.

GPB: S, s, and U Antigens

Characteristics of S, s, and U antigens include the following:

- GPB consists of 72 amino acids with 43 outside the cell membrane
- S and s antigens differ at amino acid position 29; S antigen has methionine at that position, whereas s antigen has threonine
- The U antigen is located near the membrane and is always present when S or s is inherited
- Absence of or altered GPB expression would result in red blood cells phenotyping as S–s–U–

GPB carries the same first 26 amino acid sequence as the N-antigen of the GPA structure. Inheriting S or s thus provides antigenic activity similar to N called the "N" antigen. This N-like structure may prevent N-negative individuals from forming an anti-N antibody.[35] However anti-N formed by N-negative individuals and reagent anti-N do not react with "N," because there are too few antigen copies to support agglutination.[37]

Table 6-12 Antibody Characteristics in the MNS System

ANTIBODY	IMMUNOGLOBULIN CLASS	CLINICALLY SIGNIFICANT	EFFECT OF FICIN	CHARACTERISTICS
M	IgM*	No	Removed	Rarely reported to cause HDN or HTR; stronger reactions with cells from a homozygote
N	IgM	No	Removed	Weak, cold reactive
S	IgG	Yes	Variable	
s	IgG	Yes	Variable	
U	IgG	Yes	Resistant	Reacts with all S+ or s+ red blood cells; U-negative cells are found only in the Black population

HDN, Hemolytic disease of the newborn; *HTR*, hemolytic transfusion reaction.
*Sometimes can be whole or partially IgG.[30]

Antibodies of the MNS Blood Group System

Antibodies to the antigens included in the MNS system vary in their clinical significance and serologic properties. They are summarized in Table 6-12.

Anti-M

Examples of IgM and IgG forms of anti-M have been reported. Anti-M occurs naturally and is considered a clinically insignificant antibody.[30] Examples of anti-M that react at the antiglobulin phase after a prewarming procedure should be considered clinically significant. Anti-M is rarely implicated in HDN.

Anti-M may demonstrate variable reactions with different manufacturer's panel or screening cells because of the preservative's pH.[38] Some examples of anti-M react better at a pH of 6.5. Anti-M demonstrates marked dosage, since agglutination reactions are stronger with homozygous expressions of the antigen (e.g., M+N− reagent red blood cells react stronger than M+N+ reagent red blood cells).

Anti-N

Anti-N is a rarely encountered IgM cold-reacting antibody that is not usually clinically significant. Examples of an N-like antibody have been found more frequently in dialysis patients exposed to formaldehyde-sterilized dialyzer membranes. This anti-N–like antibody is also not clinically significant and may be a result of an altered N-antigen structure on the red blood cells.[38]

Anti-S, Anti-s, and Anti-U

Anti-S, anti-s, and anti-U are clinically significant IgG antibodies that can cause decreased red blood cell survival and HDN. It is not difficult to find compatible blood for patients that have made an anti-S or anti-s. Table 6-13 shows the frequency of S and s antigens in the population. The U antigen is a high-incidence antigen, occurring in more than 99% of the population. Anti-U is rare but should be considered when serum from a previously transfused or pregnant Black person contains an antibody to a high-incidence antigen. The probability of anti-U existence can be established by showing that the person is S− and s−. U-negative blood can be found in less than 1% of the Black population and is not found in

Table 6-13 Phenotype Frequencies in the MNS System

	PHENOTYPE FREQUENCIES (%)	
Antigen	Whites	Blacks
M+	78	74
N+	72	75
S+	55	30.5
s+	89	94
U+	99.9	99

Table 6-14 Miscellaneous Blood Groups

NAME	SYMBOL	ISBT NO.	ANTIGENS	CHARACTERISTICS
Diego	DI	010	Di^a **Di^b** Wr^a **Wr^b** Wd^a Rb^a WARR	Di^a is more common in South American Indians; anti-Wr^a is commonly found with other antibodies
Cartwright	YT	011	**Yt^a** Yt^b	Variably sensitive to enzymes; sensitive to DTT
Xg	XG	012	Xg^a	Inherited on X chromosome; frequency varies with sex
Scianna	SC	013	**SC:1** SC:2 **SC:3**	
Dombrock	DO	014	Do^a Do^b **Gy^a** **Hy** **Jo^a**	Hy phenotype is found only in Blacks; anti-Do^a and anti-Do^b antibodies are rarely found as a single specificity
Colton	CO	015	**Co^a** Co^b Co3	Anti-Co^b is rarely found as a single specificity
Chido/ Rodgers	CH/RG	017	**Ch Rg**	Antigens are sensitive to enzymes and found in plasma; antibodies have HTLA characteristics
Gerbich	GE	020	**Ge2 Ge3 Ge4** Wb Ls^a An^a Dah	All antigens except for Ge4 are sensitive to enzymes
Cromer	CROM	021	**Cr^a** **Tc^a** Tc^b Tc^c **Dr^a** **Es^a** **IFC** **WES^a** WES^b **UMC**	Antigen is also found in plasma; located on decay-accelerating factor
Knops	KN	022	**Kn^a** Kn^b **McC^a** **Sl^a** **Yk^a**	Antigen depression in SLE, PNH, and AIDS; antigens are weakened by ficin treatment; antibodies have HTLA characteristics
Cost	COST	205	**Cs^a** Cs^b	Part of a blood group collection rather than a system
Vel	Vel	901. 001	**Vel**	Variable antigen expression on red blood cells; both IgG and IgM antibodies are associated with hemolytic reactions; antibodies react best with enzyme-treated red blood cells
JMH	JMH	900. 007	**JMH**	Autoanti-JMH is often found in elderly patients with absent or weak antigen expression; antibodies have HTLA characteristics; antigens are sensitive to enzymes and DTT
Sd^a	Sd^a	901. 012	**Sd^a**	Antigen found in guinea pig and human urine; antibodies are typically weak and agglutination is mixed field; reduction of Sd^a expression during pregnancy

HTLA, High-titer, low-avidity; *SLE,* systemic lupus erythematosus; *PNH,* paroxysmal nocturnal hemoglobinuria; *AIDS,* acquired immunodeficiency syndrome; *DTT,* dithiothreitol. Items in boldface indicate antigens of high incidence.

White donors. The Rare Donor Registry may need to be contacted if a patient with an anti-U needs a transfusion.

MISCELLANEOUS BLOOD GROUP SYSTEMS

This section reviews the blood groups that are less commonly encountered in routine transfusion medicine. In many of these systems the clinical significance of the antibodies associated with the system is unknown or not well documented because of the scarcity of examples. Antibodies to the antigens in these systems are infrequent because most are of either high or low frequency and others are of low immunogenicity. Table 6-14 summarizes these systems or collections. Low-frequency antigens that do not belong to a collection or system are not included. The use of molecular techniques has added to the knowledge of genetics and antigen products and in some instances has altered their classification.

CHAPTER SUMMARY

Appreciating the unique characteristics of each blood group system is helpful in understanding the serologic and clinical features of the associated antibodies. The clinical significance of the systems is summarized below.

SUMMARY OF CLINICAL SIGNIFICANCE OF BLOOD GROUP SYSTEMS*

Clinical significance	Blood group systems
Usually clinically significant	A and B; Rh; Kell; Kidd; Duffy; S, s, and U
Sometimes clinically significant	LW
Clinically significant if reactive at 37° C	A_1; H; Le^a; Lutheran; M and N; P_1
Usually clinically insignificant	Le^b

*Modified from Reid ME, Lomas-Francis C: *The blood group antigen facts book*, San Diego, 1997, Academic Press.

CRITICAL THINKING EXERCISES

◆ ***EXERCISE 6-1***

The blood bank received a call requesting 2 units of "Kell-negative" red blood cells for a patient with anti-K. Discuss why this request is incorrect. What should the request have stated?

◆ ***EXERCISE 6-2***

List the red blood cell antibodies with serologic reactivity that is usually enhanced with enzyme-treated panel cells.

◆ ***EXERCISE 6-3***

A patient has a history of the following red blood cell alloantibodies: anti-S, anti-Le^b, and anti-Jk^a. Which of these antibodies are clinically significant? How would you test for compatible red blood cell donor units? How would enzyme-treated panel cells react?

◆ ***EXERCISE 6-4***

A patient has a history of a previously identified autoanti-I. The current sample is nonreactive with screening cells when tested at room temperature. What are the implications of this result in a current request for the transfusion of 2 units of red blood cells?

◆ ***EXERCISE 6-5***

Explain how you would differentiate a Donath-Landsteiner antibody from a cold autoantibody.

◆ ***EXERCISE 6-6***

An anti-Js^b is detected in a prenatal sample. Is this antibody clinically significant? What is the most probable race of this patient? What reagents would be helpful when working up this antibody?

◆ ***EXERCISE 6-7***

A physician requests donor red blood cell units that are phenotypically matched for a very young sickle cell patient. Her phenotype is: D+, C−, E−, c+, e+, (R_or), S−, s+, M−, N+; Le(a−b−); Fy(a−b−); Jk(a−b+)
Which donor population (race) would you test to find a close match? Which antigens are not important to match because of the corresponding antibody's clinical significance?

◆ ***EXERCISE 6-8***

A patient phenotypes as Le(a−b+). Is this patient a secretor or a nonsecretor? What genes are responsible for conferring Le^a and Le^b antigens on the red blood cells?

◆ ***EXERCISE 6-9***

A patient was admitted for surgery with a history of a previous anti-U. You are directed to test this patient's siblings, since U-negative donor units are rare. No commercial antiserum is available for testing. What other source of anti-U could you use to phenotype the patient's siblings?

◆ ***EXERCISE 6-10***

Does a patient with an anti-Vel present a problem for provision of compatible donor units? How would Vel-negative units be located?

STUDY QUESTIONS

1. Which blood group system possesses the Js^b and Kp^a antigens?
   a. Duffy
   b. Lutheran
   c. Kell
   d. Kidd

2. An antibody commonly associated with delayed transfusion reactions is:
   a. anti-Lu^a
   b. anti-S
   c. anti-Jk^b
   d. anti-M

3. Which phenotype is associated with a resistance to malarial invasion?
   a. Fy(a−b−)
   b. Jk(a−b−)
   c. Le(a−b−)
   d. Lu(a−b−)

4. Enzyme-treated reagent red blood cells used in antibody identification enhances all of the following antibodies EXCEPT:
   a. anti-M
   b. anti-Le^a
   c. anti-Jk^b
   d. anti-C

5. Which of these antibodies are typically IgM?
   a. anti-K
   b. anti-S
   c. anti-U
   d. anti-N
   e. anti-Le^b
   f. anti-Jk^b
   g. anti-P_1

6. Which of the following reagents destroys the Kell system antigens?
   a. ficin
   b. albumin
   c. polyethylene glycol
   d. DTT

7. Glycophorin A and glycophorin B possess antigen sites for which blood group system?
   a. Duffy
   b. Kidd
   c. Lewis
   d. MNS

8. Select the antibody that is characteristically clinically insignificant:
   a. anti-Kp^b
   b. anti-S
   c. anti-Le^b
   d. anti-Fy^a

9. The McLeod phenotype is associated with:
   a. Rh_{null} phenotype
   b. $Kell_{null}$ phenotype
   c. U-negative phenotype
   d. absence of Kx antigens

10. Typing as Lu(a–b–) would be considered:
    a. rare in Whites but not Blacks
    b. rare in Blacks but not Whites
    c. rare in all populations
    d. common in all populations

11. Cold autoantibodies are usually of which specificity?
    a. I
    b. M
    c. P_1
    d. S

12. Individuals with the p phenotype can make:
    a. anti-P_2
    b. anti-p
    c. anti-P
    d. anti-Tj^a

13. Alleles within the Lewis system include:
    a. *Le, le*
    b. Le^a, Le^b
    c. *Le, Se, H*
    d. *Le, Le*

14. Which of the following antibodies requires the antiglobulin test for in vitro detection?
    a. anti-M
    b. anti-P_1
    c. anti-U
    d. anti-I

15. What procedure would help to distinguish between an anti-Fy^a and anti-Jk^a in an antibody mixture?
    a. lowering the pH of the patient's serum
    b. using a thiol reagent
    c. running an antibody identification panel
    d. running a ficin-treated panel

16. Anti-K1:
    a. agglutinates in indirect antiglobulin tests
    b. is usually of the IgM antibody class
    c. does not agglutinate with K+k+ panel cells
    d. loses reactivity in enzyme phases

17. Which of the following antigens is poorly expressed on cord blood cells?
    a. K1
    b. M
    c. Le^b
    d. D

18. Reagent antibody screening cells may not detect antibodies directed against low-incidence antigens. Which antibody is most likely to go undetected?
    a. Vel
    b. S
    c. Kp^a
    d. K

19. Select the disease commonly associated with the McLeod phenotype:
    a. infectious mononucleosis
    b. chronic granulomatous disease
    c. Hodgkin's disease
    d. paroxysmal cold hemoglobinuria

20. Which set of antibodies could you possibly find in a patient with no history of transfusion or pregnancy?
    a. anti-I, anti-S, and anti-P
    b. anti-M, anti-c, and anti-B
    c. anti-A, anti-I, and anti-D
    d. anti-B, anti-I, and anti-Le^a

REFERENCES

1. Lublin DM: Functional roles of blood group antigens. In Silberstein LE, editor: *Molecular and functional aspects of blood group antigens,* Bethesda, Md, 1995, American Association of Blood Banks.
2. Coombs RR, Mourant AE, Race RR: In vivo isosensitization of red cells in babies with hemolytic disease, *Lancet* 1:264, 1946.
3. Reid ME, Lomas-Francis C: *The blood group antigen facts book,* San Diego, 1997, Academic Press.
4. Levine P, Backer M, Wigod M, et al: A new human hereditary blood property (Cellano) present in 99.8% of all bloods, *Science* 109:464, 1949.
5. Allen FH, Lewis SJ: Kp^a (Penney), a new antigen in the Kell blood group system, *Vox Sang* 2:81, 1957.
6. Allen FH, Lewis SJ, Fudenberg HH: Studies of anti-Kp^b, a new alloantibody in the Kell blood group system, *Vox Sang* 3:1, 1958.
7. Gibett ER: Js, a "new" blood group system antigen found in Negroes, *Nature* 181:1221, 1958.
8. Walker RH, Argall CI, Steane EA, et al: Anti-Js^b, the expected antithetical antibody of the Sutter blood group system, *Nature* 197:295, 1963.
9. Marsh WL, Redman CM: The Kell blood group system: a review, *Transfusion* 30:158, 1990.
10. Parsons SF, Judson PA, Anstee DJ: Monoclonal antibodies against Kell glycoprotein: serology, immunochemistry, and quantitation of antigen sites, *Trans Med* 3:137, 1993.
11. Lee S, Zambas ED, Marsh WL, Redman CM: Molecular cloning and primary structure of Kell blood group protein, *Proc Natl Acad Sci USA* 88:6353, 1991.

12. Chown F, Lewis M, Kaita H: A new Kell blood group phenotype, *Nature* 180:711, 1957.
13. Issitt PD, Antsee DJ: *Applied blood group serology*, ed 4, Durham, NC, 1998, Montgomery Scientific Publications.
14. Cutbush M, Mollison PL, Parker DM: A new human blood group, *Nature* 165:188, 1950.
15. Ikin EW, Mourant AE, Pettenkoffer JH, et al: Discovery of the expected haemagglutinin, anti-Fyb, *Nature* 168:1077, 1951.
16. Sanger R, Race RR, Jack J: The Duffy blood groups of New York Negroes: the phenotype Fy(a−b−), *Br J Haematol* 1:370, 1955.
17. Albrey JA, Vincent EE, Hutchinson J, et al: A new antibody, anti-Fy3, in the Duffy blood group system, *Vox Sang* 20:29, 1971.
18. Moore S, Woodrow CF, McClelland DB: Isolation of membrane components associated with human red cell antigens Rh(D), (c), (E) and Fy, *Nature* 295:529, 1982.
19. Horuk R, Chitnis CE, Darbonne WC, et al: A receptor for the malarial parasite *Plasmodium vivax:* the erythrocyte chemokine receptor, *Science* 261:1182, 1993.
20. Donahue RP, Bias WB, Renwick JH, McKusick VA: Probable assignment of the Duffy blood group locus to chromosome 1 in man, *Proc Natl Acad Sci USA* 61:949, 1968.
21. Miller LH, Mason SJ, Dvorak JA, et al: Erythrocyte receptors for (*Plasmodium knowlesi*) malaria: Duffy blood group determinants, *Science* 189:561, 1975.
22. Allen FH, Diamond LK, Niedziela B: A new blood group antigen, *Nature* 167:482, 1951.
23. Plaut G, Ikin EW, Mourant AE, et al: A new blood group antibody, anti-Jk^b, *Nature* 171:431, 1953.
24. Pinkerton FJ, Mermod LE, Liles BA, et al: The phenotype Jk(a–b–) in the Kidd blood group system, *Vox Sang* 4:155,1959.
25. Heaton DC, McLoughlin K: Jk(a–b–) red blood cells resist urea lysis, *Transfusion* 28:197, 1982.
26. Olivès B, Mattei MG, Huet M, et al: Kidd blood group and urea transport function of human erythrocytes are carried by the same protein, *J Biol Chem* 270:15607, 1995.
27. Zelinski T, Kaita H, Coghlan G, Philipps S: Assignment of the Auberger red cell antigen polymorphism to the Lutheran blood group system: genetic justification, *Vox Sang* 61:275, 1991.
28. Parsons SF, Mallinson G, Holmes CH, et al: The Lutheran blood group glycoprotein, another member of the immunoglobulin superfamily, is widely expressed in human tissues and is developmentally regulated in human liver, *Proc Natl Acad Sci USA* 92:5496, 1995.
29. Harmening DM: *Modern blood banking and transfusion practices*, ed 3, Philadelphia, 1994, FA Davis.
30. Vengelen-Tyler V: *Technical manual*, ed 12, Bethesda, Md, 1996, American Association of Blood Banks.
31. Waheed A, Kennedy MS, Gerhan S: Transfusion significance of Lewis system antibodies: report on a nationwide survey, *Transfusion* 21:542, 1981.
32. Graham HA, Williams AN: A genetic model for the inheritance of the P, P1, and Pk antigens [Abstract], *Transfusion* 18:638, 1978.
33. Anstall HB, Blaylock RC: The P blood group system: biochemistry, genetics and clinical significance. In Moulds JM, Woods LL, editors: *Blood groups: P, I, Sda and Pr*, Arlington, Va, 1991, American Association of Blood Banks.
34. Mollison PL, Engelfriet CP, Contreras M: *Blood transfusion in clinical medicine*, ed 9, Oxford, 1993, Blackwell Scientific Publications.
35. Anstall HB, Urie PM: Transfusion therapy in special clinical situations. In Anstall HB, Urie PM: *A manual of hemotherapy*, New York, 1986, John Wiley & Sons.
36. Stroup M, Treacy M: *Blood group antigens and antibodies*, Raritan, NJ, 1982, Ortho Diagnostics.
37. Issitt P: *Applied blood group serology*, ed 3, Miami, 1985, Montgomery Scientific Publications.
38. Holliman SM: The MN blood group system: distribution, serology and genetics. In Unger PJ, Laird-Fryer B, editors: *Blood group systems: MN and Gerbich*, Arlington, Va, 1989, American Association of Blood Banks.

SUGGESTED READING

Harmening DM: *Modern blood banking and transfusion practices*, ed 4, Philadelphia, 1999, FA Davis.

ESSENTIALS OF PRETRANSFUSION TESTING

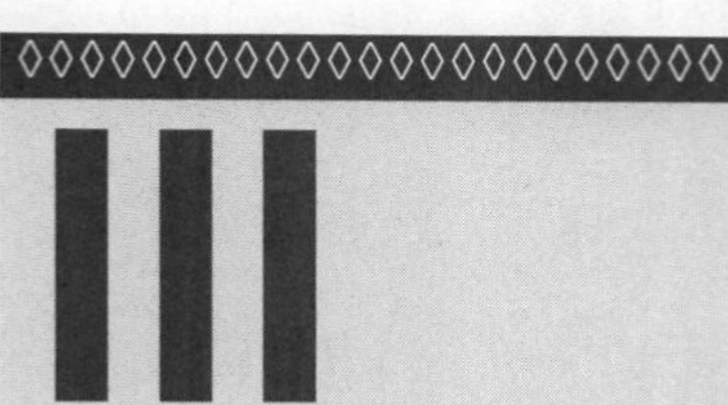

7 ANTIBODY DETECTION AND IDENTIFICATION

Kathy D. Blaney

CHAPTER OUTLINE

LEARNING OBJECTIVES

Upon completion of this chapter, the reader should be able to:

1. Define *atypical* or *unexpected antibodies* and explain how they are formed.
2. Discuss the purpose of the antibody screen and how positive results contribute to the identification process.
3. Compare and contrast the autocontrol and direct antiglobulin test.
4. Explain why patient information regarding transfusion or pregnancy history, age, race, and diagnosis helps in the process of antibody identification.
5. Describe the reagent red blood cell panel and antigram with regard to antigen configuration and ABO type.
6. Define *phase of reactions* and its significance.
7. Discuss how the reaction strength contributes to antibody resolution.
8. Describe the process of ruling out antibodies on a panel.
9. Explain the "rule of three" with regard to antibody identification.
10. List methods that may be used when working with a multiple- or high-frequency antibody or antibodies.
11. Describe the properties of a high-titer, low-avidity antibody and techniques for identifying or avoiding reactivity.
12. Explain the importance of a control when performing antibody neutralization.
13. Discuss the use of and the potential problems with the prewarm procedure.
14. List methods of enhancing weak IgG antibodies.
15. Explain the process of identifying the specificity of a cold autoantibody and techniques to avoid cold autoantibody reactivity.
16. Describe the process and limitations of adsorption techniques as they apply to warm and cold autoantibodies.
17. Define the *elution procedure* and list methods and purposes of this test.

The detection of an "atypical" or "unexpected" antibody in the screen of a patient or donor initiates the identification process that can seem like detective work. The terms *atypical* and *unexpected* refer to antibodies other than ABO antibodies. These antibodies can be made in response to a transfusion of red blood cells or exposure to fetal cells during pregnancy or delivery. Since these antibodies are directed to a nonself antigen, they are called alloantibodies. Autoantibodies are antibodies, usually formed by a disease process or medication, made to a person's own red blood cells. Determining the specificity of antibodies, or antibody identification, necessitates the knowledge of blood group antigen and antibody characteristics outlined in previous chapters and an understanding of the reagents used to enhance or eliminate reactions. Clues are often subtle and elusive, and the process must be methodical and accurate. Except for a simple antibody of one specificity, each sample is often unique and may necessitate several different approaches to reach a conclusive identification. Proficiency and confidence in antibody resolution come from experience and an understanding of basic theoretical concepts involved in the process. This chapter outlines the theory behind problem-solving techniques.

ANTIBODY DETECTION

Antibody Screen

The antibody screen determines whether an antibody to a red blood cell antigen has been made. Antibody screens are performed to detect antibodies in:

- Patients requiring transfusion
- Those who are pregnant
- Patients with suspected transfusion reactions
- Blood and plasma donors

The antibody screen involves incubating the patient's serum or plasma with screening cells and performing an indirect antiglobulin test (IAT) for the detection of IgG antibodies. Antibody screening cells are reagent red blood cells that provide a combination of antigens other than A and B antigens. These cells are tested with the patient's serum to determine whether an unexpected antibody exists. Fig. 7-1 is an example of an antigram for a two-cell screen. An antigram lists the antigens present in the reagent red blood cell suspension. A reaction to one or both of the screen cells demonstrates the presence of an atypical antibody. Some workers prefer the three-cell screen because it provides an *rr* cell and homozygous cells for the Duffy and Kidd blood groups. Most common, clinically significant antibodies react with a two- or three-cell screen. Initial conclusions regarding the type of antibody can often be made when the screen is complete. A summary of typical screen results with the tentative interpretations is listed in Fig. 7-2. Careful attention to the antibody screen results can save time when proceeding to the panel. The screen provides the initial clues that begin the antibody identification process.

Autocontrol

An autocontrol tests the patient's serum with his or her own red blood cells and includes the potentiator used in the antibody screen. It is usually incubated with the screen and read at immediate spin, after the 37° C incubation and IAT. The direct antiglobulin test (DAT) is performed on the patient's cells without serum

	Rh							MNSs				P_1	Lewis		Lutheran		Kell		Duffy		Kidd					
Cell	D	C	E	c	e	f	C^w	M	N	S	s	P_1	Le^a	Le^b	Lu^a	Lu^b	K	k	Fy^a	Fy^b	Jk^a	Jk^b				
I R1R1 (56)	+	+	0	0	+	0	0	+	+	0	+	0	+	0	0	+	+	+	+	0	+	+				
II R2R2 (89)	+	0	+	+	0	0	0	0	+	+	0	+	0	+	0	+	0	+	0	+	+	0				

Fig. 7-1 Screening cell antigram. +, Antigen present; *0,* antigen absent.

and potentiator or an incubation step. The differences and uses for both tests are explained later in this chapter. Testing an autocontrol routinely with the screen is optional; most workers prefer to perform a DAT only if the screen is positive.[1] The autocontrol and DAT provide useful information in determining whether the patient's antibody is directed against his or her red blood cells or to transfused cells.

Potentiators

Potentiators are commonly used in both antibody screening and identification to increase the speed and sensitivity of the antibody attachment to the red blood cell antigen. Chapter 1 explained the theory of each type of enhancement medium—low-ionic strength solution (LISS), bovine serum albumin (BSA), polyethylene glycol (PEG), and proteolytic enzymes. Each has its limitations and advantages that are explained in this section. Selection of potentiators and laboratory methods for antibody detection and identification is usually based on the patient population, workload, and degree of expertise in the laboratory.

The potentiator most commonly used with the screen is LISS, because it speeds the agglutination, is economical, and provides good sensitivity. Several disadvantages of LISS testing are noted here. Increasing serum in the test alters the ionic strength of a LISS procedure, thus decreasing the sensitivity of the test system. LISS also has been reported by many individuals to enhance cold autoantibodies, especially if the tubes are centrifuged at "immediate spin" and microscopic evaluations are performed.

BSA is another potentiator used in antibody detection and identification. BSA works well in enhancing the Rh-system antibodies, although increased incubation time is needed for optimal results. It does not enhance warm autoantibodies, which is beneficial in working with samples from patients with autoantibodies in their serum.

PEG increases the sensitivity of detection and identification and often detects the presence of antibodies not found with BSA or LISS. Antibodies generally considered to be of no clinical significance (IgM in nature) do not react well or at all with this potentiator. PEG has been observed to enhance warm autoantibodies, which is an important limitation of this potentiator.

Proteolytic enzymes (ficin or papain) are not usually used as potentiators in the screen, since they eliminate some antigens from the red blood cells. Enzymes can be used as additional tools for investigating complex antibody problems, but they should never be the sole methodology. Enzymes may enhance the reactions of one antibody in a mixture of antibodies or abolish the reactions, which lends important information in the solution of the problem. Enzymes enhance cold as well as warm autoantibodies. The use of enzymes is discussed in further detail later in this chapter.

Result — **Tentative interpretation**

1.

Antibody screen

Cell	IS	37° C	AHG	CC
I	0	0	0	✓
II	0	0	2+	NT

Direct antiglobulin test

Poly		IgG	C3
0	✓	NT	NT

Tentative interpretation:

1. Alloantibody
2. IgG
3. Single specificity

2.

Antibody screen

Cell	IS	37° C	AHG	CC
I	0	0	3+	NT
II	0	2+	3+	NT

Direct antiglobulin test

Poly		IgG	C3
0	✓	NT	NT

Tentative interpretation:

1. Alloantibody
2. IgG
3. Multiple specificities

3.

Antibody screen

Cell	IS	37° C	AHG	CC
I	1+	0	0	✓
II	2+	0	0	✓

Direct antiglobulin test

Poly		IgG	C3
0	✓	NT	NT

Tentative interpretation:

1. Alloantibody
2. IgM specificity
3. Single specificity showing dosage

4.

Antibody screen

Cell	IS	37° C	AHG	CC
I	1+	0	0	✓
II	1+	0	0	✓

Direct antiglobulin test

Poly	IgG		C3
2+	0	✓	1+

Tentative interpretation:

1. Autoantibody
2. IgM specificity
3. Cold autoantibody

5.

Antibody screen

Cell	IS	37° C	AHG	CC
I	0	0	2+	NT
II	0	0	2+	NT

Direct antiglobulin test

Poly	IgG	C3
2+	2+	0

Tentative interpretation:

1. Autoantibody/transfusion reaction
2. IgG
3. Warm autoantibody with possible underlying alloantibodies

Fig. 7-2 Screen interpretations. *IS*, Immediate spin; *37° C*, 37° C incubation; *AHG*, antiglobulin test; *CC*, check cells; *0*, no agglutination or hemolysis; ✓, check cells agglutinate; *NT*, not tested; *Poly*, polyspecific antiglobulin reagent; *C3*, anti-complement reagent.

Table 7-1 Comparison of Potentiators

POTENTIATOR	USE	LIMITATION
Low–ionic strength solution	Is sensitive, economical, and quick	Enhances cold autoantibodies; some weak anti-K antibodies may be missed
Bovine serum albumin	Does not enhance warm autoantibodies	Needs longer incubation; not sensitive for most antibodies except in the Rh system
Polyethylene glycol	Shows increased sensitivity	Enhances warm autoantibodies
Enzymes	Eliminate reactivity of Fy^a, Fy^b, S, M, and N antigens	Enhances cold and warm autoantibodies; should not be used as the only method

The uses and limitations of LISS, BSA, PEG, and enzymes in the screen and identification procedures are summarized in Table 7-1. Appreciating the differences and limitations of the potentiators helps the technologist select the most appropriate one for the antibody involved. The use of gel or column technology and solid phase microwell plates are alternative methods used in transfusion services and reference laboratories for screening and identification. These alternative methodologies are described in Chapter 2.

Patient History

Before beginning antibody identification procedures, it is essential to obtain a complete transfusion and pregnancy history. Transfusions within the last 3 months present the possibility of a mixed red blood cell population and recent antibody stimulation. The patient may not be aware of red blood cell antibodies, and this information may not have been transferred if he or she moved to a different hospital. Communicating with previous medical facilities where the patient may have been transfused is often helpful.

The diagnosis, race, and age of the patient should also be noted, since they offer additional clues to the nature of the antibody problem. Some diseases are associated with the development of certain antibodies. For example, a patient with lupus or carcinoma is frequently associated with a warm autoantibody, whereas pneumonia may result in a cold autoimmune process. Autoantibodies are rarely encountered in patients less than 50 years old and in blood donors. Some antibodies are associated only with certain races because of the frequency of antigens in certain populations.

ANTIBODY IDENTIFICATION

Initial Panel

Testing the serum or plasma against a panel of reagent red blood cells usually follows the detection of the antibody in the screen. A panel, like the screening cells, consists of group O reagent red blood cells that have been typed for most common antigen specificities. Manufacturers prepare panels with a variety of antigen configurations, which range from 10, 11, 15, 16, or 20 cells that can be thought of as extended antibody screens. Panels are usually initially tested using the same potentiators used in the screen. The use of an autocontrol with the panel is recommended, especially if it is not routinely tested with the screen. Some variation

BOX 7-1

Key to Reactions and Abbreviations

Key to Reactions	
0	No agglutination or hemolysis
+w	Tiny agglutinates; cloudy background
1+	Small agglutinates; cloudy background
2+	Medium agglutinates; clear background
3+	Several large agglutinates; clear background
4+	One solid agglutinate
H	Hemolysis
✓	Check cells agglutinate
NT	Not tested

Key to Abbreviations	
IS	Immediate spin
RT	Room temperature
IAT	Indirect antiglobulin test
AHG	Antihuman globulin
DAT	Direct antiglobulin test
Poly	Polyspecific antiglobulin reagent
CC	Check cells
LISS	Low–ionic strength solution
PEG	Polyethylene glycol
37	37° C incubation

exists between transfusion services and reference laboratories on antibody identification procedures. This chapter attempts to follow the most widely accepted procedures and provide brief discussions regarding alternate methods.

The panel "map" or antigram is unique to each panel lot number and is used to record and interpret the results. It is important to grade reactions consistently while following specific laboratory guidelines; procedure manuals often represent this as the "key." This allows more accurate interpretation and the ability of another technologist to review or perform additional testing. The key used for the antibody problems presented in this chapter is shown in Box 7-1.

Once results are recorded for each phase and negative reactions can be confirmed with check cells, the panel can be interpreted. The interpretation guidelines in Table 7-2 outline important concepts in evaluating panel results. These guidelines can be used in the following examples of antibody problems.

Panel Interpretation: Single Antibody Specificity

An interpretation of a single antibody is outlined in Panels 7-1 and 7-2.

Autocontrol

The autocontrol determines whether an alloantibody or autoantibody specificity exists. If the autocontrol is positive and the DAT is negative, the potentiator may be causing false positive results. In that case the panel should be repeated using a different type of potentiator or no enhancement solution. Usually a positive autocontrol or positive DAT indicates an autoantibody or an antibody produced against recently transfused red blood cells. Autoantibodies are of the cold or warm type, depending on the optimal reaction temperature; they are discussed in greater detail later in this chapter. Panel 7-1 has a negative autocontrol, which indicates an alloantibody exists only in the serum and not on the patient's red blood cells.

Phases

The phase or reaction temperature where agglutination appears is an indication that the antibody is IgG or IgM. IgM antibodies typically react at room temperature or on immediate spin. IgM antibodies such as anti-Le^a, -Le^b, -M, -N, -I, and -P_1 should be suspected if immediate spin reactions are detected. IgG antibodies

Panel 7-1 Panel: Single Antibody Specificity

	Rh							MNSs				P_1	Lewis		Lutheran		Kell		Duffy		Kidd		LISS			
Cell	**D**	**C**	**E**	**c**	**e**	**f**	**C^w**	**M**	**N**	**S**	**s**	**P_1**	**Le^a**	**Le^b**	**Lu^a**	**Lu^b**	**K**	**k**	**Fy^a**	**Fy^b**	**Jk^a**	**Jk^b**	**IS**	**37**	**AHG**	**CC**
1 R1R1 (51)	+	+	0	0	+	0	0	+	+	+	0	+	0	+	0	+	+	+	0	+	+	0	0	0	2+	
2 R1R1 (32)	+	+	0	0	+	0	+	+	0	0	+	+	0	+	0	+	0	+	0	+	+	+	0	0	0	✓
3 R2R2 (64)	+	0	+	+	0	0	0	0	+	0	+	+	+	0	0	+	+	+	0	0	+	+	0	0	2+	
4 r'r (75)	0	+	0	+	+	+	0	+	0	+	+	+	0	+	0	+	0	+	+	0	+	+	0	0	0	✓
5 r"r (87)	0	0	+	+	+	+	0	+	+	+	+	+	0	+	0	+	0	+	+	0	+	0	0	0	0	✓
6 rr (98)	0	0	0	+	+	+	0	+	+	+	+	+	+	0	0	+	0	+	+	0	+	+	0	0	0	✓
7 rr (76)	0	0	0	+	+	+	0	+	0	+	0	0	0	+	0	+	+	0	+	+	0	+	0	0	3+	
8 rr (53)	0	0	0	+	+	+	0	+	0	+	+	+	0	0	0	+	0	+	0	+	0	+	0	0	0	✓
9 rr (23)	0	0	0	+	+	+	0	+	+	+	+	0	+	0	0	+	0	+	+	+	+	0	0	0	0	✓
10 R1R1 (34)	+	+	0	0	+	0	+	0	+	+	0	+	0	+	0	+	0	+	0	+	+	0	0	0	0	✓
Patient cells																							0	0	0	✓

+, Antigen present; *0*, antigen absent.

Table 7-2 Guidelines for the Interpretation of a Panel

LOOK AT	RESULT	INTERPRETATION
Autocontrol	Negative	◆ Alloantibody
	Positive	◆ Autoantibody, or ◆ Delayed transfusion reaction; transfused cells are sensitized with antibody
Phases	Room temperature or immediate spin	◆ Cold or IgM antibody
	37° C reactions	◆ May be cold (IgM) if reactions started at room temperature, or ◆ May be warm (IgG) if reactions are not seen at room temperature but noticed at AHG
	AHG	◆ Warm or IgG antibody; clinically significant
Reaction strength	Single strength	◆ Probably one antibody specificity
	Varying strengths	◆ More than one antibody or one antibody showing dosage
Ruling out	Negative reactions	◆ If no reaction was observed, the antibody to the antigen on the panel was probably not present ◆ If the antigen on the panel is heterozygous, the antibody may be showing dosage; rule out carefully
	Positive reactions	◆ NEVER rule out positive reactions
Matching the pattern	Single antibody	◆ If the specificity is a single antibody, the pattern matches one of the antigen columns
	Multiple antibodies	◆ When more than one antibody is present, it is difficult to match a pattern unless the phases or reaction strengths are unique
Rule of three	Three positives	◆ Is the suspected antibody reactive with at least three panel cells that are antigen positive?
	Three negatives	◆ Is the suspected antibody negative with at least three panel cells that do not posses the antigen?
Phenotype the patient	Negative	◆ If the patient does not possess the antigen, it is possible to make the antibody
	Positive	◆ Transfused red blood cells are present if patient received a unit of red blood cells within 120 days ◆ Suspected antibody is incorrect

AHG, Antihuman globulin.

Panel 7-2 Ruling Out and Determining a Specificity

	Rh							MNSs				P_1	Lewis		Lutheran		Kell		Duffy		Kidd		LISS			
Cell	D	C	E	c	e	f	C^w	M	N	S	s	P_1	Le^a	Le^b	Lu^a	Lu^b	K	k	Fy^a	Fy^b	Jk^a	Jk^b	IS	37	AHG	CC
1 R1R1 (51)	+	+	0	0	+	0	0	+	+	+	0	+	0	+	0	+	+	+	0	+	+	0	0	0	2+	
2 R1R1 (32)	+	+	0	0	+	0	+	+	0	0	+	+	0	+	0	+	0	+	0	+	+	+	0	0	0	✓
3 R2R2 (64)	+	0	+	+	0	0	0	0	+	0	+	+	+	0	0	+	+	+	0	0	+	+	0	0	2+	
4 r'r (75)	0	+	0	+	+	+	0	+	0	+	+	+	0	+	0	+	0	+	+	0	+	+	0	0	0	✓
5 r"r (87)	0	0	+	+	+	+	0	+	+	+	+	+	0	+	0	+	0	+	+	0	+	0	0	0	0	✓
6 rr (98)	0	0	0	+	+	+	0	+	+	+	+	+	+	0	0	+	0	+	+	0	+	+	0	0	0	✓
7 rr (76)	0	0	0	+	+	+	0	+	0	+	0	0	0	+	0	+	+	0	+	+	0	+	0	0	3+	
8 rr (53)	0	0	0	+	+	+	0	+	0	+	+	+	0	0	0	+	0	+	0	+	0	+	0	0	0	✓
9 rr (23)	0	0	0	+	+	+	0	+	+	+	+	0	+	0	0	+	0	+	+	+	+	0	0	0	0	✓
10 R1R1 (34)	+	+	0	0	+	0	+	0	+	+	0	+	0	+	0	+	0	+	0	+	+	0	0	0	0	✓
Patient cells																							0	0	0	✓

+, Antigen present; *0,* antigen absent.

Interpretation: Anti-K. Cell 7 is homozygous for the K[1] gene. The reaction is stronger (showing dosage) with this panel cell as compared with cells 1 and 3.

react at the antiglobulin phase. Reactions at different phases may indicate more than one antibody and a combination of IgG and IgM antibodies. The example in Panel 7-1 illustrates an IgG antibody.

Reaction Strength

The strength of the reaction is a clue to the number of antibodies present. Reactions of varying strengths suggest more than one antibody. In this panel, all reactions are fairly strong and of similar strength. Antibodies such as anti-K, -D, -E, -e, -c, and -C are commonly stronger than anti-Fy^a, -Fy^b, -Jk^a, -Jk^b, -S, and -s. The strength of the reaction also varies with the antigen "dosage." If a panel cell is homozygous, a stronger reaction may be noticed. In some cases weak antibodies may not even react with heterozygous antigen expression.

Ruling Out

Rule out: to eliminate the possibility that an antibody exists in the serum based on its nonreactivity with a particular antigen.

Panel cells that give negative reactions (0) with all tested phases can be used to **rule out** antibodies. This process is illustrated in Panel 7-2. Begin with the first negative panel cell reaction, which is cell 2. Looking across the panel, place a line through the antigen specificity that is positive (+) on the panel. If an antigen-antibody reaction did not occur, the antibody did not react with the antigen on the panel cell and it can be eliminated as a possible antibody. Panel cells that are heterozygous should *not* be crossed out because the antibody may have been too weak to react. Continue ruling out using each negative cell. The process of ruling out has narrowed the antibody possibilities down to anti-K and anti-Lu^a.

Matching the Pattern

The next step in panel interpretation is to look at the reactions that are positive and match the pattern. When a single antibody is present, the pattern of reactions observed matches one of the antigen columns. In this example agglutination was observed with cells 1, 3, and 7, and the antigen K is present on these cells. Therefore the antibody identity is anti-K. The other potential antibody specificity is not ruled out; Lu^a is a low-frequency antigen (less than 5% of the population). Since the antigens are rare in the population, the probability of producing an antibody to them is uncommon. For this reason they can be ruled out without further testing.

Rule of Three

(*p*) value: probability value; value that provides a confidence limit for a particular event.

Rule of three: confirming the presence of an antibody by demonstrating three cells that are positive and three that are negative.

Identifying antibodies involves performing tests and making a conclusion based on reaction patterns. To make a scientific conclusion these reactions must be statistically greater than those in a random event. The **(*p*) value,** or probability value, must be .05 or less for identification to be considered valid.[2] To obtain this probability, at least three antigen-positive red blood cells that react and three antigen-negative red blood cells that do not react should be observed. In this example three antigen-positive cells and seven antigen-negative cells were observed. Therefore the **"rule of three"** has been met. If there were not enough cells in this panel to determine sufficient probability, additional cells from another panel would be selected for testing.

Phenotype the Patient

Individuals do not make alloantibodies to antigens they possess (self-antigens). Another way to confirm antibody identification is to test the patient's red blood cells to ensure they are negative for the antigen corresponding to the identified antibody. Testing red blood cells should be performed only if no recent transfusions have taken place. Red blood cells from transfused donor units may remain in the circulation for as long as 3 months and may cause misleading and incorrect results if different cell populations are present. Phenotyping a patient who was recently transfused would necessitate **cell separation** techniques to separate transfused and autologous red blood cells.

Cell separation: technique used to separate transfused cells from autologous or patient cells.

Multiple Antibodies

When patients have more than one antibody, additional techniques are needed to resolve the problem. Panels 7-3, 7-4, and 7-5 illustrate an approach to multiple antibody identification.

Following the guidelines outlined in Table 7-2, it can be determined that:

- The autocontrol is negative; an alloantibody should be suspected
- Reactions only at the AHG phase suggest an IgG antibody
- The reaction strength is variable, which suggests more than one antibody
- Anti-E and anti-Fy[a] cannot be ruled out after crossing out
- Matching the pattern is more difficult when more than one antibody specificity exists
- Under the rule of three, two E-positive cells were reactive, and four E-negative cells were nonreactive; six Fy[a]-positive cells reacted, and four Fy[a]-negative cells

Panel 7-3 Panel: Multiple Antibodies

	Rh							MNSs				P_1	Lewis		Lutheran		Kell		Duffy		Kidd		LISS			
Cell	**D**	**C**	**E**	**c**	**e**	**f**	**C^w**	**M**	**N**	**S**	**s**	**P_1**	**Le^a**	**Le^b**	**Lu^a**	**Lu^b**	**K**	**k**	**Fy^a**	**Fy^b**	**Jk^a**	**Jk^b**	**IS**	**37**	**AHG**	**CC**
1 R1R1 (51)	+	+	0	0	+	0	0	+	+	+	0	+	0	+	0	+	+	+	0	+	+	0	0	0	0	✓
2 R1R1 (32)	+	+	0	0	+	0	+	+	0	0	+	+	0	+	0	+	0	+	0	+	+	+	0	0	0	✓
3 R2R2 (64)	+	0	+	+	0	0	0	0	+	0	+	+	+	0	0	+	+	+	0	0	+	+	0	0	3+	
4 r'r (75)	0	+	0	+	+	+	0	+	0	+	+	+	0	+	0	+	0	+	+	0	+	+	0	0	0	✓
5 r"r (87)	0	0	+	+	+	+	0	+	+	+	+	+	0	+	0	+	0	+	+	0	+	0	0	0	2+	
6 rr (98)	0	0	0	+	+	+	0	+	+	+	+	+	+	0	0	+	0	+	+	0	+	+	0	0	2+	
7 rr (76)	0	0	0	+	+	+	0	+	0	+	0	0	0	+	0	+	+	0	+	+	0	+	0	0	2+	
8 rr (53)	0	0	0	+	+	+	0	+	0	+	+	+	0	0	0	+	0	+	0	+	0	+	0	0	0	✓
9 rr (23)	0	0	0	+	+	+	0	+	+	+	+	0	+	0	0	+	0	+	+	+	+	0	0	0	2+	
10 R1R1 (34)	+	+	0	0	+	0	+	0	+	+	0	+	0	+	0	+	0	+	0	+	+	0	0	0	0	✓
Patient cells			0																0				0	0	0	✓

+, Antigen present; *0*, antigen absent.
Interpretation: Anti-Fy[a] and anti-E.

Panel 7-4 Selected Cell Panel

	Rh							MNSs				P_1	Lewis		Lutheran		Kell		Duffy		Kidd		LISS		
Cell	**D**	**C**	**E**	**c**	**e**	**f**	**C^w**	**M**	**N**	**S**	**s**	**P_1**	**Le^a**	**Le^b**	**Lu^a**	**Lu^b**	**K**	**k**	**Fy^a**	**Fy^b**	**Jk^a**	**Jk^b**	**IS**	**37**	**AHG**
1 r'r (22)	0	+	0	+	+	0	0	+	+	+	0	+	0	+	0	+	+	+	0	+	+	0			
2 R1R1 (72)	+	+	0	0	+	0	+	+	0	0	+	+	0	+	0	+	0	+	0	+	+	+			
3 R2R2 (45)	+	0	+	+	0	0	0	0	+	0	+	+	+	0	0	+	+	+	0	0	+	+	0	0	3+
4 r"r (28)	0	0	+	+	+	+	0	+	0	+	+	+	0	+	0	+	0	+	+	0	+	+			
5 rr (88)	0	0	0	+	+	+	0	+	+	+	+	+	0	+	0	+	0	+	0	0	+	0			
6 rr (38)	0	0	0	+	+	+	0	+	+	+	+	+	+	0	0	+	0	+	+	0	+	+			
7 rr (74)	0	0	0	+	+	+	0	+	0	+	0	0	0	+	0	+	+	0	+	+	0	+			
8 rr (21)	0	0	0	+	+	+	0	+	0	+	+	+	0	0	0	+	0	+	0	+	0	+			
9 rr (67)	0	0	0	+	+	+	0	+	+	+	+	0	+	0	0	+	0	+	+	+	+	0			
10 R2R2 (92)	+	0	+	+	0	0	0	0	+	+	0	+	0	+	0	+	0	+	0	+	+	0	0	0	3+

+, Antigen present; *0*, antigen absent.
Interpretation: Selected cells for determining that an anti-E was present in the serum along with the anti-Fy[a].

Panel 7-5 Ficin-Treated Panel

	Rh							MNSs				P_1	Lewis		Lutheran		Kell		Duffy		Kidd		LISS			Ficin	
Cell	**D**	**C**	**E**	**c**	**e**	**f**	**C^w**	**M**	**N**	**S**	**s**	**P_1**	**Le^a**	**Le^b**	**Lu^a**	**Lu^b**	**K**	**k**	**Fy^a**	**Fy^b**	**Jk^a**	**Jk^b**	**37**	**AHG**	**CC**	**AHG**	**CC**
1 R1R1 (51)	+	+	0	0	+	0	0	+	+	+	0	+	0	+	0	+	+	+	0	+	+	0	0	0	✓	0	✓
2 R1R1 (32)	+	+	0	0	+	0	+	+	0	0	+	+	0	+	0	+	0	+	0	+	+	+	0	0	✓	0	✓
3 R2R2 (64)	+	0	+	+	0	0	0	0	+	0	+	+	+	0	0	+	+	+	0	0	+	+	0	3+		3+	
4 r'r (75)	0	+	0	+	+	+	0	+	0	+	+	+	0	+	0	+	0	+	+	0	+	+	0	2+		0	✓
5 rr (87)	0	0	+	+	+	+	0	+	+	+	+	+	0	+	0	+	0	+	+	0	+	0	0	2+		3+	
6 rr (98)	0	0	0	+	+	+	0	+	+	+	+	+	+	0	0	+	0	+	+	0	+	+	0	2+		0	✓
7 rr (76)	0	0	0	+	+	+	0	+	0	+	0	0	0	+	0	+	+	0	+	+	0	+	0	2+		0	✓
8 rr (53)	0	0	0	+	+	+	0	+	0	+	+	+	0	0	0	+	0	+	0	+	0	+	0	0	✓	0	✓
9 rr (23)	0	0	0	+	+	+	0	+	+	+	+	0	+	0	0	+	0	+	+	+	+	0	0	2+		0	✓
10 R1R1 (34)	+	+	0	0	+	0	+	0	+	+	0	+	0	+	0	+	0	+	0	+	+	0	0	0	✓	0	✓
Patient cells																							0	0	✓	0	✓

+, Antigen present; *0*, antigen absent.
Interpretation: Ficin treatment of panel cells removed the Fy^a antigen. Retesting the ficin-treated cells eliminated the reactions with the anti-Fy^a antibody. The treated panel more clearly shows the anti-E antibody.

were nonreactive; one cell (cell 5) is positive for both E and Fy^a, which cannot be included, and therefore two more E-positive and Fy^a-negative panel cells need to be tested

- The phenotype shows the patient is E negative and Fy^a negative

Multiple Antibody Resolution

Selected cells: cells chosen from another panel to confirm or eliminate the possibility of an antibody.

Selected cells are often used to complete the requirements for the "rule of three" to confirm the antibody specificities that are initially suspected. Cells may be "selected" from other panels without running the entire panel. In this example, Panel 7-4 shows another panel that can be used to select additional E-positive, Fy^a-negative cells. Cells 3 and 10 are E positive and Fy^a negative. If the same panel manufacturer is used to select more cells, it is important to check that the "donor number or code" is not the same as the cell used in the original panel. This number is usually indicated in the first column of the panel. The donor codes for the selected cells used in this example are 45 and 92, which are not the same as the original cells. If the number were the same, it would mean that the same cell is being repeated. It is also important to remember that the screening cells that had been initially tested may provide additional selected cells.

Multiple Antibodies: Additional Techniques

Proteolytic enzymes can be used to eliminate or enhance antibody activity. The Fy^a, Fy^b, S, M, and N antigenic activity is eliminated using enzyme methods. The antibodies to antigens of the Rh, Kidd, and Lewis systems, however, are greatly enhanced using enzymes in the test system. Enzymes act by removing the sialic acid residues from the red blood cell membrane, thus eliminating some antigens while exposing others. Two procedures can be used for enzyme treatment:

One-stage enzyme technique: antibody identification technique that requires the addition of the enzyme to the cell and serum mixture.

Two-stage enzyme technique: treatment of the red blood cells with an enzyme before the addition of the serum.

- **One-stage enzyme technique:** simultaneous incubation of test serum, enzyme (papain), and red blood cells.
- **Two-stage enzyme technique:** panel or screening cells are pretreated with enzymes (ficin or papain), washed, and then used without other enhancement media in the antiglobulin test. Enzyme-treated red blood cells can be prepared before use and are also available commercially.

Following enzyme treatment red blood cells are retested with the serum to determine whether the antibody or mixture of antibodies is still reacting. In the example shown in Panel 7-5, the following conclusions can be made:

- If there is no agglutination following enzyme treatment, it can be concluded that the antibody was specific for one of the antigens removed by enzymes. Panel cells 4, 6, 7, and 9 were not reactive following ficin treatment because the anti-Fy^a reactivity was eliminated.
- Cell 5 could then be used to confirm the anti-E specificity. The Fy^a antigen was eliminated with ficin, and the reaction became stronger following enzyme treatment and retesting because of the anti-E antibody.

When using an enzyme-treated cell, observing agglutination only at the antihuman globulin (AHG) phase is recommended to avoid false positive reactions. Since enzymes denature some antigens, it should not be used as the only antibody detection or identification method.

Antibodies to High-Frequency Antigens

An antibody to high-frequency or high-incidence antigens presents another type of identification challenge. If an antigen occurs in the population at a 98% or higher frequency, it is considered high frequency or high incidence. Typical reaction patterns are illustrated in Panel 7-6. Once again, by using the panel interpretation guidelines (see Table 7-2), several conclusions can be made to give direction for additional testing:

- The autocontrol is negative; an alloantibody should be suspected
- The phases show the reactions are occurring only at the AHG phase, which suggests an IgG antibody
- The reaction strengths are the same, which suggests one specificity
- Since only one negative cell exists on the panel, anti-D, -C, -e, -M, -N, -S, -P_1, -Le^b, -Lu^a, -K, -Fy^b, and -Jk^a can be ruled out, which leaves anti-E, -c, -s, -Le^a, -k, -Fy^a, and -Jk^b as possible antibodies in the sample

Panel 7-6 Antibody to a High-Frequency Antigen

	Rh							MNSs				P_1	Lewis		Lutheran		Kell		Duffy		Kidd		LISS			
Cell	D	C	E	c	e	f	C^w	M	N	S	s	P_1	Le^a	Le^b	Lu^a	Lu^b	K	k	Fy^a	Fy^b	Jk^a	Jk^b	IS	37	AHG	CC
1 R1R1 (51)	+	+	0	0	+	0	0	+	+	+	0	+	0	+	0	+	+	+	0	+	+	0	0	0	3+	
2 R1R1 (32)	+	+	0	0	+	0	+	+	0	0	+	+	0	+	0	+	0	+	0	+	+	+	0	0	3+	
3 R2R2 (64)	+	0	+	+	0	0	0	0	+	0	+	+	+	0	0	+	+	+	0	0	+	+	0	0	3+	
4 r'r (75)	0	0	+	+	+	+	0	+	0	+	+	+	0	+	0	+	0	+	+	0	+	+	0	0	3+	
5 r"r (87)	0	0	+	+	+	+	0	+	+	+	+	+	0	+	0	+	0	+	+	0	+	0	0	0	3+	
6 rr (98)	0	0	0	+	+	+	0	+	+	+	+	+	+	0	0	+	0	+	+	0	+	+	0	0	3+	
7 rr (76)	0	0	0	+	+	+	0	+	0	+	0	0	0	+	0	+	+	0	+	+	0	+	0	0	0	✓
8 rr (53)	0	0	0	+	+	+	0	+	0	+	+	+	0	0	0	+	0	+	0	+	0	+	0	0	3+	
9 rr (23)	0	0	0	+	+	+	0	+	+	+	+	0	+	0	0	+	0	+	+	+	+	0	0	0	3+	
10 R1R1 (34)	+	+	0	0	+	0	+	0	+	+	0	+	0	+	0	+	0	+	0	+	+	0	0	0	3+	
Patient cells																							0	0	0	✓

+, Antigen present; *0*, antigen absent.
Interpretation: Anti-k.

Table 7-3 Clues for Identifying High-Frequency Antibodies

Clue	Antibodies affected
Room-temperature reactions	I, H, P, P_1, PP_1P^k
Negative with ficin-treated cells	Ch, Rg, JMH
Negative with DTT-treated cells	JMH, Yt^a, Js^b, Kp^b, k, LW
Weakened with DTT-treated cells	Lu^b, Do^b, Kn^a
Weak reactions at AHG	Lu^b, Ch, Rg, Cs^a, Kn^a, McC^a, Sl^a, JMH
Negative or weak on cord blood cells	Sd^a, Ch, Rg, Lu^b, I, Vel, Le^a, Le^b
Stronger on cord blood cells	i, LW
Variable expression on red blood cells	Lu^b, Kn^a, Sl^a, I, P_1, Sd^a, Ch, Rg, McC^a, JMH, Vel
Race association: Black	U, Js^b, Sl^a, At^a, Hy, Tc^a, Cr^a
Race association: White	Kp^b, Lan

DTT, Dithiothreitol; *AHG,* antihuman globulin.

- In matching the pattern, the anti-k fits the pattern under the k-antigen column when looking across at the potential specificities; since it was not ruled out, the tentative antibody identification is an anti-k
- Under the rule of three, two additional k-negative cells need to be "selected" from other panels and tested to conclude that an anti-k exists
- In phenotyping the patient, the frequency of the k antigen in the population is less than 1 in 500; if the patient is k negative, the specificity is probably anti-k

Additional Testing

Although the antibody specificity determined in Panel 7-6 is probably an anti-k after testing the two additional k-negative selected cells, the antibodies that were not ruled out still need to be investigated. Additional k-negative selected cells should be tested. Phenotyping the patient cells for the antigens corresponding to the antibodies not ruled out could also be done, since k-negative panel cells are not common.

Eliminating the antigen reactivity by dithiothreitol (DTT) treatment is another approach to working with anti-k.[3] DTT is a reagent that can be used to denature the Kell system antigens on red blood cells. It works by disrupting the tertiary structure of proteins, which makes them unable to bind with the specific antibody. Treating k-positive cells with DTT, followed by retesting, would eliminate the anti-k agglutination. Potential antibodies "underlying" the anti-k could then be investigated.

Additional clues when working with antibodies to high-frequency antigens are summarized in Table 7-3. The potential of multiple antibodies underlying the high-frequency antibody adds to the challenge. Rare reagent cells used to identify an antibody to a high-incidence antigen and rule out underlying antibodies are not commonly found on panels. Samples may need to be referred to an immunohematology reference laboratory, where an inventory of frozen rare red blood cells is available for further testing.

High-Titer, Low-Avidity Antibodies

Some antibodies to high-incidence antigens may have the characteristic "high-titer, low-avidity" (HTLA) reaction pattern. These antibodies are typically weak (low avidity) and can often be diluted out to relatively high titer despite the weak reaction strengths. HTLA antibodies react at the AHG phase, are inconsistent, and are not usually enhanced with other potentiators such as PEG, increased incubation time, or the addition of more serum. They have not been implicated in causing transfusion reactions or hemolytic disease of the newborn (HDN). It is not important to identify the specificity of the HTLA antibody. Clinically significant antibodies may be masked by the HTLA reactions. Box 7-2 and Table 7-4 summarize some characteristics of the different HTLA antibodies and provide techniques for investigation and identification.[4]

BOX 7-2

Characteristics of High-Titer, Low-Avidity Antibodies

- Weak reactions at antiglobulin phase
- Variable reactions among panel cells
- Inconsistent reactions that are sometimes not reproducible
- Reactions may be weaker on older red blood cells
- Nonreactive with autologous cells
- Not usually enhanced with polyethylene glycol, low–ionic strength solution, or enzymes
- Often found with other antibodies
- Not clinically significant

Antibodies to Low-Frequency Antigens

Patients who make antibodies to multiple antigen specificities often make antibodies to antigens of low incidence. Antibodies to low-incidence antigens can also sometimes occur alone and may be suspected when the screen is negative and the crossmatch is positive. A panel with only one reactive cell suggests this type of antibody. Identification of the antibody is limited to the available cells and should never be a reason to delay transfusion. The "special type" column

Table 7-4 Identifying High-Titer, Low-Avidity Antibodies

HTLA ANTIBODY	ENZYMES	INHIBITED WITH PLASMA?	DTT	OTHER CLUES
Ch	0	Yes	+	
Rg	0	Yes	+	
Yk[a]	Variable*	No	+	
Cs[a]	+	No	+	
JMH	0	No	0	Can be an autoantibody; occurs in older patients
Kn[a]	+	No	0	
McC[a]	+	No	0	
Sl[a]	+	No	Weak/0	Antigen is less frequent in the Black population
Hy	+	No	0	
Yt[a]	Variable*	No	0	
Gy[a]	+	No	0	

HTLA, High-titer, low-avidity; *DTT*, dithiothreitol; +, antigen present; *0*, antigen absent.
*Can be enhanced, weakened, or negative.

found on panels can be used to find additional selected cells for identification. An "extended cell profile" is often available from most reagent manufacturers that lists in greater detail the less common specificities found on panel cells. Box 7-3 lists some common low-incidence antigens.

The more common antibodies to low-incidence antigens include anti-C[w], -Wr[a], -V, -Co[b], -Bg[a], -Kp[a], and -Lu[a]. When blood is needed, crossmatching for compatibility through the AHG phase is acceptable. Using reagent antisera to screen red blood cells for transfusion is not necessary and in most cases antisera are not available. If a low-frequency antibody is identified in a pregnant woman, testing the serum against the father's red blood cells can predict the possibility of incompatibility with the fetus (assuming the parents are ABO compatible). Titration studies to determine a rise in titer during pregnancy can then be performed using the father's cells.

BOX 7-3

Low-incidence Antigens

Lu[a]	Kp[a]	V	VS
C[w]	Wr[a]	Bg[a]	Co[b]

Enhancing Weak IgG Antibodies

Weak IgG antibodies are sometimes difficult to identify because the reaction patterns may not fit probable specificities. Repeating the panel with a different enhancement medium, increasing the serum-to-cell ratio, or increasing the incubation time may be necessary. Panel 7-7 illustrates this concept. The antibody (anti-c) reacted only with homozygous cells in the panel tested with LISS. Repeating the panel using PEG enhanced the anti-c reactions significantly. If the serum-to-cell ratio or incubation time is altered to enhance reaction strength, the package inserts for the enhancement media should be reviewed for specific limitations. Reagent red blood cells from different manufacturers may also give variable results because of preservatives and slight differences in the pH of the red blood cell suspension. If this is suspected, washing the panel cells once before use may eliminate the problem. Using panels before the expiration date is important as well, since some antigens deteriorate with storage. Obtaining a fresher sample from the patient may also enhance the antibody activity. Determining the identity of weak reacting antibodies is especially important if a suspected transfusion reaction has occurred and an antibody is beginning to develop.

Panel 7-7 PEG Enhancement

	Rh							MNSs				P_1	Lewis		Lutheran		Kell		Duffy		Kidd		LISS			PEG	
Cell	D	C	E	c	e	f	C^w	M	N	S	s	P_1	Le^a	Le^b	Lu^a	Lu^b	K	k	Fy^a	Fy^b	Jk^a	Jk^b	37	AHG	CC	AHG	CC
1 R1R1 (51)	+	+	0	0	+	0	0	+	+	+	0	+	0	+	0	+	+	+	0	+	+	0	0	0	✓	0	✓
2 R1R1 (32)	+	+	0	0	+	0	+	+	0	0	+	+	0	+	0	+	0	+	0	+	+	+	0	0	✓	0	✓
3 R2R2 (64)	+	0	+	+	0	0	0	0	+	0	+	+	+	0	0	+	+	+	0	0	+	+	0	1+		2+	
4 r'r (75)	0	+	0	+	+	+	0	+	0	+	+	+	0	+	0	+	0	+	+	0	+	+	0	0	✓	2+	
5 r"r (87)	0	0	+	+	+	+	0	+	+	+	+	+	0	+	0	+	0	+	+	0	+	0	0	+w		2+	
6 rr (98)	0	0	0	+	+	+	0	+	+	+	+	+	+	0	0	+	0	+	+	0	+	+	0	+w		2+	
7 rr (76)	0	0	0	+	+	+	0	+	0	+	0	0	0	+	0	+	+	0	+	+	0	+	0	1+		2+	
8 rr (53)	0	0	0	+	+	+	0	+	0	+	+	+	0	0	0	+	0	+	0	+	0	+	0	1+		2+	
9 rr (23)	0	0	0	+	+	+	0	+	+	+	+	0	+	0	0	+	0	+	+	+	+	0	0	1+		2+	
10 R1R1 (34)	+	+	0	0	+	0	+	0	+	+	0	+	0	+	0	+	0	+	0	+	+	0	0	0	✓	0	✓
Patient cells																							0	0	✓	0	✓

+, Antigen present; *0,* antigen absent; *PEG,* polyethylene glycol.
Interpretation: Anti-c, which may have been misidentified without PEG enhancement.

Panel 7-8 Cold-Reacting Alloantibody

	Rh							MNSs				P_1	Lewis		Lutheran		Kell		Duffy		Kidd		LISS			
Cell	D	C	E	c	e	f	C^w	M	N	S	s	P_1	Le^a	Le^b	Lu^a	Lu^b	K	k	Fy^a	Fy^b	Jk^a	Jk^b	IS	37	AHG	CC
1 R1R1 (51)	+	+	0	0	+	0	0	+	+	+	0	+	0	+	0	+	+	+	0	+	+	0	2+	1+	+w	
2 R1R1 (32)	+	+	0	0	+	0	+	+	0	0	+	+	0	+	0	+	0	+	0	+	+	+	2+	1+	+w	
3 R2R2 (64)	+	0	+	+	0	0	0	0	+	0	+	+	+	0	0	+	+	+	0	0	+	+	0	0	0	✓
4 r'r (75)	0	+	0	+	+	+	0	+	0	+	+	+	0	+	0	+	0	+	+	0	+	+	2+	1+	+w	
5 r"r (87)	0	0	+	+	+	+	0	+	+	+	+	+	0	+	0	+	0	+	+	0	+	0	1+	1+	+w	
6 rr (98)	0	0	0	+	+	+	0	+	+	+	+	+	+	0	0	+	0	+	+	0	+	+	0	0	0	✓
7 rr (76)	0	0	0	+	+	+	0	+	0	+	0	0	0	+	0	+	+	0	+	+	0	+	2+	1+	+w	
8 rr (53)	0	0	0	+	+	+	0	+	0	+	+	+	0	0	0	+	0	+	0	+	0	+	0	0	0	✓
9 rr (23)	0	0	0	+	+	+	0	+	+	+	+	0	+	0	0	+	0	+	+	+	+	0	0	0	0	✓
10 R1R1 (34)	+	+	0	0	+	0	+	0	+	+	0	+	0	+	0	+	0	+	0	+	+	0	1+	1+	+w	
Patient cells																							0	0	0	✓

+, Antigen present; *0,* antigen absent.
Interpretation: anti-Le^b.

Cold Alloantibodies

"Cold" or IgM antibodies typically react at immediate spin, room temperature, and sometimes 37° C phases. These antibodies are usually clinically insignificant, since they do not cause red blood cell destruction if antigen-positive red blood cells are transfused. When the crossmatch is performed, the antibody activity often has to be avoided to find serologically compatible blood.

The specificities of the antibodies are anti-P_1, -M, -N, -Le^a, and -Le^b. The antibody is usually identified by noting reactions at immediate spin that may not carry through to the AHG phase, although 37° C reactions are sometimes seen. Panel 7-8 is an example of a "typical" anti-Le^b identification panel. Antibodies to P_1, M, and N sometimes do not react with all antigen-positive cells, since variability often exists in antigen strength. Anti-M and anti-N demonstrate dosage. Anti-P_1 reactions vary greatly with the age of the cells used and may not always react with all P_1-positive panel cells. To enhance weak reactions or reactions not fitting the expected pattern, incubation at or below room temperature is recommended. Techniques to avoid the reactivity are used to identify underlying anti-

BOX 7-4 ***Prewarm Technique***

1. Incubate serum and one drop of cells to be tested (panel, screen, or crossmatch) separately at 37° C for 10 minutes.
2. Add serum to cells and incubate for a minimum of 30 minutes. Polyethylene glycol, also warmed to 37° C, may be added to increase sensitivity.
3. Wash three times with saline warmed to 37° C.
4. Add IgG antihuman globulin. Centrifuge and read.
5. Add check cells to negative reactions.

Table 7-5 Neutralization of Anti-Le^b

	Control	Neutralization	
Selected Cells	Serum + Saline	Serum + Le Substance	
1 Le(a−b+)	1+	0	✓
2 Le(a−b+)	1+	0	✓
3 Le(a−b+)	1+	0	✓

1+, Small agglutinates, clear background; *0*, no agglutination or hemolysis, ✓, check cells agglutinate.
Interpretation: Serum was neutralized; no underlying antibodies exist. The control indicates that the addition of the Le substance did not dilute the serum, causing the antibody to be undetected.

bodies and perform a crossmatch. Neutralization or inhibition, enzymes, and prewarming techniques are useful procedures for working with these antibodies. It is important when performing a neutralization procedure that controls are tested. The control indicates that the negative reactions after neutralization are due to the elimination of antibody reactivity and not simply dilution. These techniques are outlined in Table 7-5 and Box 7-4.[5]

AUTOANTIBODIES

The first section of this chapter explained the detection and identification process involving alloantibodies. As previously discussed, the initial investigation of an antibody includes a DAT or autocontrol which, if positive, may be caused by a cold autoantibody, warm autoantibody, or delayed transfusion reaction. This section reviews the process of differentiating an alloantibody and autoantibody, determining the most probable specificity, and avoiding autoantibody interference. Serologic techniques to remove the autoantibody from the serum by adsorption are briefly discussed, and readers are referred to the suggested reading list for a more detailed discussion of advanced techniques. (Adsorption, in the sense used in this chapter, involves the attachment of antibody to red blood cell antigens and the subsequent removal from the serum.) A discussion regarding the clinical manifestations and transfusion support for these patients is covered in Chapter 14.

The first clue to an autoantibody is a positive DAT or autocontrol with serum antibodies that are reactive with most or all cells tested. The causes for a positive DAT are summarized in Table 7-6. The patient diagnosis and medication history are important to obtain, since this information helps to determine the classification and direction of an autoantibody investigation. Performing a DAT on a clotted specimen may result in a false positive complement reaction with anti-C3 and polyspecific AHG reagent.[6] Samples collected in EDTA anticoagulant are preferred for performing a DAT to avoid unnecessary testing.

This section discusses the recognition of cold and warm autoantibodies and provides techniques in avoiding their reactivity and determining clinically insignificant underlying alloantibodies.

Cold Autoantibodies

Example number 4 in Fig. 7-2 illustrates the initial screen and DAT for a "typical" cold autoantibody problem. Panel 7-9 further illustrates the nonspecificity of the reactions, phase, and fairly consistent reaction strengths. Complement-coated

Table 7-6 Interpreting a Positive Direct Antiglobulin Test

ASSOCIATED WITH	SPECIFICITY	SERUM ANTIBODY
Transfusion reaction	IgG	Specific alloantibody
Warm autoimmune disease	IgG (C3)	Reacts with all cells at antihuman globulin phase
Cold autoimmune disease; pneumonia	C3	Reacts with all cells at colder temperatures
Drug interaction	IgG	Serum may be nonreactive
Clot tube stored at 4° C	C3	None
Hemolytic disease of the newborn; maternal antibodies on baby's red blood cells	IgG	Alloantibody or ABO antibody from mother on baby's cells

Panel 7-9 Cold Autoantibody

	Rh							MNSs				P_1	Lewis		Lutheran		Kell		Duffy		Kidd		LISS			
Cell	**D**	**C**	**E**	**c**	**e**	**f**	**C^w**	**M**	**N**	**S**	**s**	**P_1**	**Le^a**	**Le^b**	**Lu^a**	**Lu^b**	**K**	**k**	**Fy^a**	**Fy^b**	**Jk^a**	**Jk^b**	**IS**	**37**	**AHG**	**CC**
1 R1R1 (51)	+	+	0	0	+	0	0	+	+	+	0	+	0	+	0	+	+	+	0	+	+	0	2+	1+	+w	
2 R1R1 (32)	+	+	0	0	+	0	+	+	0	0	+	+	0	+	0	+	0	+	0	+	+	+	2+	1+	1+	
3 R2R2 (64)	+	0	+	+	0	0	0	0	+	0	+	+	+	0	0	+	+	+	0	0	+	+	2+	1+	+w	
4 r'r (75)	0	+	+	+	+	+	0	+	0	+	+	+	0	+	0	+	0	+	+	0	+	+	2+	1+	+w	
5 r"r (87)	0	0	+	+	+	+	0	+	+	+	+	+	0	+	0	+	0	+	+	0	+	0	1+	1+	+w	
6 rr (98)	0	0	0	+	+	+	0	+	+	+	+	+	+	0	0	+	0	+	+	0	+	+	1+	1+	+w	
7 rr (76)	0	0	0	+	+	+	0	+	0	+	0	0	0	+	0	+	+	0	+	+	0	+	2+	1+	+w	
8 rr (53)	0	0	0	+	+	+	0	+	0	+	+	+	0	0	0	+	0	+	0	+	0	+	2+	1+	+w	
9 rr (23)	0	0	0	+	+	+	0	+	+	+	+	0	+	0	0	+	0	+	+	+	+	0	2+	1+	1+	
10 R1R1 (34)	+	+	0	0	+	0	+	0	+	+	0	+	0	+	0	+	0	+	0	+	+	0	1+	1+	+w	
Patient cells																							2+	1+	1+	

+, Antigen present; *0*, antigen absent.

patient red blood cells and panel cells that react at room temperature are the most significant clues in recognizing a cold autoantibody. A DAT performed with monospecific anti-C3 detects complement attachment. An ABO discrepancy caused by cold autoantibodies in the serum may also be detected in patients who are not group O. Patients may have a history of mild anemia, *Mycoplasma pneumoniae* infection, or infectious mononucleosis. Hemolytic cold antibodies found in cold agglutinin syndrome may necessitate transfusion support. A wide range of degree in serologic manifestations of cold autoantibodies exists, which contributes to the difficulty in problem resolution. Determining the specificity of the cold autoantibody is helpful to ascertain that additional techniques are reliable. Locating red blood cells that are negative for the antigen corresponding to the cold antibody is not necessary.

Specificity

A "cold panel" is a set of selected cells that aids in the identification of a suspected cold autoantibody (Fig. 7-3). The most common cold autoantibody specificities are anti-I, -H, and -IH. The I antigen is not well developed at birth. Therefore cord blood cells (I negative) can be used to determine the specificity. Hospitals with neonatal units usually have access to group O cord samples, which can be used

A

	SC I	SC II	AC	Cord	Cord	A_1	A_2
4° C	3+	3+	3+	0	0	NT	NT

B

	SC I	SC II	AC	Cord	Cord	A_1	A_2
4° C	3+	3+	3+	1+	1+	1+	2+

Fig. 7-3 Mini-cold panel. ***A,*** Typical cold autoanti-I in a group "O" individual. Cord cells are negative (no I antigen). A cells were not tested, since the serum of a type "O" individual has anti-A. ***B,*** Typical cold autoanti-IH in a group "A" individual. Cord cells are weakly positive because of the presence of H antigen. A cells are positive, although weaker than the "O" screening cells. Group O cells have more H antigen than A cells.

for this purpose. Some manufacturers also have these available. Autoanti-H and anti-IH are more commonly found in the serum of Group A_1 and A_1B individuals, since their red blood cells have the least amount of H antigen.

Avoiding Cold Autoantibody Reactivity

Once it has been determined that the cold autoantibody is of I, IH, or H specificity, serologic techniques that avoid the reactivity of the anti-I and determine the presence of an underlying alloantibody should be selected (summarized in Table 7-7). The following section outlines the reasons for this approach:

- The use of IgG antiglobulin reagent rather than polyspecific reagent may help eliminate the cold autoantibody reactions at the AHG phase, since this reagent does not detect the attachment of complement. Many laboratories routinely use this reagent for this reason.[7]
- By skipping the immediate spin or room temperature reaction phases, the attachment of weak cold autoantibodies can be avoided. Some laboratories do this routinely to avoid detection of cold autoantibodies in testing.
- Using 22% albumin as an enhancement instead of LISS avoids some cold autoantibodies that are enhanced by LISS. If albumin is used, an extended incubation is suggested.
- If the procedures listed above still do not eliminate a cold autoantibody that is carrying through to the AHG phase, the prewarm technique may be necessary. Box 7-4 outlines this technique. Warming the serum and cell suspension to 37° C in separate tubes avoids the antibody attachments that occur at or below room temperature.[8] This technique should be used with care, since it may lessen the strength of clinically significant alloantibodies that may be masked by the cold autoantibody.[9] Washing with warm saline and not using an enhancement can lessen the sensitivity of the antiglobulin test.

Adsorption Techniques

If the cold autoantibody still persists after implementing the above techniques, the cold antibody needs to be adsorbed from the serum. If the patient has not been transfused in the last 3 months, an **autoadsorption** can be performed. If the patient has been transfused, the use of **allogeneic** red blood cells or **rabbit stroma** for adsorption is necessary. Table 7-8 compares the adsorption

Table 7-7 Cold Autoantibodies

Problem	Technique
Avoiding cold antibodies	1. Use anti-IgG instead of polyspecific antihuman globulin 2. Eliminate the immediate spin screen
After a cold antibody has been identified	1. Repeat testing without low–ionic strength solution or enzymes 2. Perform a prewarm technique 3. Perform adsorption techniques

Anti-IgG, Anti–immune globulin G.

Autoadsorption: attachment of the patient's antibodies to the patient's own red blood cells and subsequent removal from the serum.
Allogeneic: blood or tissue from the same species that is not genetically identical.
Rabbit stroma: red blood cell membranes from rabbits used for adsorption of I antigen.

Table 7-8 Adsorption Techniques

ADSORPTION TECHNIQUE	DESCRIPTION	LIMITATION
Rabbit erythrocyte stroma	Removes cold autoantibodies with I or IH specificity	May adsorb anti-B
Cold autoadsorption	Patient red blood cells are used to remove cold autoantibodies to determine if alloantibodies are present	Do not use if recently transfused
Warm autoadsorption	Patient red blood cells are used to remove warm autoantibodies to determine if alloantibodies are present	Do not use if recently transfused
Differential (allogeneic) adsorption	Uses known phenotyped red blood cells to separate specificities: warm autoantibodies from alloantibodies or several separate alloantibody specificities	May adsorb a high-frequency alloantibody

techniques. Once the cold autoantibody is adsorbed, the adsorbed serum is retested with a panel to determine whether underlying alloantibodies exist in the serum.[10]

Warm Autoantibodies

Warm autoantibodies are more common than cold autoantibodies. As with cold autoantibodies the clinical significance and serologic manifestations can vary greatly. Warm autoimmune hemolytic anemia (WAIHA) can be idiopathic with no underlying disease process or it may be a result of a pathologic disorder or medications used to treat various diseases. The patient diagnosis, medication history, and transfusion history are important in determining whether a warm autoantibody has been detected and what the best approach is to resolving the problem.

The initial antibody screen and DAT results commonly found in a patient with a warm autoantibody are found in example number 5 of Fig. 7-2. A typical panel may react as shown in Panel 7-10. Panel cells are usually all reactive with the patient's serum, crossmatches, and screening cells. The patient's cells are usually coated with IgG antibodies. Complement can also sometimes be detected. The typical initial serologic and clinical description of a warm autoantibody is outlined in Table 7-9. Since warm autoantibodies react best with LISS, PEG, and enzymes, retesting with 22% albumin as an enhancement often eliminates the reactivity.

The goal in testing a sample with a suspected warm autoantibody is to determine whether an underlying alloantibody exists. Although laboratories may have various resources to perform autoantibody workups, understanding the theory of the procedures is important. This section describes some of the procedures used when working with a warm autoantibody.

Specificity

The specificity of a warm autoantibody is sometimes directed to the Rh system, especially to the e antigen. When this occurs, the patient serum appears to be anti-e, although the patient's red blood cells are e-positive and have a positive DAT. In the case of an autoantibody with anti-e specificity, testing e-negative panel cells

Panel 7-10 Warm Autoantibody

	Rh							MNSs				P_1	Lewis		Lutheran		Kell		Duffy		Kidd		LISS			
Cell	D	C	E	c	e	f	C^w	M	N	S	s	P_1	Le^a	Le^b	Lu^a	Lu^b	K	k	Fy^a	Fy^b	Jk^a	Jk^b	IS	37	AHG	CC
1 R1R1 (51)	+	+	0	0	+	0	0	+	+	+	0	+	0	+	0	+	+	+	0	+	+	0	0	0	3+	
2 R1R1 (32)	+	+	0	0	+	0	+	+	0	0	+	+	0	+	0	+	0	+	0	+	+	+	0	0	3+	
3 R2R2 (64)	+	0	+	+	0	0	0	0	+	0	+	+	+	0	0	+	+	+	0	0	+	+	0	0	3+	
4 r'r (75)	0	+	0	+	+	+	0	+	0	+	+	+	0	+	0	+	0	+	+	0	+	+	0	0	3+	
5 r"r (87)	0	0	+	+	+	+	0	+	+	+	+	+	0	+	0	+	0	+	+	0	+	0	0	0	3+	
6 rr (98)	0	0	0	+	+	+	0	+	+	+	+	+	+	0	0	+	0	+	+	0	+	+	0	0	3+	
7 rr (76)	0	0	0	+	+	+	0	+	0	+	0	0	0	+	0	+	+	0	+	+	0	+	0	0	3+	
8 rr (53)	0	0	0	+	+	+	0	+	0	+	+	+	0	0	0	+	0	+	0	+	0	+	0	0	3+	
9 rr (23)	0	0	0	+	+	+	0	+	+	+	+	0	+	0	0	+	0	+	+	+	+	0	0	0	3+	
10 R1R1 (34)	+	+	0	0	+	0	+	0	+	+	0	+	0	+	0	+	0	+	0	+	+	0	0	0	3+	
Patient cells																							0	0	3+	

+, Antigen present; *0*, antigen absent.

Interpretation: an autoantibody is typically reactive at the AHG phase with all panel cells and the autocontrol. A similar reaction strength is usually observed with panel cells, screen cells, and crossmatches.

can be performed to determine whether an underlying specificity exists. Crossmatching e-negative units provides serologically compatible blood. If chronic hemolysis exists, providing e-negative blood may increase the red blood cell survival.[10]

Elution

IgG antibody complexes on red blood cells can be dissociated and placed into a solution to test the specificity. This process is called an elution, and the recovered antibody is an **eluate.** Various elution methods are listed in Table 7-10. Acid elutions are the most commonly used because of their availability in a commercially prepared kit and reliability in antibody recovery. The acid elution reduces the pH, which results in antibody disassociation from the red blood cell membrane. Organic solvents denature antigens by dissolving the red blood cell bilipid layer.[11] Heat produces conformational changes to red blood cells and antibody molecules. The freeze-thaw elution method lyses red blood cells to disrupt antigen-antibody bonds. The freeze-thaw and heat elution should be used only when testing for ABO antibodies on red blood cells, since their sensitivity is limited. In summary, elution methods work by disturbing the antigen and antibody bond, allowing the antibody to be removed from the red blood cell membrane.[11]

Once the eluate is prepared, it is tested against panel cells in a method similar to serum testing to determine the specificity. The eluate is usually reactive with all panel cells tested when working with a warm autoantibody. This observation helps to confirm the presence of a warm autoantibody.

When the DAT is positive because of IgG attached to the red blood cell, an elution should be performed. Eluates prepared from patients who have been recently transfused and are experiencing a delayed hemolytic reaction usually demonstrate the antibody causing the reaction. An eluate prepared from a newborn's red blood cells that have a positive DAT demonstrates an antibody that was passed to the baby by the mother during pregnancy. Identification of this antibody is important if HDN is suspected. Testing the eluate against a panel of red blood cells therefore helps determine the antibody specificity causing a positive DAT.

Eluate: antibody recovered in a solution for further testing by an antibody identification technique.

Table 7-9 "Typical" Warm Autoantibody Characteristics

TESTS	RESULTS
Screen and panel	All screen cells, panel cells, and crossmatches reactive at antihuman globulin phase, unless the autoantibody is specific for a medication
DAT	Positive because of IgG; C3 also may be positive
Eluate	Usually reactive with all cells tested, unless the autoantibody is specific for medications
Hb/Hct	Low Hb/Hct, usually requiring transfusion support, may be chronic or acute
Compatibility test	Determine if there is an underlying alloantibody before transfusion

DAT, Direct antiglobulin test; *Hb/Hct,* hemoglobin/hematocrit.

Table 7-10 Elution Methods

METHOD	ANTIBODY REMOVAL	BENEFITS	LIMITATIONS
Glycine acid	Lower pH	Rapid and sensitive; commercially available	
Ether Methylene chloride Chloroform	Organic solvent	Sensitive; inexpensive	Hazardous, carcinogenic, or flammable
Heat Freeze-thaw	Physical	Rapid; effective for ABO antibodies; inexpensive	Not sensitive for antibodies other than ABO

Nonreactive eluates may also be associated with warm autoantibodies. Antibodies to medications and nonspecific binding of proteins to red blood cell membranes can cause a positive DAT and a negative eluate. Evaluation of patients' medications and clinical symptoms should be considered in determining whether a warm autoantibody exists when the eluate is nonreactive. In addition, patients who show serologic evidence of warm autoimmune disease may not always demonstrate the same reactions in the serum and eluate with each transfusion request.

Adsorption

As discussed in the section describing cold autoantibodies, adsorption procedures may be necessary to remove the warm autoantibody specificity from the serum to determine whether an underlying alloantibody exists. This may be accomplished through an autologous adsorption. Initial pretreatment of the patient's red blood cells with DTT is necessary to remove as many of the in vivo–attached autoantibodies as possible. In addition, treating the red blood cells with enzymes increases the capacity to adsorb more antibodies. After treatment of the red blood cells the patient's serum is combined with his or her red blood cells and incubated for 30 to 60 minutes to remove the nonspecific warm antibody.

The serum is removed from the red blood cells and retested with reagent red blood cells. If the patient has been transfused within the last 3 months, transfused red blood cells may exist in the patient's circulation. An autoadsorption is not appropriate in this circumstance, since the transfused cells may adsorb the alloantibody necessary to identify.

Differential adsorption: adsorption or attachment of antibodies in the serum to specific known antigens, usually to different aliquots of red blood cells.

For patients who have been transfused within the preceding 3 months, a **differential**, or allogeneic, **adsorption** technique should be performed to investigate underlying alloantibodies. An allogeneic adsorption uses known red blood cell types that either match the patient's phenotype or represent a combination of antigens that "selectively remove" certain known antibody specificities. As in the autoadsorption procedure, enzyme pretreatment of red blood cells enhances antibody uptake. Fig. 7-4 outlines the autologous adsorption and differential adsorption procedures. After incubation of the patient serum with the allogeneic red blood cells, the serum is removed and retested against screening or panel cells to determine whether underlying alloantibodies exist.

Crossmatching with adsorbed serum should be performed with discretion. Adsorption techniques may dilute the serum and increase the risk of sample errors because of transference of serum or mislabeling of tubes. Individual laboratory policies must be followed with regard to using adsorbed serum for crossmatching.

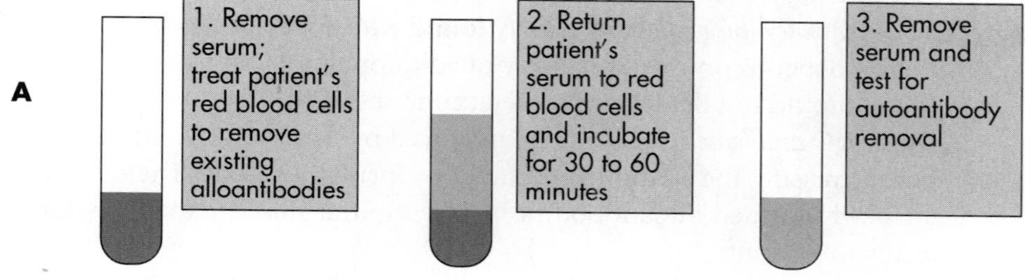

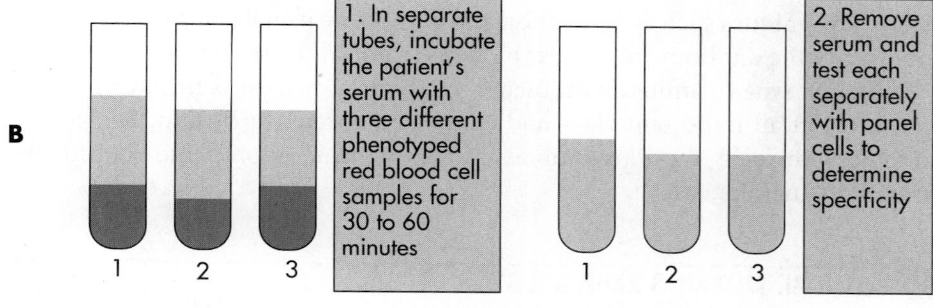

Fig. 7-4 Adsorption procedure outline, showing, *A*, autoadsorption and *B*, differential (allogeneic) adsorption.

Warm autoantibodies represent the more complicated of the antibody identification procedures. Patients with WAIHA may require frequent transfusions, which further complicates the serologic results. Good communication with the physician responsible for the patient must be initiated early to assess alternatives to transfusion and monitor the clinical symptoms associated with immune red blood cell destruction.

CHAPTER SUMMARY

Identification of alloantibodies and resolving complex autoantibody problem is a process that becomes easier and more interesting with experience. Box 7-5, which incorporates an acronym for the words "BLOOD BANK," outlines some of the clues in antibody identification that are helpful in resolving the problems. The use of case studies is a good way to develop and enhance the problem-solving process necessary in becoming proficient in antibody identification. Antibody problems generally fall into the following categories:

1. *Single antibody specificity* has a pattern easily identifiable with a panel following the rules of panel interpretation. Confirmation that the patient or donor is negative for the corresponding antigen helps confirm the specificity.
2. *Multiple antibodies* necessitate the use of carefully selected cells and antibody techniques such as enzymes. Distinguishing multiple specificities necessitates attention to detail and a good understanding of antibody characteristics. Phenotyping the patient's cells is also useful.

BOX 7-5

Rules of Antibody Identification

B Blood typing problem?
L Last transfusion or pregnancy?
O Observe reactions at each phase
O 0.05 probability
D Dosage

B Black or White race?
A Autocontrol
N Negatives for ruling out
K Know your reagents

3. *Antibodies to high-incidence antigens* should be suspected if all panel cells are positive. Identification depends on locating cells that are negative for high-incidence antigens, and determining if underlying antibodies exist.
4. *Low-frequency antibodies* are usually found with other antibodies. Identification depends on the availability of additional cells for testing. Transfusions should not be delayed to determine specificity.
5. *Weak IgG antibodies* often can be enhanced by using a different potentiator, increasing the serum-to-cell ratio, or incubation time. The detection of newly formed alloantibodies in recently transfused patients is especially important.
6. *Cold alloantibodies* are usually clinically insignificant. Avoiding the reactions or using neutralization or prewarm techniques to eliminate agglutination is sometimes necessary.
7. *Autoantibodies* are either of the cold or warm type, and they should be suspected if the autocontrol or DAT is positive. Determining the existence of underlying alloantibodies is important to avoid additional hemolysis. Techniques such as adsorption and elution are usually performed to identify the antibody on the red blood cell and in the serum.

In each type of antibody problem a methodical process is necessary to take into account all important clues and reach an accurate conclusion. Being comfortable with many types of antibody situations is an appreciable goal for the immunohematologist.

◊ CRITICAL THINKING EXERCISES

◆ *EXERCISE 7-1*

A donor sample from a 55-year-old White male demonstrated a positive antibody screen during routine processing testing. Results of testing with an antibody identification panel are shown below. Refer to the panel to answer the following questions:

	Rh							MNSs				P_1	Lewis		Lutheran		Kell		Duffy		Kidd		LISS			
Cell	D	C	E	c	e	f	C^w	M	N	S	s	P_1	Le^a	Le^b	Lu^a	Lu^b	K	k	Fy^a	Fy^b	Jk^a	Jk^b	IS	37	AHG	CC
1 R1R1	+	+	0	0	+	0	0	+	+	+	0	+	0	+	0	+	+	+	0	+	+	0	0	0	1+	
2 R1R1	+	+	0	0	+	0	+	+	0	0	+	+	0	+	0	+	0	+	0	+	+	+	0	0	0	✓
3 R2R2	+	0	+	+	0	0	0	0	+	0	+	+	+	0	0	+	+	+	+	0	+	+	0	0	0	✓
4 r"r	0	0	+	+	+	+	0	+	0	+	+	+	0	+	0	+	0	+	+	0	+	+	0	0	2+	
5 rr	0	0	0	+	+	+	0	+	+	+	+	+	0	+	0	+	0	+	0	0	+	0	0	0	2+	
6 rr	0	0	0	+	+	+	0	+	+	+	+	+	+	0	0	+	0	+	+	0	+	+	0	0	2+	
7 rr	0	0	0	+	+	+	0	+	0	0	0	0	0	+	0	+	+	+	+	+	0	+	0	0	0	✓
8 rr	0	0	0	+	+	+	0	+	0	+	+	+	0	0	0	+	0	+	0	+	0	+	0	0	2+	
9 rr	0	0	0	+	+	+	0	+	+	+	+	0	+	0	0	+	0	+	+	+	+	0	0	0	2+	
10 R1R1	+	+	0	0	+	0	+	0	+	0	+	+	0	+	0	+	0	+	0	+	+	0	0	0	0	✓
Patient cells																							0	0	0	✓

1. At what phase are the reactions occurring?
2. What does the phase of the reaction suggest regarding the immunoglobulin class of antibody?
3. Is this an alloantibody or an autoantibody?
4. What is the most likely antibody specificity?

5. Are there antibodies that cannot be ruled out on this panel?
6. What additional testing should be performed to verify the specificity?
7. What caused the production of this antibody in this donor?
8. Referring to the antigram, which cell(s) is or are homozygous for the Fy^a antigen?
9. Which cell is probably U negative?

◆ *EXERCISE 7-2*

A sample from a 25-year-old obstetric patient was referred to the hospital for antibody identification. One of the antibody screening cells was weakly positive using LISS enhancement. A panel was tested and results are shown below:

	Rh							MNSs				P_1	Lewis		Lutheran		Kell		Duffy		Kidd		LISS			
Cell	D	C	E	c	e	f	C^w	M	N	S	s	P_1	Le^a	Le^b	Lu^a	Lu^b	K	k	Fy^a	Fy^b	Jk^a	Jk^b	IS	37	AHG	CC
1 R1R1	+	+	0	0	+	0	0	+	+	+	0	+	0	+	0	+	+	+	0	+	+	0	1+	0	0	✓
2 R1R1	+	+	0	0	+	0	+	+	0	0	+	+	0	+	0	+	0	+	0	+	+	+	2+	2+	1+	
3 R2R2	+	0	+	+	0	0	0	0	+	0	+	+	+	0	0	+	+	+	0	0	+	+	0	0	0	✓
4 r'r	0	+	0	+	+	+	0	+	0	+	+	+	0	+	0	+	0	+	+	0	+	+	3+	2+	1+	
5 rr	0	0	0	+	+	+	0	+	+	0	+	+	0	+	0	+	0	+	0	0	+	0	1+	0	0	✓
6 rr	0	0	0	+	+	+	0	+	+	+	+	+	+	0	0	+	0	+	+	0	+	+	1+	0	0	✓
7 rr	0	0	0	+	+	+	0	0	+	+	0	0	0	+	0	+	+	0	+	+	0	+	0	0	0	✓
8 rr	0	0	0	+	+	+	0	+	0	+	+	+	0	0	0	+	0	+	0	+	0	+	3+	2+	1+	
9 rr	0	0	0	+	+	+	0	+	+	+	+	0	+	0	0	+	0	+	+	+	+	0	1+	0	0	✓
10 R1R1	+	+	0	0	+	0	+	0	+	+	0	+	0	+	0	+	0	+	0	+	+	0	0	0	0	✓
Patient cells																							0	0	0	✓

1. At what phase are the reactions the strongest?
2. What does the phase suggest about the immunoglobulin class of this antibody?
3. Is this an alloantibody or an autoantibody?
4. Could this antibody cross the placenta?
5. What is the most likely identity of the demonstrating antibody?
6. If the panel cells were treated with enzymes and retesting followed, what would be the expected reactions?
7. Is this antibody usually clinically significant? Define *clinically significant.*

◆ *EXERCISE 7-3*

A sample from a 65-year-old White male was submitted for a 2-unit crossmatch. He is to be transfused as an outpatient at the cancer clinic. A transfusion history indicated that he received 2 units of red blood cells 4 months ago. Results of the ABO/Rh and antibody screen follow:

Anti-A	Anti-B	Anti-D	A_1 cells	B cells	ABO/Rh interpretation
4+	0	3+	0	3+	A positive

	LISS		
	IS	37° C	AHG
SC I	0	0	2+
SC II	0	0	2+

1. Is it possible to make an initial interpretation regarding the type of antibody present in this patient's serum?
2. What additional testing should be performed?
3. What types of medical history questions are important with this type of patient?

◆ ***Additional Testing***

The laboratory's policy is to perform a DAT only on samples with a positive screen, unless specifically ordered. Results are as follows:

Polyspecific AHG: 3+ Anti-IgG: 3+ Anti-C3: 0

4. Based on the DAT results, what type of antibody problem should be suspected?
5. When a DAT is positive, what procedure can be performed to identify the antibody attached to the red blood cells?

◆ ***Panel Results***

An antibody panel was performed using LISS and observing reactions at all phases. All cells were positive (2+) by the IAT. The autocontrol was 3+. An elution was performed, and the eluate reacted 3+ with all panel cells (the last wash was negative).

6. What is the specificity of the antibody?
7. What additional procedures are necessary before releasing units?
8. Would different procedures be necessary if the patient had been transfused within the last 3 months?

◆ ***EXERCISE 7-4***

A specimen from a 70-year-old White female was submitted for pretransfusion workup for hip surgery in 1 week. Two units of autologous red blood cells were reserved. Since the physician anticipated the need for additional units, routine compatibility testing procedures were performed. The patient had no recent transfusions. Results of the ABO/Rh and antibody screen follow:

Anti-A	Anti-B	Anti-D	A_1 cells	B cells	ABO/Rh interpretation
0	0	3+	4+	4+	O positive

	LISS		
	IS	37° C	AHG
SC I	2+	1+	+w
SC II	2+	2+	+w

1. Based on the antibody screen results, what type of antibody is demonstrated?
2. Is this an alloantibody or an autoantibody?
3. What additional testing should be performed to determine the answer to question 2?

◆ ***Additional Testing***

The DAT results are as follows:

Polyspecific AHG: 1+ Anti-IgG: 0 (check cells 2+) Anti-C3: 1+

4. Do the results of the DAT confirm your suspicions?
5. What additional testing should be performed to confirm the antibody specificity?

◆ *Additional Testing*

A "mini-cold panel" was tested and gave the following results:

	SC I	SC II	CORD 1	CORD 2	AUTO
4° C	3+	3+	0	0	3+

6. What is the probable specificity of the antibody?
7. What procedures could be performed to avoid the reactivity?

STUDY QUESTIONS

1. The antibody screen:
   a. detects most clinically significant antibodies
   b. detects all low-frequency antibodies
   c. helps distinguish between an alloantibody and autoantibody
   d. can be omitted if the patient has no history of antibodies

2. HTLA antibodies:
   a. typically react at room temperature
   b. can be enhanced with PEG
   c. are usually clinically insignificant
   d. are associated with HDN

3. Which of the following statements is associated with anti-I?
   a. it has weaker reactions with stored blood
   b. it can be neutralized with commercially prepared substance
   c. it reacts best at 37°C
   d. it does not react with cord blood cells

4. A multiple antibody problem was resolved using enzymes. One of the antibody reactions was eliminated after treatment. Which of the following antibodies was probably present?
   a. anti-c
   b. anti-I
   c. anti-Jk^a
   d. anti-Fy^a

5. An antibody demonstrating dosage would mean that:
   a. homozygous cells were stronger
   b. heterozygous cells were stronger
   c. cells reacted best with PEG
   d. cells reacted best at 4°C

6. The neutralization technique was performed on a sample containing an anti-Le^b. The control and the Lewis-neutralized serum were both negative when retested with panel cells. How should this test be interpreted?
   a. the anti-Le^b was successfully neutralized and no underlying antibodies were found
   b. the panel cells were not washed sufficiently
   c. the sample was probably diluted
   d. the antibody originally identified was probably not anti-Le^b

7. The rule of three used in antibody identification ensures which (p) value?
   a. .09
   b. .02
   c. .05
   d. .15

8. A DAT performed on a clotted sample stored at 4°C may demonstrate:
   a. in vivo complement attachment
   b. in vivo IgG attachment
   c. in vitro complement attachment
   d. in vitro IgM attachment

9. The prewarm technique may weaken IgG reactions because:
   a. samples are not read at the immediate spin phase
   b. warm saline washes may detach IgG antibodies
   c. the 37°C readings are omitted
   d. polyspecific IgG is not recommended

10. The procedure that removes intact antibodies from the red blood cell membranes is:
    a. autoadsorption
    b. neutralization
    c. enzyme pretreatment
    d. elution

11. The removal of an antibody from serum or plasma using the individual's own cells is:
    a. autoadsorption
    b. differential adsorption
    c. neutralization
    d. elution

12. An antibody was detected in the screen at 37°C and did not react at the AHG phase. Which of the following should be suspected?
    a. anti-S
    b. anti-E
    c. anti-N
    d. anti-Jk^a

13. Antigen typing on red blood cells should not be performed if the patient has been transfused within the following:
    a. 30 days
    b. 2 months
    c. 3 months
    d. 6 months

14. DTT is useful in evaluating a sample when which antibody is suspected?
    a. anti-Js^b
    b. anti-Kp^b
    c. anti-k
    d. all of the above

15. The purpose of additional procedures when working up a warm autoantibody is to:
    a. identify the warm autoantibody specificity in the serum
    b. find red blood cells that are compatible with the autoantibody
    c. identify potential underlying alloantibodies
    d. identify the antibodies coating the red blood cell

REFERENCES

1. Judd WJ, Barnes BA, Steiner EA, et al: The evaluation of a positive direct antiglobulin test (autocontrol) in pretransfusion testing revisited, *Transfusion* 26:220, 1986.
2. Vengelen-Tyler V, editor: *Technical manual,* ed 12, Bethesda, Md, 1996, American Association of Blood Banks.
3. Branch DR, Muensch HA, Sy Siok Hian S, Petz LD: Disulfide bonds are a requirement for Kell and Cartwright (Yt^a) blood group integrity, *Br J Haematol* 54:573, 1983.
4. Moulds MK: Selection of procedures for problem solving weak reactions in the antiglobulin phase. In Wallace ME, Green TS, editors: *Selection of procedures for problem solving,* Arlington, Va, 1996, American Association of Blood Banks.
5. Judd WJ: *Methods in immunohematology,* ed 2, Durham, NC, 1994, Montgomery Scientific Publications.
6. Petz LD, Branch DR: Serological tests for the diagnosis of immune hemolytic anemia. In McMillan R, editor: *Methods in hematology: immune cytopenias,* New York, 1983, Churchill Livingstone.
7. Pierce SR: Anomalous blood bank results. In Dawson RB, editor: *Troubleshooting the crossmatch,* Washington DC, 1997, American Association of Blood Banks.
8. Mallory D: Controversies in transfusion medicine. Prewarmed tests: pro—why, when, and how—not if, *Transfusion* 35:268, 1995.
9. Judd WJ: Controversies in transfusion medicine. Prewarmed tests: con, *Transfusion* 35:271, 1995.
10. Branch DR: Blood transfusion in autoimmune hemolytic anemia, *Lab Med* 15:402, 1984.
11. Judd WJ: Antibody elution form red cells. In Bell CA, editor: *Seminar on antigen antibody reactions revisited,* Arlington, Va, 1982, American Association of Blood Banks.

8 COMPATIBILITY TESTING

Sarah L. Dopp

CHAPTER OUTLINE

LEARNING OBJECTIVES

Upon completion of this chapter, the reader should be able to:

1. Define *compatibility testing.*
2. Define *crossmatching* and distinguish between the major and minor crossmatch.
3. List the procedures included in the routine compatibility test and explain their purpose.
4. Explain the American Association of Blood Banks' *Standards for Blood Banks and Transfusion Services* as it relates to compatibility testing.
5. Discuss the selection of crossmatch-compatible whole blood, red blood cells, plasma, platelets, and cryoprecipitate for transfusion.
6. Discuss strategies for transfusion when compatible blood cannot be located.
7. Discuss limitations of the crossmatch.
8. Describe how crossmatching is handled in the massive transfusion situation.
9. Discuss the advantages and issues related to the electronic (computer) crossmatch.
10. Explain the performance of the immediate spin crossmatch and antiglobulin crossmatch and when they would be performed.
11. Explain the elements of patient identification and their importance in compatibility testing.
12. Explain the use of a type and screen protocol and a Maximum Surgical Blood Order Schedule.
13. Explain how compatibility testing is carried out for an infant less than 4 months old.
14. Discuss the principles in crossmatching autologous blood.

Compatibility testing is a term that has often been considered synonymous with crossmatching.[1] Currently a broader view of the term is taken, and compatibility testing is understood to include recipient identification, sample collection and handling, and pretransfusion testing required to ensure the greatest compatibility (no adverse reactions from transfused blood) technically possible between the donor unit and the proposed recipient. Compatibility testing thus encompasses these steps:

- Accurate patient identification
- Proper sample collection and handling
- Review of the recipient's past blood bank records
- Careful ABO/Rh determinations and other testing on the donor units
- Careful ABO/Rh determination and antibody screening of the recipient; crossmatch of the recipient's sample with the donor units
- If a recipient is determined to possess a clinically significant antibody, donor units are screened and found negative for the corresponding antigen and crossmatched
- The actual transfusion and careful observation of the recipient's vital signs and posttransfusion hematocrit and hemoglobin levels (or other more precise measures) must be considered the final and most important part of compatibility testing[2]

Crossmatching is routinely performed only with donor products containing red blood cells. Because the antibody screen, ABO and Rh determination, and donor testing are discussed elsewhere in this book, this chapter concentrates on the issues related to crossmatching, a component of compatibility testing.

Compatibility testing: all steps in the identification and testing of a potential transfusion recipient and donor blood before transfusion in an attempt to provide a blood product that survives in vivo and provides its therapeutic effect in the recipient.

DEFINITIONS

The concept of major and minor crossmatching was debated until the mid-1960s, when the minor crossmatch was finally eliminated as a suggested or required test.[3] Though obsolete the terms *major* and *minor* are helpful in understanding the two sides of safe blood transfusion from both the donor side and recipient side. A minor crossmatch involves the mixing of serum or plasma from the donor with red blood cells from the recipient. A major crossmatch involves the mixing of serum or plasma from the recipient with red blood cells from the donor (Fig. 8-1). Hemolysis or agglutination at any phase or step of the process indicates the presence of antibodies interacting with red blood cell antigens and thus a mismatch between donor and recipient (Box 8-1). The term *crossmatch* implies a crossway mixing of donor and recipient blood components. This definition is still retained by general medical dictionaries, although the minor crossmatch is no longer performed.[4] As donor antibody screening became standard and comprehensive in donor centers, the justification for minor crossmatching disappeared. Furthermore, it became more universal to transfuse blood as a packed red blood cell preparation with most of the plasma removed rather than as whole blood containing more than 50% plasma by volume. Even with blood components containing large volumes of plasma (frozen plasma or pooled platelet concentrates), a crossmatch is considered unnecessary if thorough donor testing is first performed. The thought exists that an infusion of antibody-containing plasma from a donor (if an antibody should go undetected) into the large blood volume of the recipient results in sufficient dilution to render the antibody less dangerous in terms of red blood cell destruction. However, an

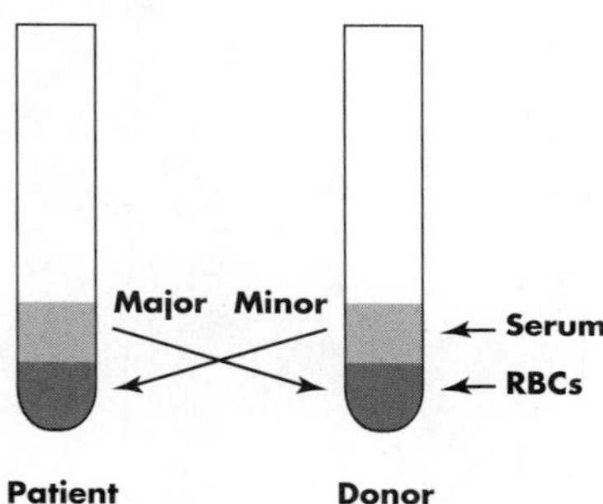

Fig. 8-1 Major versus minor crossmatch. Major: Patient serum crossmatched with donor red blood cells. Minor: Donor serum crossmatched with patient red blood cells. *RBCs*, Red blood cells.

BOX 8-1

Compatible versus Incompatible Crossmatches

Crossmatch Interpretation: COMPATIBLE
No agglutination and no hemolysis present

Crossmatch Interpretation: INCOMPATIBLE
Agglutination or hemolysis present

antibody present in the circulation of the recipient could swiftly lessen red blood cell survival in a donor unit containing the corresponding antigen.

HISTORICAL OVERVIEW OF CROSSMATCHING

The history of blood bank testing and transfusion practices is fascinating, and an interesting progression of events in the compatibility testing area can be observed. The first human venous transfusions became possible once William Harvey discovered the circulation of the blood in 1628. The first in vivo transfusion was attempted with animal blood, and later human blood, using a quill or a metal apparatus introduced into a recipient's vein. Early recipients often died, since no understanding existed of ABO principles (elucidated by Landsteiner in 1900) or of other blood group system alloantibodies. Carrel and Crile performed direct transfusions again in the first decade of this century with some success, despite lack of compatibility testing. Progress from the era of no testing to a century of rapid discoveries led to a proliferation of testing protocols that peaked in the 1960s. A movement existed for the discovery and characterization of every possible blood group antigen and the detection of every corresponding antibody. Over the past several decades, however, the forces of cost containment, practicality, and safety have abbreviated, and ultimately eliminated, many of the previous testing protocols from routine practice. The blood banking community has proposed the elimination of in vitro crossmatching under certain defined circumstances (see the section on the electronic crossmatch later in this chapter).

A crossmatch procedure was first attempted in 1907 in New York by Weil and Ottenberg. Sera of recipient and donor were separately subjected to lengthy room temperature incubation with red blood cells from the opposite sources to detect hemolysins. Major and minor crossmatching were in vogue. Around the time of World War I, Ewing conceived the idea of mixing citrated drops of donor and recipient whole blood on slides and observing them microscopically for agglutination. This method had been recognized as comparable to hemolysis for detection of incompatibilities; it also eliminated the lengthy incubation and cumbersome crossmatching procedure. During World War I group O blood was often transfused as a universal donor in battlefield conditions, since the Rh blood group system was not yet recognized. Since soldiers were usually transfused on an emergency (rather than long-term) basis in acute bleeding or surgical episodes, this practice did not lead to much of a practical problem from anti-D production in the D-negative individuals. A man ahead of his time, a Canadian surgeon in World War I named L. B. Robertson, advocated the use of ABO-identical blood with no crossmatch. He administered small test doses of donor blood and observed for adverse reactions before proceeding with the balance of the transfusion.

Through the 1920s and 1930s various techniques for reading tests and performing major and minor crossmatches were devised using tiles. Debate continued on whether both crossmatch tests were needed. Despite these relatively advanced techniques, some fatal reactions continued to occur because of lack of comprehensive antibody detection or knowledge of Rh and other blood group systems. Around 1939 Riddell began suggesting that only the major crossmatch was needed, but since antibody screening as such did not become routine until the late 1950s to mid-1960s, the concept of minor crossmatching remained for many years. The American Association of Blood Banks (AABB) made the minor crossmatch optional in the 1960s and "unnecessary" in 1976.[5]

Wiener began to suggest the use of tubes instead of slides for testing in the 1940s. Until that time crossmatch methodologies detected only IgM, room temperature antibodies. The discovery of the Rh factor in 1940 acknowledged the importance of IgG antibody detection and introduced enhancement techniques (the addition of bovine albumin and 37° C incubations) and an antiglobulin phase to the crossmatch. At first experts like Grove-Rasmussen recommended the antiglobulin phase crossmatch only if an antibody had already been detected in the screen, but it was later advocated as a universal step of the crossmatch procedure. In 1947 proteolytic enzymes were introduced as a further enhancer of agglutination.

Debate about the role of complement prevailed throughout the decades following World War II. Two aspects were discussed: the presence or absence of complement in the recipient's serum sample, and the need for an anticomplement component to the polyspecific antihuman globulin (AHG) reagent. Advocates for complement believed it was important to detect and identify complement-dependent hemolytic antibodies. Detractors claimed that the presence of complement promoted hemolysis and therefore interfered with the detection of agglutination. They also argued that complement enhanced unwanted nonspecific agglutination, which complicated testing. Stratton stressed the importance of complement in 1965, and the AABB continued to require that complement be active in the test serum. By 1976 Garratty and Petz reported that complement-only antibodies were exceedingly rare.[6] Beck and Marsh bolstered this view, and in 1978 the AABB removed the requirement from its *Standards for Blood Banks and Transfusion Services.*

Other significant historical developments in crossmatching include the following:

- Introduction of potentiators such as polybrene, polyethylene glycol (PEG), and low-ionic strength solution (LISS)
- Movement in the 1980s toward the abbreviated, or immediate spin, crossmatch (immediate spin phase in the absence of antibodies in the current antibody screen or the patient's past record)
- Development in the 1990s of electronic (or computer) crossmatches

Fig. 8-2 summarizes important historical events in crossmatching.

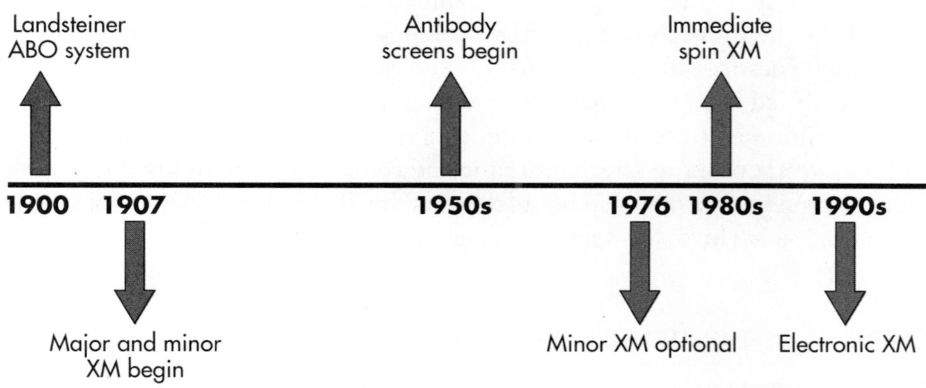

Fig. 8-2 Important events in compatibility testing. *XM,* Crossmatch.

PURPOSES OF CROSSMATCHING

The purposes of crossmatching are to:

- Prevent life-threatening or uncomfortable transfusion reactions
- Maximize in vivo survival of transfused red blood cells

The procedure attempts to fulfill these purposes in the following ways:

- The crossmatch serves as a double check of ABO errors caused by patient misidentification or donor unit mislabeling
- If the recipient possesses a clinically significant antibody or a history of one, the crossmatch provides a second means of antibody detection and checks the results of the antibody screen

A recipient might possess an antibody directed against a low-incidence antigen not contained in the commercial screening cells, and a crossmatch might detect this situation. On the other hand, an antibody detected with screening cells might not react with a weak expression of the antigen on donor cells in a crossmatch. Commercial high-titered antiserum is necessary when selecting compatible donor units. In other words, the antibody screen and the major crossmatch have inherent limitations as separate tests and therefore should be used in tandem.

The crossmatch, designed to detect and eliminate those donor units unlikely to survive normally once transfused, must be kept rapid and simple enough to be practical. Actual measurement of the survival rates of transfused red blood cells may be considered to constitute the best crossmatch. This technique can be performed directly through the use of radioisotope labeling, but this is impractical for regular use. Posttransfusion hematocrit or hemoglobin values are often performed to provide a working measure of successful transfusion. One unit of transfused red blood cells should increase the hematocrit by 3% and the hemoglobin by 1 g/dl.

LIMITATIONS OF TESTING

The performance of acceptable compatibility testing does not guarantee a successful transfusion outcome. Adverse transfusion reactions may still occur. The risks of viral transmission, allergic reactions, and white blood cell reactions are several complications that may be consequences of transfusions. These adverse complications of transfusions are further discussed in Chapter 12.

Compatibility also does not guarantee the optimal survival of red blood cells. Aspects of the patient's clinical course (bleeding, red blood cell sequestration, etc.) may limit the benefit of the transfusion. A delayed transfusion reaction could occur if a preexisting, undetectable recipient antibody is boosted in strength by the infusion of the corresponding antigen in the donor unit and in turn rapidly destroys those donor red blood cells.

Even if red blood cell destruction does not take place, a recipient may become alloimmunized to the donor antigen(s), thus rendering subsequent compatibility workups more time consuming and complicated. Non–life-threatening transfusion reactions may also occur, thus making the transfusion uncomfortable for the recipient (hives, low-grade fever, chills, itching, etc.).

Antibodies can be missed in compatibility testing if:

- The corresponding antigen is absent from screening cells
- The antibody is so weak that it detects only homozygous expressions of the antigen (dosage effect)
- The antibody is detectable only by a method not routinely employed (e.g., in the presence of a particular enhancement medium)
- Past testing history is unknown

OVERVIEW OF THE STEPS IN COMPATIBILITY TESTING

Recipient Blood Sample

Safe and accurate pretransfusion testing begins with the recipient's blood sample, properly collected and labeled with accurate patient identification procedures. Patient samples for compatibility testing may be serum or plasma. Plain tubes with a red top (no anticoagulant), yellow top (acid citrate dextrose, or ACD, formula B), purple top (ethylenediaminetetraacetic acid, or EDTA), or blue top (citrate) are all acceptable sample types. At one time any form of anticoagulated blood sample was discouraged for compatibility testing because of the anticomplementary properties of anticoagulants and the possible presence of fibrin in plasma. Most clinically significant antibodies are now recognized to not depend solely on the presence of complement for their detection. Considerable time can be saved in emergencies in not waiting for a blood specimen to clot, especially when the vast majority of crossmatches are performed on immediate spin where fibrin is less likely to interfere.

Samples should be collected within 3 days (with the date of draw being day 0) of the transfusion if the patient has been transfused or pregnant in the previous 3 months or the history is unclear or unknown.[7] If a reliable history exists of no recent pregnancy or transfusion, or of no current or past unexpected antibodies, the sample may be kept and reused. This allows preoperative testing before a patient's surgical procedure and crossmatching at the time of need. In some settings, where patients are being repeatedly transfused, new samples may be required for these patients (e.g., every other day). This decision must be made after considering the volume of extra work and expense entailed compared with the number of new transfusion-induced antibodies detected.

Serum or plasma hemolyzed during the collection process is not an acceptable specimen and should be recollected. Mechanical hemolysis may be caused by the use of small-gauge needles, trauma to a small vein, the forcing of blood into the tube through a small needle, or the further addition of blood to a partially clotted sample. Mechanical hemolysis can mask the detection of antibody-induced hemolysis (a positive reaction in some examples of ABO, P_1, Lewis, Kidd, or Vel system antibodies). Samples potentially diluted with IV fluids (e.g., Ringer's lactate) are also unacceptable because of the chance of missing a weak antibody or the inducement of false-positive reactions caused by the molecules in the IV fluid. Therefore samples for compatibility should always be collected from below an IV, preferably from a different vein and ideally from the other arm. If the IV site is the only site for drawing blood, the IV should be turned off and flushed with saline, and the first 5 to 10 ml of blood should be discarded.

Minimum labeling requirements are defined in the AABB *Standards*.[7] The patient first must be positively identified by comparing the requisition and sample label to the identification band attached to the patient (not to the wall or the bed). The patient should also state his or her name without prompting from the phlebotomist. A caregiver may identify the patient if the patient is incoherent or a language barrier exists. Commercial banding systems are available whereby a number on the patient's band is also attached to the specimen, request form, and eventual blood product to be transfused. The sample must be labeled at the bedside. To prevent a possible sample mix-up, prelabeled tubes should never be used. The label must include first and last name of recipient, unique identification number, date of collection, and signature, initials, or a method to identify the phlebotomist. The label must also be legible and indelible (Fig. 8-3).

Information on the label must match the request form. This request form must also include the type(s) of blood product being ordered and the requesting physician's name. The request form is, in effect, a prescription. Other useful information on the request form includes the location of the patient, sex, diagnosis, date of the proposed transfusion, and priority indicator (routine, stat, transfuse on date, preoperative, standby, etc.).

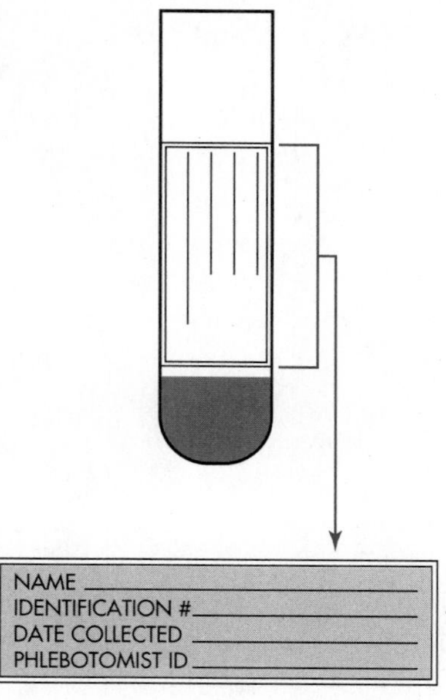

Fig. 8-3 Recipient sample labeling.

Comparison with Previous Records

The AABB *Standards* requires comparison of results of current blood typing with ABO and Rh typing performed over the past 12 months. It also mandates that all previous records be consulted for typing anomalies, presence of clinically significant antibodies, significant transfusion reactions, and special transfusion requirements. Inconsistencies or problems must be investigated and resolved before proceeding with transfusion.

Repeat Testing of Donor Blood

The transfusing facility is responsible for confirming the correct ABO labeling of all donor blood (whole blood or red blood cells) received from the donor center if the units were not previously confirmed. AABB's *Standards* dictates that the ABO phenotype must be retested on all units, and that the Rh typing must be retested on all units labeled "negative." For instance, if an Rh-negative unit were mislabeled "Rh-positive," the unit would be transfused to an Rh-positive person and no clinical harm would result. However, if an Rh-positive unit were mislabeled "Rh-negative," the unit would be selected for an Rh-negative recipient and could effect an immunization to the D antigen in this individual. Testing for the weak-D antigen is not required in repeat testing of donor blood. Retyping is performed by making a red blood cell suspension of the donor blood from a **segment** attached to the donor bag. Records of these repeat tests must be kept for 5 years. Any discrepancy with the typing on the label must result in rejection of the unit and notification to the collecting facility. Plasma and platelet products do not require retyping.

Segment: sealed piece of integral tubing from the donor unit bag that contains a small aliquot of donor blood; used in the preparation of red blood cell suspensions for crossmatching.

Standards and Regulations Governing the Crossmatch

The AABB and the Food and Drug Administration (FDA) are the two principal organizations applying standards to the blood banking and transfusion service communities in the United States. The College of American Pathologists and the Joint Commission on the Accreditation of Healthcare Organizations also inspect blood establishments. The AABB *Standards* provides the most inclusive summary of crossmatch standards. It requires that a crossmatch procedure always be performed using the recipient's serum or plasma and a sample of donor cells taken from a segment originally attached to the blood product bag. The exception is the emergency situation in which blood may be released for transfusion before crossmatch. The crossmatch defined by the AABB *Standards* is a technique that "shall use methods that demonstrate ABO incompatibility and clinically significant antibodies to red (blood) cell antigens and shall include an antiglobulin test."[7] Again, an exception is provided. If no clinically significant antibodies were detected in the current sample or in the patient's past records, an immediate spin crossmatch is permitted to fulfill the requirement of detecting ABO incompatibility. The AABB provision for a computer crossmatch as an alternative to these requirements is presented later in this chapter.

Crossmatching Procedures

Abbreviated or Immediate Spin Crossmatch

The abbreviated or immediate spin crossmatch may be used for recipients with no evidence of clinically significant antibody or antibodies in the current sample and in the historical record. In this procedure recipient serum or plasma and donor cell suspensions are added to a tube, and the tube is immediately centrifuged. This procedure fulfills the AABB standard for detecting ABO incompatibility.

Antiglobulin Crossmatch

In the event that the patient demonstrates a clinically significant antibody in the current antibody screen or has done so in the past, antigen-negative units should be crossmatched by the antiglobulin crossmatch procedure. The antiglobulin crossmatch procedure includes an immediate spin phase, a 37° C incubation, and an antiglobulin phase. Enhancement media used in the antibody screen are usually added to the crossmatch tubes to mirror the conditions in which the antibody was detected.

Autoabsorbed serum may be used for crossmatching to eliminate the reactivity of an autoantibody, which may be masking the alloantibody or alloantibodies. These autoantibodies may be either the cold-reactive type (stronger at room temperature or immediate spin) or the warm-reactive type (stronger at 37°C or in an antiglobulin phase).

Electronic (Computer) Crossmatch

An electronic crossmatch uses a computer to make the final check of ABO compatibility in the selection of appropriate units for transfusion instead of a serologic immediate spin procedure. The same prerequisite pertains to the electronic crossmatch and the immediate spin method, in that the recipient does not possess clinically significant antibody or antibodies in the current or any previous sample. The computer program should provide a flag indicating the recipient's eligibility or ineligibility for electronic crossmatch. The AABB *Standards* contains the required provisions for an acceptable electronic crossmatch.[7] Box 8-2 summarizes criteria for the electronic crossmatch.

Keystroke errors are easy to make when using a computer. Therefore the system must alert the user to nonsense entries or mismatches with hard-coded ABO logic tables and require confirmation points along the way, which forces the user to verify or accept crucial conclusions with an additional entry. The bar coding of blood components and recipient specimens adds another measure of safety.

BOX 8-2 ***Electronic Crossmatch Requirements***

- Computer system validation on site and assurance that ABO incompatibilities are detected; incompatible blood product(s) not released
- Computer validation must be submitted to the Food and Drug Administration
- Two identical ABO interpretations have been made on recipient
- ABO has been performed on a current sample
- The second ABO interpretation may be a retype of same current sample or separate current sample or a typing in the historical record
- Individual facility determines whether ABO typing is performed by two technologists or if two samples must be collected at different times
- Computer system includes the donor unit information: product name, ABO and Rh type, unique number, and interpretation of ABO confirmation test
- Computer system includes recipient ABO and Rh typing
- Logic to alert user to ABO incompatibility between donor unit and recipient and between donor unit label and ABO confirmation test
- Method to verify the correct entry of all data

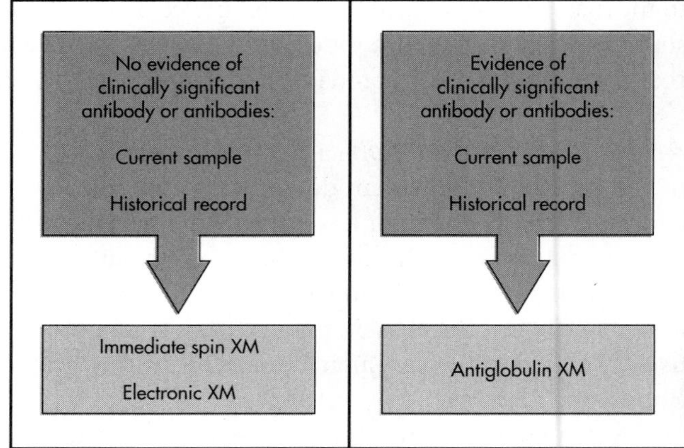

Fig. 8-4 Comparison of immediate spin, electronic, and antiglobulin crossmatch requirements. *XM*, Crossmatch.

The first large-scale implementation of an electronic crossmatch protocol took place in 1992 at the University of Michigan Hospital's Blood Bank, under an AABB exemption that still met FDA requirements for alternative compatibility procedures.[8] Though the electronic crossmatch is defined and governed by the AABB *Standards,* and this functionality is now provided by most blood bank software vendors, the procedure is not yet widely used and is considered by the FDA as an "alternative procedure" as the immediate spin crossmatch once was. The FDA's *Code of Federal Regulations* (640.120) requires that transfusion services seek approval for its use in writing.

Electronic crossmatching has a number of advantages:

- Increased efficiency of time
- Reduced volume of sample needed on large crossmatch orders
- Greater flexibility in staffing
- Better management of blood bank inventory
- Potential for a centralized transfusion service

Fig. 8-4 compares immediate spin, electronic, and antiglobulin crossmatching requirements.

Tagging, Inspecting, and Issuing Blood Products

Once the appropriate compatibility testing has been completed and the unit or units determined to be suitable for transfusion, a tag is produced and attached to each unit. The tag must clearly state the patient's full name and identification number, name of the product, donor number, expiration date and ABO and Rh type of the unit, interpretation of the crossmatching test (if performed), and identity of the person doing the testing or selection of the unit (Box 8-3). If compatibility testing is incomplete or shows incompatibility, but the unit has to be issued regardless, this must be indicated in bold on the tag.

A physician's order for blood or a blood product must be on file for the transfusion to occur. Ideally the person requesting the donor unit presents a form to the blood bank staff indicating the product desired and the patient for whom it is intended. This form is checked carefully and independently by both persons against the unit tag, and the unit tag information is also checked against the unit label. The expiration date is carefully checked to ensure that outdated units are not issued. The unit is visually checked for discoloration, clots, or other abnormal appearance. These checks are documented with the name of the person issu-

BOX 8-3 Tagging the Donor Unit

Patient's full name and identification number
Name of blood product
Unique donor unit number
Unit's expiration date and ABO and Rh typing
Interpretation of crossmatch
Technologist's identification

BOX 8-4 Issuing the Donor Unit

Physician's order
Requisition form: patient name and blood product
Compare requisition form with donor unit tag
Compare donor unit tag with blood product label
Blood product's expiration date
Visual check of unit: Discoloration? Clot? Abnormal appearance?
Documentation of person issuing and person receiving donor unit
Date and time of issue, unit destination

ing the unit and the person picking it up. The date and time of issue and the unit's ultimate destination are also documented (Box 8-4). After the transfusion is complete, a copy of the tag is attached to the patient's chart.

Patient identification is crucial for safe transfusion and ultimately resides with the nursing or medical personnel who hang the unit. A wristband with the patient's full name and identification number must be on the patient and exactly match the information on the unit tag. Commercial transfusion identification tagging systems use a separate wristband with special numbers to be attached to the patient specimen and any units prepared on the basis of that specimen. This system can be useful to ensure correct patient identification, and bar-coding features and handheld scanners provide even greater accuracy.

Once issued for transfusion, blood products may be returned to the transfusion service for storage if they are not going to be used immediately. Unmonitored refrigerators in patient care areas should never be used for storage of blood products. Reissuing of blood products from the transfusion service is permitted if the closure has not been entered and the unit has not exceeded the upper or lower temperature conditions for that product (1° to 10° C for red blood cells). Red blood cells, if not stored in a monitored refrigerator, should be returned to the transfusion service within 30 minutes to allow reissue.

PROBLEM-SOLVING INCOMPATIBLE CROSSMATCHES

Since compatibility testing encompasses antibody screening and identification and crossmatching, interpreting incompatibilities in conjunction with the results of these tests is important. Table 8-1 summarizes the causes of incompatible crossmatches in the immediate spin crossmatch and presents suggestions for resolutions. Since the antiglobulin crossmatch is more commonly performed in the presence of a clinically significant antibody or previous history of one, problem solving has revolved around the identification of the antibody's specificity and the location of antigen-negative donor units. An incompatible antiglobulin crossmatch may occasionally be detected. Often the primary reason for this incompatibility is the presence of a preexisting positive direct antiglobulin test (DAT) in the donor unit.

Table 8-1 Unexpected Incompatibilities in the Immediate Spin Crossmatch

PROBLEM	CAUSES	RESOLUTIONS
ABO typing errors	Patient identification error	Repeat ABO testing
	Sample labeling error	Redraw patient
Unexpected antibodies	Cold alloantibody (M, P_1)	Test panel cells
	Anti-A_1 in an A_2 patient	Test A_2 cells
	Cold autoantibody (I, IH)	Determine clinical significance

SPECIAL TOPICS

Emergency Release of Uncrossmatched Blood

Provision must be made by the transfusion service to expedite the release of blood in cases of life-threatening hemorrhage before completion of the usual compatibility tests. If possible a pretransfusion sample obtained from the patient and a recent transfusion history are highly desirable. However, obtaining such a sample is complicated if the patient received donor units that were ABO compatible (group O Rh negative, etc.) but not identical at another facility. Because the chaotic atmosphere of an emergency situation increases the likelihood of making errors and mislabeling or suboptimal specimens, personnel responsible for obtaining the blood bank sample must remain focused on the task of proper identification of the patient and acquisition of an adequate specimen.

Once the specimen is in the blood bank, the most important test to complete is the ABO and Rh typing so that blood can be issued. The recipient's past records should also be consulted at the outset to provide a check on the ABO and Rh typing and to acquaint the personnel with knowledge of any antibodies. Records alone (without current typing) may not be used as a basis for issuing blood. While these procedures are being performed, only group O Rh-negative red blood cells or AB plasma should be issued. If group O Rh-negative red blood cells are in short supply, they should be reserved preferentially for emergency release to women below or of childbearing age. Group O Rh-positive red blood cells may be substituted for emergency release to males and to females over childbearing age. Once the phenotype is determined and confirmed, ABO identical blood products should be issued. If an antibody is noted in the record, and if time permits, the red blood cell products should be screened for the corresponding antigen before being issued.

The second most important test to complete is the antibody screen. Crossmatching may be initiated simultaneously. If a positive reaction is noted at any step of the antibody screen, antibody identification procedures and antiglobulin crossmatches (on the issued units as well as additional ones) should be initiated at once and the patient's physician advised of the problem. Further transfusion should be delayed if possible until the problem is identified and safe units can be provided, but the patient's physician must make this decision. The AABB *Technical Manual* states: "The risk that the transfused unit might be incompatible may be judged to be less than the risk of depriving the patient of oxygen-carrying capacity."[9]

The AABB *Standards* stipulates that detailed records be kept of the emergency release of blood products. These records must include the patient's full name, hospital identification number, ABO and Rh typing, list of all units issued, name of the person who issued them, and the name of the physician who requested emergency release of blood (Box 8-5). The AABB *Standards* and the *Code of Fed-*

BOX 8-5

Emergency Release Requirements

- Release signed by physician
- Tag on donor unit indicating emergency release: uncrossmatched
- Patient name and identification
- Donor unit number(s), ABO and Rh typing, expiration date
- Retain segments from units for crossmatching
- Name of person issuing units

eral Regulations (606.151) require that the physician sign a release. Although this can wait until after the emergency, the physician should understand that it is his or her ultimate responsibility. In addition the tag or label on each unit that was issued uncrossmatched must include a conspicuous indication that the unit was issued that way. Segments must be pulled from the donor bags as soon as possible before they are issued and must be placed in tubes labeled with the donor unit number for subsequent crossmatching.

During the acute emergency, the blood bank personnel should "stay ahead" by crossmatching additional red blood cell units, preparing platelets, and thawing cryoprecipitate and frozen plasma in anticipation of need by (and in consultation with) the team caring for the patient. If the patient dies as a result of the emergency, remaining compatibility testing may be waived or abbreviated at the discretion of the transfusion service physician. Testing should be complete enough to show that the death was unrelated to the transfusion of uncrossmatched blood.

Massive Transfusion

A massive transfusion is defined as a total volume exchange of blood through transfusion within a 24-hour period, whether in an infant or an adult patient. In other words the blood products transfused in 24 hours approximate or exceed the recipient's original blood volume (approximately 10 to 12 units of whole blood in an average adult male). At that point the recipient's circulation contains almost entirely transfused blood and essentially no autologous blood. The original patient's sample no longer represents the circulating blood of the patient. The transfusion service physician should have a policy clearly in place dictating what is done under these circumstances and at what point a new "recipient" sample is required. Some policies indicate that serologic immediate spin crossmatching is eliminated for a time, and ABO-identical donor units are simply tagged and issued. If an electronic crossmatch protocol were in place, this would not be necessary. When clinically significant antibodies are involved, all units issued must be negative for antigens, but an immediate spin crossmatch still could be used.

The other consideration in massive transfusion is the availability first of group O Rh-negative and then of ABO-identical blood. Once the blood group is established, group-specific blood should be transfused to protect the supply of group O Rh-negative blood. However, if ABO-identical blood begins to run out, ABO-compatible blood may be used. In the case of group AB, A, or B recipients, group O red blood cells may always be substituted. Group AB recipients could receive As or Bs but not both; group A typically would be used because of greater availability. Refer to Table 4-6 in Chapter 4 for a review of these concepts. In the selection of the Rh type, females negative for the D antigen with childbearing potential should receive only Rh-negative blood. Other Rh-negative recipients may receive Rh-positive blood. However, approximately 50% to 70% subsequently develop anti-D,[10] which sharply diminishes flexibility in a subsequent bleeding episode.

Only one way exists that determines the safe point of switching the patient back to the original ABO phenotype. A new "recipient" sample must be obtained and used to determine whether the level of **passively transfused** anti-A, anti-B, or anti-A,B is sufficient to cause incompatibility with group A, B, or AB donors.

Passively transfused: when an antibody is transferred to the recipient from the plasma portion of a blood product during transfusion.

Maximum Surgical Blood Order Schedule

Many transfusion services use a philosophy for preparing blood for scheduled surgery that is based on statistical measures of average blood use for certain surgical procedures in their own facility. A list of all surgical procedures performed in the facility is first drawn up, and then actual usage figures for each procedure are compiled. The average number of blood units used is then determined. The surgeons, anesthesiologists, and blood transfusion physician agree on this number as the standard blood order for the stated procedure. For example, a procedure for a total hip replacement is determined to require a preoperative order of 5 units of red blood cells. Such a list is called the Maximum Surgical Blood Order Schedule (MSBOS). The MSBOS may also be used as a guide for the number of autologous units the patient may donate before surgery.

Type and Screen Protocols

If the average use for a particular surgical procedure is less than 1 unit of red blood cells, many transfusion services decide that these are the cases where only a type and screen (T/S) is performed (unless clinically significant antibodies are found). If blood is subsequently needed, the T/S specimen is retrieved and a unit(s) is crossmatched by the immediate spin or electronic crossmatch technique. Some institutions initially perform only a T/S on all preoperative patients and crossmatch (immediate spin or electronic) only when the blood is ordered. This policy allows greater inventory availability. The physician must be able to trust that blood is always issued quickly if the T/S protocol is used. If clinically significant antibodies are or were ever present, antigen-negative units should be identified and reserved or crossmatched.

These approaches are intended to conserve blood inventory by not "tying up" excess numbers of units unlikely to be transfused. Sufficient blood supply to cover unexpected needs must, of course, be readily available, though units may not be crossmatched until the time of issue.

Crossmatching Autologous Blood

Autologous blood is blood donated by the prospective recipient for later use, usually in the context of elective surgery. Special procedures must exist (whether manual or computerized) to ensure that these units be found and transfused to the intended recipient. The extent of pretransfusion testing for autologous units varies in individual facilities.

A system must exist to ensure that the autologous units are transfused before any directed or allogeneic donor units. Computerized tracking makes this easier, but it can be done manually when necessary. If autologous units are donated, many issues of liability arise if these units are not made available and allogeneic units are given instead, particularly if subsequent antibody production is stimulated or a disease is transmitted.

Crossmatching of Infants Less than 4 Months Old

Infants less than 4 months old are unable to produce their own antibodies. Antibodies detected in the circulation of a newborn are maternal in origin. At 4 to 6 months of age infants begin producing their own ABO antibodies and become capable of producing antibodies if immunologically challenged through transfusion.

Initial compatibility testing in an infant must include pretransfusion ABO and Rh typing. Since serum ABO antibodies are not present, no reason exists for serum testing. ABO and Rh typing does not need to be repeated for the duration of the current admission. An initial antibody screen needs to be performed on either the infant's or mother's sample. If clinically significant antibodies are found, the blood for transfusion needs to be antigen negative or compatible in an antiglobulin crossmatch. Crossmatching continues until maternal antibody is no longer detectable in the infant's serum. If the antibody screen is negative, however, no crossmatches or repeat screens are needed during the current admission as long as red blood cells are used that are ABO compatible with the infant and Rh identical (or D negative).

Donor centers customarily prepare pediatric units for infants by dividing a full unit of red blood cells into sterile portions. The transfusing facility may further subdivide these "pedipacks" if necessary. The use of syringes for transfusions to infants is also a common practice. This method transfuses the same donor blood repeatedly to the infant if multiple transfusions are needed, thus limiting the exposures to undetected diseases and immunologic stimuli from donor blood.

PRETRANSFUSION TESTING FOR NON–RED BLOOD CELL PRODUCTS

Frozen plasma, platelet concentrates, and **cryoprecipitate** contain almost no red blood cells and do not need to be crossmatched. **Platelets pheresis** and especially **granulocyte concentrates** may contain red blood cells, but they need be crossmatched only if the unit contains more than 2 ml of red blood cells.

It is assumed that the serum or plasma of the donors of non–red blood cell products has been thoroughly screened for antibodies. Therefore repeat screening and ABO and Rh testing of these products by the transfusing facility are not required. Products containing a large volume of plasma must be selected on the basis of ABO serum compatibility with the recipient. Cryoprecipitate and platelet concentrates may be transfused with combinations of ABO-compatible units and units that are not ABO compatible if the cumulative volume is not large. For example, a group A recipient may receive a mixture of group A and O platelets for transfusion. The transfusion of platelets with the same ABO phenotype as the patient may increase platelet survival rates in vivo.

Frozen plasma: blood component prepared from whole blood that contains only the plasma portion of whole blood and is frozen after separation.
Platelet concentrates: platelets obtained from a whole blood donation; contain a minimum of 5.5×10^{10} platelets.
Cryoprecipitate: blood component recovered from a controlled thaw of fresh frozen plasma; the cold-insoluble precipitate is rich in coagulation Factor VIII, von Willebrand factor, Factor XIII, and fibrinogen.
Platelets pheresis: a pheresis procedure in which the platelets are removed from a donor and the remaining red blood cells and plasma are returned.
Granulocyte concentrates: blood component collected by cytapheresis; contain a minimum of 1.0×10^{10} granulocytes.

CHAPTER SUMMARY

This chapter emphasizes that the process of compatibility testing extends beyond the boundaries of the transfusion service. The procedure begins and ends with the most important individual in the process: the recipient of the transfusion. Responsibilities of blood bank personnel include evaluating, monitoring, and following transfusion procedures and policies to meet the needs of these patients. An overview of compatibility testing is shown below.

SUMMARY: PROCESS OF COMPATIBILITY TESTING

Patient: Accurate identification

Patient: Proper sample collection and handling

Patient: Review of past blood bank records

Patient: ABO and Rh typing, antibody screen, crossmatch

SUMMARY: PROCESS OF COMPATIBILITY TESTING—CONT'D

Donor:	ABO and Rh typing and other testing
Donor:	Double check of unit's ABO and Rh label
Patient:	Tagging, inspecting, and issuing blood products
Patient:	Accurate reidentification and monitoring of transfusion

CRITICAL THINKING EXERCISE

◆ ***EXERCISE 8-1***

A 60-year-old woman with anemia is admitted to the hospital. Her hematocrit is 17%, and she has been experiencing subtle gastrointestinal bleeding over many weeks. Her physician requests 4 units of red blood cells for transfusion. The patient's red blood cells phenotype as group AB Rh positive. Her antibody screen is negative on the sample drawn in the emergency room, but her records indicate a previously detected anti-E. Three group AB Rh-positive red blood cell units are available in the blood bank.

1. What ABO phenotype should be selected for the fourth donor unit? State your reasons for this choice.
2. What type of crossmatches should be performed?
3. Is any additional screening required on the donor units before crossmatching?

◆ ***Additional Testing***

After screening the 4 units of red blood cells, one of the group AB Rh-positive units is E positive.

4. How many donor units should be screened to find the 4 units ordered, plus 2 more to hold in reserve for the patient?

◆ ***Additional Testing***

Having located 6 E-negative donor units, you perform crossmatching on the units. One of the units is incompatible in the antiglobulin phase (2+ reactivity). The physician is becoming insistent on beginning the transfusion, since the patient is having some shortness of breath.

5. How do you respond to the physician's request?
6. List several reasons to explain the one incompatible donor unit.
7. What additional testing do you perform?

◆ ***Additional Testing***

Antibody-identification testing reveals no detectable antibodies, and the autologous control is also negative. Additional testing revealed a positive DAT on the donor unit.

8. What is the usual transfusion service policy on donor units with a positive DAT?

STUDY QUESTIONS

1. Detection of serologic incompatibility between donor red blood cells and recipient serum is performed in the:
   a. antibody screen
   b. crossmatch
   c. direct antiglobulin test
   d. autologous control

2. What incompatibilities are detected in the antiglobulin phase of a crossmatch?
   a. IgM alloantibodies in recipient's serum
   b. ABO incompatibilities
   c. IgG alloantibodies in recipient's serum
   d. room temperature incompatibilities

3. Which of the following statements is true regarding compatibility testing for infants under 4 months of age?
   a. a direct antiglobulin test is required
   b. a crossmatch is needed when the antibody screen is negative
   c. maternal serum can be used for the crossmatch
   d. testing for ABO antibodies is required for the infant

4. What tests are included in compatibility testing?
   a. blood typing of recipient
   b. antibody screening of recipient
   c. crossmatch
   d. all of the above

5. A group B Rh-positive unit of red blood cells is received in the transfusion service. What repeat testing is required on this unit?
   a. ABO typing only
   b. ABO and Rh typing
   c. ABO, Rh, and weak D typing
   d. ABO and Rh typing; antibody screen

6. What ABO and Rh type is selected for red blood cell units issued to a patient in emergency release?
   a. group O Rh positive
   b. group O Rh negative
   c. group A Rh positive
   d. group AB Rh negative

7. What antibodies are detected in the immediate spin crossmatch?
   a. Rh antibodies
   b. high-titer, low-avidity antibodies
   c. ABO antibodies
   d. Kell antibodies

For Questions 8 and 9, use the following information. Current pretransfusion testing on John Smith reveals a negative antibody screen with a previous history of anti-K. He is group A Rh positive.

8. Which of the following crossmatch procedures is performed to identify compatible units?
   a. immediate spin crossmatch
   b. electronic crossmatch
   c. antiglobulin crossmatch
   d. none of the above

9. Which of the following donor units could be selected to run in the crossmatch?
   a. group A Rh positive, K+k+
   b. group A Rh negative, K−k+
   c. group O Rh positive, K+k−
   d. group O Rh negative, K+k−

10. What information is sufficient for a properly labeled blood sample for the blood bank?
    a. name, unique identification number
    b. name, unique identification number, date of collection
    c. name, unique identification number, date of collection, physician's name
    d. none of the above

True or False

___ 11. The electronic crossmatch is an easy policy to establish in the blood bank.

___ 12. A crossmatch detects most errors in the identification of antigens on patient's cells.

___ 13. A crossmatch demonstrating a 2+ agglutination is interpreted as compatible.

___ 14. An immediate spin crossmatch of a D-positive recipient with a D-negative donor unit is incompatible.

___ 15. The electronic crossmatch requires two ABO and Rh typings on the recipient.

___ 16. A crossmatch prevents the immunization of the recipient to blood group antigens.

___ 17. A type and screen protocol provides a mechanism to increase the number of uncrossmatched donor units in inventory.

___ 18. The only component that requires crossmatching is a unit of red blood cells.

___ 19. Group O plasma is considered the universal donor of plasma products.

___ 20. The recipient sample must be labeled with full name, unique identifying number, date, and some means of identifying the phlebotomist.

REFERENCES

1. Guy LR, Huestis DW, Wilson LR: *Technical methods and procedures,* ed 4, Chicago, 1966, American Association of Blood Banks.
2. Petz LD, Swisher SN: *Clinical practice of blood transfusion,* New York, 1981, Churchill Livingstone.
3. Oberman HA: The crossmatch, a brief historical perspective, *Transfusion* 21:645, 1981.
4. Spraycar M, editor: *Stedman's medical dictionary,* ed 26, Baltimore, 1995, Williams & Wilkins.
5. Oberman HA, editor: *Standards for blood banks and transfusion services,* ed 8, Washington, DC, 1976, American Association of Blood Banks.
6. Garratty G, Petz LD: The significance of red cell bound complement components in development of standards and quality assurance for the anti-complement components of antiglobulin sera, *Transfusion* 16:297, 1976.
7. Menitove JE, editor: *Standards for blood banks and transfusion services,* ed 19, Bethesda, Md, 1999, American Association of Blood Banks.
8. Butch SH, Oberman HA: The computer or electronic crossmatch, *Transfus Med Rev* 11:256, 1997.
9. Vengelen-Tyler V, editor: *Technical manual,* ed 12, Bethesda, Md, 1996, American Association of Blood Banks.
10. Issitt PD, Anstee DJ: *Applied blood group serology,* ed 4, Durham, NC, 1998, Montgomery Scientific Publications.

SUGGESTED READINGS

Cooper ES: *Accreditation information manual,* Bethesda, Md, 1997, American Association of Blood Banks.

Harmening D: *Modern blood banking and transfusion practices,* ed 4, Philadelphia, 1999, FA Davis.

Mollison PL: *Blood transfusion in clinical medicine,* ed 9, Oxford, 1993, Blackwell Scientific Publications.

Sazama K: *Accreditation requirements manual,* ed 6, Bethesda, Md, 1995, American Association of Blood Banks.

Blood Collection, Testing, and Components

IV

9 DONOR SELECTION AND PHLEBOTOMY

Carol J. Grant

CHAPTER OUTLINE

Donor Screening
Registration
Preinterview Educational Materials
Health History Interview
Physical Examination
Confidential Unit Exclusion
Informed Consent
Phlebotomy
Identification
Bag Labeling
Arm Preparation and Venipuncture
Adverse Donor Reactions
Postdonation Care
Special Blood Collection
Autologous Donations
Directed Donations
Hemapheresis
Therapeutic Phlebotomy

LEARNING OBJECTIVES

Upon completion of this chapter, the reader should be able to:

1. Describe the required donor registration information.
2. Discuss the donor medical history criteria for protecting the donor.
3. List some of the donor questions that are asked to protect the recipient.
4. Describe the physical criteria required for allogeneic donors.
5. Describe the confidential unit exclusion procedure and the reason for its use.
6. Explain the informed consent process for blood donation.
7. List possible adverse donor reactions.
8. Compare and contrast allogeneic and autologous donor criteria.
9. Describe various forms of autologous donations.
10. Describe the apheresis procedure and the products collected.
11. Discuss the reason for and criteria for directed donation.
12. Define *therapeutic phlebotomy* and state the conditions for which it is used.

Blood centers and transfusion services are responsible for providing an adequate blood supply to the patients they serve. This process begins with educating the public about the need for volunteer donations. After recruiting donors the safety of the blood supply depends on a thorough and accurate donor screening and processing or testing of each unit collected. This chapter covers donor screening, and Chapter 10 covers the processing performed on donated blood.

DONOR SCREENING

The screening of each donor can be divided into three phases: registration, health history interview, and physical examination.

Registration

The donor registration process includes documenting information that fully identifies the donor on an individual donation registration record. These records must be retained indefinitely to make it possible to notify donors of any necessary information.[1] Questions regarding name changes or nicknames are important for correct identification. Registration should also include prescreening for the donor eligibility status. With the exception of first-time donors, access to past donation history, usually through computerized databases, allows the staff to confirm that:

- Donor information is correct
- Sufficient time has passed since the last donation
- The donor has not been deferred from a donation based on previous history questions or test results

Correct identification of the donor is essential to ensure accuracy of the following required donor information:

- Donor's full name
- Permanent address
- Home and business telephone numbers
- Date of birth (donor must be at least 17 years old; if the state considers 17-year-olds to be minors, parental consent is required)
- Gender
- Date of last donation (whole blood donors must wait 56 days between donations, whereas plasmapheresis, plateletpheresis, or leukapheresis donors must wait at least 48 hours before donating whole blood; a physician may request more frequent donations from a single donor for a specific patient)
- Written informed consent to proceed with the donation process

Additional useful information includes:

- Social Security or driver's license number
- Positive identification: this usually entails photo identification
- Race: this can be useful in selecting donor units for patients with certain antibodies
- Intended use of the donation: **allogeneic, directed, autologous,** or **apheresis.** These "special donation" processes are described later in this chapter.

Allogeneic donation: donation for use by the general patient population.
Directed donation: donation reserved for use by a specific patient.
Autologous donation: donation by a donor reserved for the donor's later use.
Apheresis donation: donation of a specific component of the blood; parts of the whole blood that are not retained are returned to the donor.

Preinterview Educational Materials

Before donating, all prospective donors must be given educational materials describing the risks of infectious diseases transmitted by blood transfusion, including the signs, symptoms, and high-risk behaviors associated with the human immunodeficiency virus (HIV) and acquired immunodeficiency syndrome (AIDS).[2] The prospective donors should be given ample opportunity to read the material and ask questions, and they are excluded from donating blood if they have experienced any of the signs or symptoms explained in the material. This preinterview material also describes the possible side effects and risks associated with the donation process.

Health History Interview

The health history is used to protect both the donor during the donation process and the patient receiving the blood. Questions are asked in an environment that provides confidentiality and encourages the donor to answer truthfully. The interviewer should document and evaluate all responses to determine suitability for donation.

The criteria used to accept donors are regulated by the Food and Drug Administration (FDA) and accrediting bodies such as the American Association of Blood Banks (AABB). Although the use of a uniform donor history questionnaire developed by AABB is recommended, **medical directors** have the option to modify the questions as appropriate for their center based on demographics. The use of local vernacular is recommended.

Medical directors: designated physicians responsible for the medical and technical policies of the blood bank.

Questions generally can be divided into two categories: those intended to protect the donor and those intended to protect the recipient. An explanation of some of the questions from the AABB Uniform Donor History Questionnaire[3] (Table 9-1) follows.

Questions for Protection of the Donor

Properly trained staff are required to ask specific questions to determine donor eligibility, such as those regarding general health, previous surgeries, heart and lung disease, bleeding problems, and pregnancy. Donors with cold or influenza symptoms, headache, or nausea should be temporarily deferred. Donors who are currently pregnant or have been pregnant in the last 6 weeks should also be deferred. A 12-month deferral is required for donors who have had surgery requiring a transfusion of blood or blood products.[3] An evaluation by the medical director regarding donors with a history of cancer is necessary, although individuals who have been free of the disease for at least 5 years are usually acceptable. Permanent deferral because of leukemia or lymphoma is required. A tendency for abnormal bleeding usually necessitates deferral to avoid complications following donation.

Deferring donors for any reason should be handled tactfully. Donors should be provided with a full explanation of the reason for the deferral and information on whether they can donate in the future.

Questions for Protection of the Recipient

Donors are thoroughly questioned regarding possible exposure to diseases that may be transmitted through the blood supply. Medications, vaccinations, and high-risk activities are carefully evaluated to protect recipients of blood transfusions from risks. The list of donor questions in this category is updated frequently to reflect current knowledge of blood-borne pathogen and medication issues.

Although viral marker testing has increased the safety of the blood supply, questions to determine potential exposure to certain transmissible diseases are also necessary. Many viral markers may be below detectable limits on donation,

Text cont'd on p. 216

Table 9-1 American Association of Blood Banks Uniform Donor History Questionnaire

DONOR HISTORY QUESTIONS	AMERICAN ASSOCIATION OF BLOOD BANKS	FOOD AND DRUG ADMINISTRATION	COMMENTS
1. Have you ever donated or attempted to donate blood using a different (or another) name here or anywhere else?	No specific requirement.	A record shall be available from which unsuitable donors may be identified so that products from such individuals will not be distributed. [21 CFR 606.160(e) April 1997]	Identifying information should be obtained from the donor.
2. In the past 8 weeks, have you given blood, plasma, or platelets here or anywhere else?	Frequency of blood donation is every 8 weeks. (Standard B2.000)	Frequency of blood donation is every 8 weeks unless otherwise approved by the medical director. [21 CFR 640.3(f) April 1997]	Infrequent plasma donors can donate every 4 weeks. (FDA Memos 3/10/95[1] and 12/14/95[2])
3. Have you for any reason been deferred or refused as a blood donor or told not to donate blood?	No specific requirement.	No specific requirement.	
4. Are you feeling well and healthy today?	The prospective donor shall appear to be in good health. (Standard B2.000)	Donor must be determined to be in general good health. [21 CFR 640.3(b) April 1997]	Requires "yes" answer that tests donor's attention to question content. Initiates sequence of personal health history questions (4-13).

Standards referred to are from the 18th edition of *Standards for Blood Banks and Transfusion Services,* effective January 1, 1998, and for this publication, were reviewed against the 19th edition.

1. Food and Drug Administration: *Memorandum: revision of FDA Memorandum of August 27, 1982: Requirements for infrequent plasma donors,* Rockville, Md, March 10, 1995, Congressional and Consumer Affairs.
2. Food and Drug Administration: *Memorandum: donor deferral due to red blood cell loss during collection of source plasma,* Rockville, Md, Dec 14, 1995, Congressional and Consumer Affairs.
3. Food and Drug Administration: *Memorandum: revised recommendations for the prevention of HIV transmission by blood and blood products,* Rockville, Md, April 23, 1992, Congressional and Consumer Affairs.
4. Food and Drug Administration: *Exemptions to permit persons with a history of viral hepatitis before the age of eleven years to serve as donors of whole blood and plasma: alternative procedures, 21 CFR 640.120,* Rockville, Md, April 23, 1992, Congressional and Consumer Affairs.
5. Food and Drug Administration: *Memorandum: donor suitability related to laboratory testing for viral hepatitis and a history of viral hepatitis,* Rockville, Md, Dec 22, 1993, Congressional and Consumer Affairs.
6. Food and Drug Administration: *Memorandum: recommendations for deferral of donors for malaria risk,* Rockville, Md, July 26, 1994, Congressional and Consumer Affairs.
7. Food and Drug Administration: *Memorandum: Deferral of blood and blood and plasma donors based on medications,* Rockville, Md, July 28, 1993, Congressional and Consumer Affairs.
8. Food and Drug Administration: *Memorandum: revised guideline for the collection of platelets, pheresis,* Rockville, Md, Oct 7, 1988, Congressional and Consumer Affairs.
9. Food and Drug Administration: *Memorandum: revised precautionary measures to reduce the possible risk of transfusion of Creutzfeldt-Jakob disease (CJD) by blood and blood products,* Rockville, Md, Dec 11, 1996, Congressional and Consumer Affairs.
10. Food and Drug Administration: *Memorandum: revised recommendations for testing whole blood, blood components, source plasma and source leukocytes for antibody to hepatitis C virus encoded antigen (anti-HCV),* Rockville, Md, April 23, 1992, Congressional and Consumer Affairs.
11. Food and Drug Administration: *Memorandum: clarification of FDA recommendations for donor deferral and product distribution based on the results of syphilis testing,* Rockville, Md, Dec 12, 1991, Congressional and Consumer Affairs.
12. Food and Drug Administration: *Memorandum: interim recommendations for deferral of donors at increased risk for HIV-1 group O infection,* Rockville, Md, Dec 11, 1996, Congressional and Consumer Affairs.
13. American Association of Blood Banks: *Association bulletin 97-5, FDA Accepts AABB changes to HIV-1 group O donor questions,* Aug 1, 1997.
14. Food and Drug Administration: *Memorandum: recommendations for the deferral of current and recent inmates of correctional institutions as donors of whole blood, blood components, source leukocytes, and source plasma,* Rockville, Md, June 8, 1995, Congressional and Consumer Affairs.
15. American Association of Blood Banks: *Association bulletin 99-5, Donor question of Soriatane, Bethesda, Md,* 1999, American Association of Blood Banks.

(Note: After the above Uniform History Questionnaire was approved by the FDA in May 1998, information on a new drug came to the attention of the FDA and the AABB. Donors who are taking, or who in the last 3 years have taken, acitretin [Soriatane, Roche Pharmaceuticals, Nutley, NJ] for psoriasis therapy must be deferred.)

Table 9-1 American Association of Blood Banks Uniform Donor History Questionnaire—cont'd

DONOR HISTORY QUESTIONS	AMERICAN ASSOCIATION OF BLOOD BANKS	FOOD AND DRUG ADMINISTRATION	COMMENTS
5. In the past 12 months have you been under a doctor's care or had a major illness or surgery?	No specific requirement.	Persons who have received a transfusion of whole blood or a blood component within the past 12 months should not donate blood or blood components. (FDA Memo 4/23/92[1])	
6. Have you ever had chest pain, heart disease, recent or severe respiratory disease?	Prospective donors with diseases of the heart or lungs shall be excluded unless determined to be suitable to donate by a blood bank physician. (Standard B1.700)	Donor must be free of acute respiratory disease. [21 CFR 640.3(b)(4) April 1997]	
7. Have you ever had cancer, a blood disease, or a bleeding problem?	Prospective donors with a history of cancer or abnormal bleeding tendency shall be excluded unless determined to be suitable to donate by a blood bank physician. (Standard B1.700)	Persons with hemophilia or related clotting disorders who have received clotting factor concentrates must not donate blood or blood components. (FDA Memo 4/23/92[3])	
8. Have you ever had yellow jaundice, liver disease, viral hepatitis, or a positive test for hepatitis?	Prospective donors with diseases of the liver shall be excluded unless determined to be suitable to donate by a blood bank physician. (Standard B1.700) Donors with a history of hepatitis after their 11th birthday or a confirmed positive test for HBsAg or a repeatedly reactive test for HBc are indefinitely deferred. (Standard B2.711)	No individual with a history of hepatitis shall be a source of whole blood donation. [21 CFR 640.3(c) April 1997] Exemptions for history of hepatitis before age 11. (FDA Memos 4/23/92[4] and 12/22/93[5])	
9. Have you ever had malaria, Chagas' disease, or babesiosis?	Prospective donors who have had a diagnosis of malaria shall be deferred for 3 years after becoming asymptomatic. (Standard B2.741) A history of babesiosis or Chagas' disease shall be cause for indefinite deferral. (Standard B2.750)	Prospective donors who have had malaria should be deferred for 3 years after becoming asymptomatic. (FDA Memo 7/26/94[6])	
10. A. Have you ever taken etretinate (Tegison) for psoriasis?	A. People who have received etretinate (e.g., Tegison) shall be indefinitely deferred (B2.530)	A. A donor who has taken or is taking Tegison should be permanently deferred. (FDA Memo 7/28/93[7])	A. Potentially teratogenic. May be present up to 3 years after last use.
B. In the past 3 years, have you taken acetretin (Soriatane)?	B. Donor is to be deferred from date of last use (Proposed for 19th ed. Standards, to be published 1999, B2.520)	B. Donor is to be deferred for 3 years from date of last dose (per manufacturer's insert)	B. Potentially teratogenic. May be present up to 3 years after last use.

Table 9-1 American Association of Blood Banks Uniform Donor History Questionnaire—cont'd

DONOR HISTORY QUESTIONS	AMERICAN ASSOCIATION OF BLOOD BANKS	FOOD AND DRUG ADMINISTRATION	COMMENTS
C. In the past 3 days have you taken piroxicam (Feldene), aspirin, or anything that has aspirin in it?	C. Ingestion within 3 days of donation of medications known to irreversibly damage platelet function (e.g., aspirin-containing medications) or that inhibit platelet function and have a prolonged half-life should preclude the use of a donor as the sole source of platelets for a recipient. (Standard B2.510)	C. No specific requirement for whole blood donation. Donors who have recently taken medication containing aspirin, especially within 36 hours, may not be suitable donors for platelet pheresis. (FDA Guidelines 10/7/88[8])	C. Preferred time varies. May be mandated by state health and safety code.
D. In the past month have you taken isotretinoin (Accutane) or finasteride (Proscar) (Propecia)?	D. For Accutane or Proscar, donor is to be deferred for 1 month after receipt of last dose. (18th ed. Standards B2.520) For Propecia, donor is to be deferred for 1 month after receipt of last dose. (Proposed for 19th ed. Standards, to be published 1999, B2.520)	D. A donor taking Accutane or Proscar should be deferred from donating blood for at least 1 month after receipt of the last dose. (FDA Memo 7/28/93[7]) 1 month deferral. (FDA telephone communication to AABB, January 1998.)	D. Medication questions grouped.
E. In the past 4 weeks have you taken any pills or medications?	E. Drug therapy shall be evaluated by a qualified person to determine suitability to donate blood. (Standards, B1.900)	E. Facility medical director to determine donor acceptability or deferral based on medications. (FDA memo 7-28-93)	E. Medication questions grouped.
11. In the past 4 weeks, have you had any shots or vaccinations?	Donors must be queried about vaccines and immunizations. (Standards B2.610, B2.620, B2.630)	No specific requirement.	
12. In the past 12 months, have you been given rabies shots?	Donor is deferred for 12 months after vaccine treatment for rabies. (Standard B2.640)	No specific requirement.	
13. Female donors: In the past 6 weeks, have you been pregnant or are you pregnant now?	Existing pregnancy or pregnancy in past 6 weeks is cause for deferral. (Standard B1.800)	No specific requirement.	
14. In the past 3 years, have you been outside the United States or Canada?	Residents of countries in which malaria is not considered endemic but who have been in an area in which malaria is considered endemic may be accepted as regular blood donors 1 year after return irrespective of the receipt of antimalarial prophylaxis. (Standard B2.743) Immigrants, refugees, or citizens coming from a country in which malaria	Travelers to an area considered endemic for malaria should not be accepted as donors of whole blood and blood components prior to 1 year after departure. After 1 year, donors free of unexplained symptoms suggestive of malaria may be accepted whether or not they have received antimalarial chemoprophylaxis. Immigrants, refugees, and citizens of	Initiates sequence of exposure-type questions (14-30).

Table 9-1 American Association of Blood Banks Uniform Donor History Questionnaire—cont'd

DONOR HISTORY QUESTIONS	AMERICAN ASSOCIATION OF BLOOD BANKS	FOOD AND DRUG ADMINISTRATION	COMMENTS
	is considered endemic may be accepted as blood donors 3 years after departure. (Standard B2.742)	endemic countries should not be accepted as donors prior to 3 years after departure. After 3 years, donors free of unexplained symptoms suggestive of malaria may be accepted. (FDA Memo 7/26/94[6])	
15. A. Have you ever received human pituitary-derived growth hormone? B. Have you received a dura mater (or brain covering) graft? C. Have you or any of your blood relatives ever had Creutzfeldt-Jakob disease or have you ever been told that your family is at an increased risk for Creutzfeldt-Jakob disease?	Prospective donors who have a family history of Creutzfeldt-Jakob disease or who have received tissue or tissue derivatives known to be a possible source of the Creutzfeldt-Jakob agent (e.g., dura mater, pituitary growth hormone of human origin) shall be deferred indefinitely. (Standard B2.410)	A. The FDA recommends that any donor who has received injections of pit-hGH be permanently deferred. (FDA Memo 7/28/93[7]) B. The FDA recommends that persons who have received transplants of dura mater be permanently deferred from donation. (FDA Memo 12/11/96[8]) C. The FDA recommends that persons with a family history of Creutzfeldt-Jakob disease be permanently deferred from donation unless increased risk is excluded based on specialized testing. (FDA Memo 12/11/96[9])	
16. In the past 12 months, have you had close contact with a person with yellow jaundice or viral hepatitis, or have you been given Hepatitis B Immune Globulin (HBIG)? 17. In the past 12 months, have you taken (snorted) cocaine through your nose?	Close contact with a person who has viral hepatitis is a 12-month deferral. (Standard B2.724)	Close contact with person who has viral hepatitis is a 12-month deferral. (FDA Memo 4/23/92[10])	Close contact generally refers to cohabitation or sexual contact. The medical director should establish a policy for these potential donors.
18. In the past 12 months, have you received blood or had an organ or a tissue transplant or graft?	Prospective donors who, during the preceding 12 months, received blood, blood components or derivatives, or other human tissues known to be possible sources of blood-borne pathogens, shall be excluded. (Standard B2.420)	Persons who have received a transfusion of whole blood or a blood component within the past 12 months should not donate blood or blood components. (FDA Memo 4/23/92[3])	Includes immunization with red blood cells.

Table 9-1 American Association of Blood Banks Uniform Donor History Questionnaire—cont'd

DONOR HISTORY QUESTIONS	AMERICAN ASSOCIATION OF BLOOD BANKS	FOOD AND DRUG ADMINISTRATION	COMMENTS
19. In the past 12 months, have you had a tattoo applied, ear or skin piercing, acupuncture, accidental needlestick, or come in contact with someone else's blood?	Prospective donors shall be deferred from donating blood or blood components for transfusion who, within the preceding 12 months, have a history of: 1) A tattoo. 2) Mucous membrane exposure to blood. 3) Nonsterile skin penetration with instruments or equipment contaminated with blood or body fluids. 4) Sexual or household contact with an individual with viral hepatitis. 5) Sexual contact with an individual with HIV or at high risk of HIV infection. (Standards B2.721, B2.722, B2.723, B2.724, B2.275)	Persons who have had any contact with blood and body fluids through percutaneous inoculation (such as injury or accidental needlestick) or through contact with an open wound, nonintact skin, or mucous membrane during the preceding 12 months should be deferred. (FDA Memo 4/23/92[3])	Donors should be questioned about ear piercing, skin piercing, electrolysis, and acupuncture to make sure that single-use equipment, disposals, or properly sterilized needles were used. Health care workers should be carefully evaluated to determine if they have had a needlestick injury or other type of percutaneous or mucosal exposure to patient's blood or an unknown source. Exposure to another person's blood through broken skin or intact mucosal surface is cause for 12-month deferral from the time the exposure occurred.
20. A. In the past 12 months, have you had a positive test for syphilis? B. In the past 12 months, have you had or been treated for syphilis or gonorrhea?	A history of syphilis or gonorrhea, treatment for either, or a confirmed reactive screening test for syphilis shall be cause for deferral for 12 months after completion of therapy. (Standard B2.340)	Persons who have had, or have been treated for, syphilis or gonorrhea during the preceding 12 months should not donate blood or blood components. Persons with a positive (STS) test should be deferred for 12 months. (FDA Memo 12/12/91[11])	
21. In the past 12 months, have you given money or drugs to anyone to have sex with you?	Donor must be given educational material on AIDS high-risk activity, and such at-risk persons should refrain from donating blood. (Standards B3.100, B2.730)	Men and women who have engaged in sex for money or drugs since 1977 and persons who have engaged in sex with such people during the preceding 12 months should not donate blood or blood components. (FDA Memo 4/23/92[3])	
22. A. At any time since 1977, have you taken money or drugs for sex? B. In the past 12 months, have you had sex, even once, with anyone who has taken money or drugs for sex?	Refer to question #21.	Men and women who have engaged in sex for money or drugs since 1977 and persons who have engaged in sex with such people during the preceding 12 months should not donate blood or blood components. (FDA Memo 4/23/92[3])	

Table 9-1 American Association of Blood Banks Uniform Donor History Questionnaire—cont'd

DONOR HISTORY QUESTIONS	AMERICAN ASSOCIATION OF BLOOD BANKS	FOOD AND DRUG ADMINISTRATION	COMMENTS
23. A. Have you ever used a needle, even once, to take drugs that were not prescribed for you by a doctor?	A. Stigma of narcotic habituation is permanent deferral. (Standard B2.330)	A. Donor must be free from skin punctures or scars indicative of addiction to self-injected narcotics. [21 CFR 640.3(b)(7) April 1997] Past or present intravenous drug users should not donate blood or blood components. (FDA Memo 4/23/92[3])	
B. In the past 12 months, have you had sex, even once, with anyone who has used a needle to take drugs not prescribed by a doctor?	B. Refer to question #21.	B. Persons who have had sex with any person who is a past or present intravenous drug user should not donate blood or blood components for 12 months. (FDA Memo 4/23/92[3])	
24. Male donors: Have you had sex with another male, even once, since 1977?	Refer to question #21.	Men who have had sex with another man even one time since 1977 should not donate blood or blood components permanently. (FDA Memo 4/23/92[3])	
25. Female donors: In the past 12 months, have you had sex with a male who has had sex, even once, since 1977 with another male?	Refer to question #21.	Persons who have had sex with men who have had sex with another man even one time since 1977 should not donate blood or blood components for 12 months. (FDA Memo 4/23/92[3])	
26. A. Have you ever taken clotting factor concentrates for a bleeding problem such as hemophilia?	No specific requirement.	A. Persons with hemophilia or related clotting disorders who have received clotting factor concentrates should not donate blood or blood components. (FDA Memo 4/23/92[3])	
B. In the past 12 months, have you had sex, even once, with anyone who has taken clotting factor concentrates for a bleeding problem such as hemophilia?		B. Persons who have had sex with any person with hemophilia or related clotting disorders who have received clotting factor concentrates should not donate blood or blood components for 12 months. (FDA memo 4/23/92[3])	
27. A. Do you have AIDS or have you had a positive test for the AIDS virus?	Refer to question #21.	A. Persons with clinical or laboratory evidence of HIV infection must not donate blood or blood components. (FDA Memo 4/23/92[3])	

Table 9-1 American Association of Blood Banks Uniform Donor History Questionnaire—cont'd

DONOR HISTORY QUESTIONS	AMERICAN ASSOCIATION OF BLOOD BANKS	FOOD AND DRUG ADMINISTRATION	COMMENTS
B. In the past 12 months, have you had sex, even once, with anyone who has AIDS or has had a positive test for the AIDS virus?		B. Persons who have had sex with persons with clinical or laboratory evidence of HIV infection should not donate blood or blood components for 12 months. (FDA Memo 4/23/92[3])	
28. Are you giving blood because you want to be tested for HIV or the AIDS virus?	No specific requirement.	No specific requirement.	Direct questions to further evaluate donation motive.
29. Do you understand that if you have the AIDS virus, you can give it to someone else even though you may feel well and have a negative AIDS test?	No specific requirement.	Donors should be informed that there is an interval during early infection when the HIV antibody test may be negative although the infection may still be transmitted. (FDA Memo 4/23/92[3])	Queries donor's understanding of "Important Information for Donors." Alternative testing site information should be offered.
30. A. Were you born in, have you lived in, or have you traveled to any African country since 1977?	(Association Bulletin 97-5[11])	(FDA Memo 12/11/96[12])	A. If "no," proceed to the questions about sexual contact. If "yes," the donor should be asked to name the specific country(ies). If the donor identifies an African country *not* listed in the FDA Memo, proceed to question C. If one or more of the countries listed in the FDA Memo is named by the donor, determine if the donor was born in, lived in, or traveled to the country(ies) named by the donor. If the donor was born in or lived in any of the FDA-identified countries, defer him/her indefinitely; questioning stops here. If travel was the donor's risk, ask questions. The Central African Republic was named the Central African Empire in the late 1970s. None of the other countries listed in the FDA Memo have undergone a change in name since 1977. Blood establishments should critically evaluate the potential donor's history

Table 9-1 American Association of Blood Banks Uniform Donor History Questionnaire—cont'd

DONOR HISTORY QUESTIONS	AMERICAN ASSOCIATION OF BLOOD BANKS	FOOD AND DRUG ADMINISTRATION	COMMENTS
			and statements, and decide whether the individual could have been in the country long enough to have encountered those local conditions related to risk, such as use of unsterile needles or sexual contact. When donors report demographic HIV-1 Group O risk, no followup actions regarding previously donated blood are necessary.
B. When you traveled to <country(ies)> did you receive a blood transfusion or any other medical treatment with a product made from blood?			B. If "no," proceed to question C. If "yes," defer indefinitely.
C. Have you had sexual contact with anyone who was born in or lived in any African country since 1977?			C. If "no," or the donor names a country not identified in the FDA Memo, no deferral. If "yes," ask the donor to specify which country(ies). If donor names a country listed in the FDA Memo, defer him/her indefinitely.
31. In the past 12 months, have you been in jail or prison?	Donors are deferred for 12 months if, in the preceding 12 months, they have been incarcerated in a correctional institution (jail or prison) for more than 72 consecutive hours. (Standard B2.726)	Individuals who have been incarcerated for more than 72 consecutive hours during the previous 12 months should be deferred as donors for 12 months from the last date of incarceration. (FDA Memo 6/8/95[14])	
32. Have you read and understood all the donor information presented to you, and have all your questions been answered?	No specific requirement.	Information should be written in language that ensures that the donor understands the definition of high-risk behavior and the importance of self-exclusion. Donors should not be considered suitable unless information about risks can be communicated in the language appropriate to them and is constructed to be culturally sensitive to promote comprehension. (FDA Memo 4/23/92[4])	

and with some blood-borne diseases, an available screening test may not currently exist.

A history of yellow jaundice, liver disease, viral hepatitis, IV drug use, or a positive test for hepatitis generally necessitates a permanent deferral of the donor. Potential contact with hepatitis from body piercing, tattoos, or living with a person with symptomatic viral hepatitis necessitates a 12-month deferral.[2] Table 9-2 lists potential hepatitis exposures necessitating deferral.

Malaria, Chagas' disease, and babesiosis are parasitic infections that can be transmitted through transfusion. Malaria is caused by several species of the protozoan genus *Plasmodium*. Chagas' disease is endemic in South and Central America and is caused by the parasite *Trypanosoma cruzi*. An enzyme-linked immunosorbent assay test for antibodies to *T. cruzi* is currently being used in blood centers where the number of immigrants from endemic areas is high. Infected deer ticks in the northeastern United States can spread the parasite *Babesia microti,* which causes human babesiosis. The primary method of screening for these diseases is by questioning donors regarding travel or immigration from endemic areas. Donors who have had malaria are deferred for 3 years. Donors with a history of having babesiosis or Chagas' disease would be deferred indefinitely.[4]

Certain medications may cause some deferrals based on the nature of the disease process they are being used for and not because of the drug's properties. Antibiotics, anticonvulsants, anticoagulants, digitalis, insulin, vasodilators, or antiarrhythmic drugs are prescribed for conditions that would generally exclude donors. Exceptions include etretinate (Tegison), which necessitates a permanent deferral, and isotretinoin (Accutane) and finasteride (Proscar or Propecia), which necessitate a one-month deferral.[5] Box 9-1 partially lists medications commonly accepted for blood donation.[4]

Table 9-2 Temporary Deferrals

DEFERRAL TIME	REASON FOR DEFERRAL
2 weeks	Measles (rubeola) vaccine Mumps vaccine Polio (oral) vaccine Typhoid (oral) vaccine Yellow fever vaccine
4 weeks	German measles (rubella) vaccine Varicella-zoster (chickenpox) vaccine
6 weeks	Conclusion of pregnancy
12 months	Hepatitis B immune globulin Tattoo Mucous-membrane or skin-penetration exposure to blood Sexual contact with an individual at high risk for human immunodeficiency virus Incarceration in a correctional institution for more than 72 hours Return from a malarial-endemic area Completion of therapy for syphilis Transfusion of blood, components, or derivatives Human diploid cell–rabies vaccine following an animal bite Victims of rape
3 years	Asymptomatic after diagnosis of malaria

BOX 9-1

Medications Commonly Accepted for Blood Donation

- Hypnotics used at bedtime
- Blood pressure medications (if patient is free of side effects and cardiovascular symptoms)
- Over-the-counter bronchodilators
- Decongestants
- Oral contraceptives
- Replacement hormones
- Weight-reduction drugs
- Mild analgesics
- Vitamins
- Tetracyclines and other antibiotics taken for acne

Aspirin and aspirin-containing medications depress platelet function. For this reason donors who are the only source of platelets for a patient (such as apheresis donors) are deferred for 36 hours.[6]

Donors receiving vaccinations that are prepared from toxoids or killed organisms do not require deferral if the donor is free of symptoms. The use of attenuated viral and bacterial vaccines generally necessitates a temporary deferral as indicated in Table 9-2. Recombinant vaccines such as hepatitis B do not necessitate deferral. A 12-month deferral is necessary if the donor was exposed to an animal that resulted in the need for a rabies vaccination.

Human pituitary growth hormone (pit-hGH) has been associated with transmission of Creutzfeldt-Jakob (CJD) disease. Since the potential exists for transmission of CJD through a transfusion, pit-hGH recipients must not donate. A history of familial CJD or dura matter transplants from brain surgery is also reason for permanent deferral.[7]

A 12-month deferral is necessary if a prospective donor has had a positive test for syphilis or has been treated for syphilis or gonorrhea.[8] Although transmitting syphilis through a transfusion is unlikely, the potential high-risk behavior that makes transmission of other infectious diseases more likely is the main reason for deferral.

Verbal questions regarding high-risk behavior associated with transmission of the HIV virus are required.[2] Donors must understand the activities that may be considered high risk, and they must be deferred if they are donating for the purpose of HIV testing. Alternate site testing should be offered to individuals seeking HIV testing. Donors must also be informed of local requirements and policies that necessitate notification to governmental agencies of the donor's HIV status. Deferral is required for donors who have had sexual contact with anyone who:

- Has used a needle to take drugs not prescribed by a doctor
- Has taken clotting factor concentrates for a bleeding problem
- Has AIDS or has had a positive test for the AIDS virus

In addition males who have had sex with another male since 1977 are permanently deferred. Females who have had sexual contact with a male who has had sex with another male are deferred for 12 months. The donor's responses to these questions could lead to additional questions or to a temporary or permanent deferral from donating. See Table 9-2 and Box 9-2.

BOX 9-2

Conditions for Indefinite Deferral

- History of viral hepatitis
- Confirmed positive test for hepatitis B surface antigen
- Repeatedly reactive test to antibodies to hepatitis B core
- Clinical or laboratory evidence of human T cell lymphotropic virus
- Clinical or laboratory evidence of human immunodeficiency virus
- Family history of Creutzfeldt-Jakob disease
- Recipient of dura mater or human pituitary growth hormone
- Treatment with etretinate (Tegison)
- History of babesiosis or Chagas' disease

Physical Examination

General Appearance

The prospective donor should appear to be in generally good health. Donors should be deferred if alcohol or drug use is suspected.

Hemoglobin or Hematocrit Determination

Blood for the hemoglobin or hematocrit test is obtained from venipuncture, finger stick, or earlobe stick. For whole blood donation the minimum hemoglobin level is 12.5 g/dl (125 g/L) or minimum hematocrit of 38%.[9] This ensures a sufficient hemoglobin level to allow the removal of a maximum of 525 ml, including samples drawn for testing without harming the donor.

The spun hematocrit is determined by centrifugation of a capillary tube filled with blood. The hemoglobin can be estimated by the use of copper sulfate ($CuSO_4$) or determined by spectrophotometric methods. The $CuSO_4$ method is based on the fact that blood dropped into a $CuSO_4$ solution becomes encased in a sac of copper proteinate and the specific gravity of the drop is not changed for about 15 seconds. If the specific gravity of the blood is higher than that of the solution, the drop sinks within 15 seconds. If the specific gravity of the blood is less than that of the $CuSO_4$, it remains suspended or rises to the top. A specific gravity of 1.053 corresponds to a hemoglobin concentration of 12.5 g/dl.

Temperature

Body temperature should not exceed 37.5° C (99.5° F).[9] An elevated temperature could indicate a possible infection in the donor, which could pose a danger to the recipient.

Blood Pressure

Systolic pressure: contraction of the heart; the first sound heard while taking a blood pressure.
Diastolic pressure: filling of the heart chamber; the second sound heard while taking a blood pressure.

Systolic pressure should be no greater than 180 mm Hg, and the **diastolic pressure** should be no greater than 100 mm Hg.[9] Elevated blood pressure or abnormal differences in the systolic and diastolic pressures could indicate health problems.

Pulse

The pulse should be between 50 and 100 beats per minute and exhibit no pathologic irregularities.[9] Lower rates may be acceptable if the donor is an athlete.

Table 9-3 Physical Examination Requirements

Criteria checked	Acceptable limit
Appearance	In good health
Hemoglobin	≥12.5 g/dl (125 g/L)
Hematocrit	≥38%
Blood pressure	Systolic: <180 mm Hg; Diastolic: <100 mm Hg
Temperature	≤37.5° C (99.5° F)
Pulse	Between 50 to 100 beats/min
Weight	≥110 lb (50 kg)

Weight

Donors weighing a minimum of 110 lb (50 kg) can tolerate a maximum withdrawal of 525 ml, including samples drawn for processing. Donors who weigh less are not restricted from donating, but a proportionally smaller amount of blood should be removed. The formula for reducing the anticoagulant in proportion to the volume collected is found in Chapter 11, Box 11-2. The physical examination criteria for blood donation are summarized in Table 9-3.

Confidential Unit Exclusion

Confidential Unit Exclusion: method that allows donors to exclude their unit from the general inventory following donation in a confidential manner.

In many blood centers donors are given an opportunity to request that their unit be discarded after donation. **Confidential Unit Exclusion** (CUE) provides donors with a confidential way to inform the blood center, without specifics, that their blood may not be safe to transfuse.

Confidential exclusion can be accomplished in various ways. One way is to give the donor two bar code labels that only a computer scanner can read. One confirms that the unit of blood "should be used for transfusion," and the other instructs the blood center to "discard the blood after testing." One bar code is affixed to the donation form and the other is discarded (Fig. 9-1). Since the donor room staff cannot read the stickers, the donation process continues regardless of which sticker is selected. After the donor leaves, the sticker is read to determine whether the blood should be labeled and made available for transfusion. Testing the unit is optional if the unit is not used.

Informed Consent

The donor must sign a written informed consent to allow blood to be collected and used. The donor is asked to read and sign a statement that shows an under-

CONFIDENTIAL SAFETY CHECK FOR DONORS

PLEASE STICK ONE OF THESE LABELS ON YOUR MEDICAL HISTORY QUESTIONNAIRE.

- Place the ***OK TO USE MY BLOOD*** label on your form if you believe your donation would be safe for patient use.
- Affix the ***THROW MY BLOOD AWAY*** label if you believe for any reason that your donation would be unsafe for a patient. Your blood will be tested, however use of this label permanently excludes you as a future donor.

• SOME PEOPLE MAY FEEL THE NEED TO DONATE BECAUSE OF PRESSURE FROM FRIENDS, RELATIVE OR CO-WORKERS. DON'T TAKE THE CHANCE OF HURTING A PATIENT IF YOU FEEL THAT YOUR BLOOD MAY NOT BE SAFE.

OK TO USE MY BLOOD

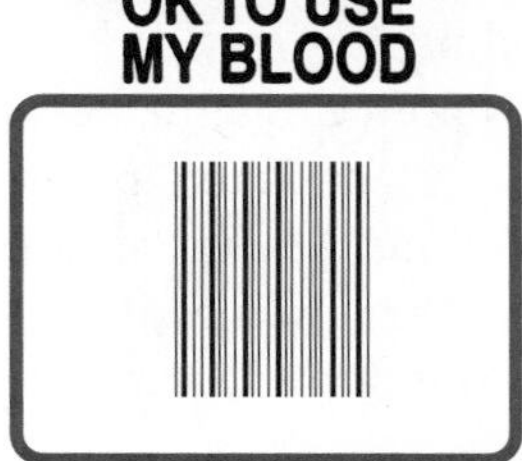

THROW MY BLOOD AWAY

ONLY A COMPUTER SCANNER WILL BE ABLE TO READ YOUR REPLY.
TO MAINTAIN THIS CONFIDENTIALITY, PLEASE DISCARD THE REMAINING PORTION OF THIS FORM.

Central Florida Blood Bank, Inc. **4/93**

Fig. 9-1 Confidential Unit Exclusion.
Courtesy of Central Florida Blood Bank, Inc., Orlando, Fla.

standing of all the donor information presented, including what high-risk behaviors are included. The donor is also asked if he or she has additional questions.[9] The donor is then informed about the infectious disease tests to be run on the blood, and that he or she will be notified if testing indicates that the blood presents a risk for transmitting disease; his or her name is then placed on a list to defer future donations.

PHLEBOTOMY

Identification

The donor's identity should be confirmed at each step of the donation process. The phlebotomist is often different from the person taking the donor's health history; therefore he or she needs to confirm the identity of the donor before beginning the venipuncture. Next, the antecubital area of both donor arms needs to be inspected. This gives the phlebotomist the opportunity to select the arm with the best vein and the ability to check for skin lesions and intravenous drug use.

Bag Labeling

The primary bag used for blood collection, all attached satellite bags, sample tubes, and the donor registration form must be labeled with a unique identification number. The label consists of both numbers (or letters) readable by the phlebotomist and bar codes used for computer scanning. The use of identical numbers allows the collected blood, prepared components, and the blood samples used for testing to be traced back to the original donor registration record.

Arm Preparation and Venipuncture

After an appropriate vein has been selected, the skin needs to be prepared for the venipuncture. Skin cannot be sterilized, but several methods are acceptable for disinfecting the drawing site.

The venipuncture site is scrubbed with a 70% aqueous scrub solution of iodophor compound to remove surface dirt and bacteria and begin germicidal action. Next a prep solution of 10% PVP-iodine is applied beginning at the intended venipuncture site and continuing outward in a concentric spiral. The area is allowed to air dry for 30 seconds before being covered with sterile gauze. Green soap (Exidine) should be used for donors sensitive to iodine.[4]

A tourniquet or blood pressure cuff inflated to 40 to 60 mm Hg makes the vein more prominent for venipuncture. A 16-gauge needle attached to a primary blood bag is inserted into a large firm vein free of skin lesions. The usual donation time for a unit of whole blood is 8 to 12 minutes. After the needle is removed, pressure is applied to the venipuncture site and the donor's arm is elevated. Two to four tubes to be used for testing are filled.

Adverse Donor Reactions

Donors usually tolerate the donation process, but adverse reactions do occur. Most reactions are vasovagal, which may include sweating, rapid breathing, dizziness, nausea, and syncope (fainting). Whether caused by the actual loss of blood or the sight or thought of donating blood, the tourniquet and needle are removed and immediate treatment is initiated at the first sign of a reaction. Instructions for handling donor reactions, including procedures for emergency medical treatment, must be available to the staff and part of their training.[4] Table 9-4 summarizes possible donor reactions and appropriate treatment.[4]

Postdonation Care

The donor is given postphlebotomy instructions to:

- Avoid alcohol and smoking immediately after leaving
- Drink more fluids than usual for 3 days
- Be cautious of dizziness or fainting that may occur

Table 9-4 Adverse Donor Reactions and Appropriate Treatment

SYMPTOMS	TREATMENT
Weakness, sweating, dizziness, pallor, nausea and vomiting	Remove needle and tourniquet Raise feet above head Apply cold compresses to forehead and back of neck
Syncope (fainting)	Apply aromatic spirits of ammonia
Twitching, muscle spasms	Have donor rebreathe into a paper bag
Hematoma	Apply pressure for 7 to 10 minutes; apply ice to area for 5 minutes
Convulsions	Call for help Prevent donor from falling from the donor chair or injuring himself or herself Make sure the donor's airway is adequate
Cardiac difficulties	Begin cardiopulmonary resuscitation; call for emergency help

◆ Inform the blood center if any symptoms persist

Postdonation fluid replacement begins in the donor room. Total fluid volume replacement is usually restored within 72 hours of donation. Iron replacement takes substantially longer; therefore the whole blood donor is eligible to donate again after 56 days.

SPECIAL BLOOD COLLECTION

Autologous Donations

A voluntary donation of blood for use by the general patient population is called *allogeneic*. Any donation of blood reserved for the donor's own use at a later time, which is the safest transfusion possible, is considered an *autologous* donation. Risk of disease transmission, transfusion reactions, or alloimmunization to red blood cells, platelets, white blood cells, or plasma proteins is significantly reduced. Physicians encourage autologous donations for patients undergoing planned surgery who are well enough to undergo the donation process. Requirements for autologous donors are significantly different from allogeneic donors and are described in the following section. Advantages and disadvantages of autologous donations are summarized on Box 9-3.

Four general types of autologous procedures exist: preoperative collection, intraoperative hemodilution, intraoperative collection, and postoperative collection. Preoperative autologous donation is the most common and necessitates careful tracking and handling to ensure units are available for surgery. Each category is summarized below.

BOX 9-3

Autologous Donations: Advantages and Disadvantages

ADVANTAGES

Prevention of transfusion-transmitted diseases
Prevention of alloimmunization
Supplementing the blood supply
Prevention of febrile and allergic reactions
Reassurance of patient

DISADVANTAGES

Inventory control
Postponement of surgery
Increased cost
High wastage
Adverse reactions to donations

Preoperative Collection

In preoperative collection the blood is drawn and stored before the anticipated transfusion. This procedure, used for stable patients scheduled for surgical procedures likely to necessitate blood transfusion, is especially useful for patients with antibodies that make crossmatching allogeneic units difficult or for patients whose religious beliefs do not allow allogeneic transfusions. Prospective autologous donors being treated for bacteremia are ineligible.

The preoperative blood collection process begins with a written order from the patient's physician. Informed consent must be obtained from the patient (donor) with written notification that all test results are released to their physician. Criteria for donor selection do not include high-risk questions. The collecting facility's medical director establishes guidelines concerning the autologous donor's health for donation eligibility. Donors are not restricted by age; the ability for younger patients to donate is determined more by the size of the patient. For patients weighing less than 110 lb (50 kg), the volume of blood collected and the amount of anticoagulant used should be proportionately less. The hemoglobin concentration should be no less than 11 g/dl. The hematocrit should be no less than 33%.[9] Blood is not typically drawn more frequently than every 72 hours and not drawn within 72 hours of surgery. In addition to the routine labeling of the blood bag, the patient's name, transfusion facility, unique patient identifier (Social Security number, birthdate, hospital number, etc.), and an "autologous use only" or "autologous donor" statement are included.[4]

ABO and Rh typing must be determined at the collecting facility. If the blood is transfused outside the collecting facility, tests for hepatitis B surface antigen,

HIV-1 antigen, antibodies to HIV-1/2, antibodies to hepatitis C, antibodies to hepatitis B core, and a serologic test for syphilis must be performed before shipping. These tests must be performed on at least the first unit shipped within each 30-day period.[9] A repeatedly reactive viral test does not necessarily mean that the unit is destroyed as allogeneic units are. With permission of the patient's physician and the receiving facility's transfusion service, units can ship after a biohazard label has been affixed.[9]

The AABB *Standards* prohibits unused units collected for autologous donation to crossover to allogeneic transfusion, since this crossover does not fit the "volunteer donor" requirement.[9]

Intraoperative Hemodilution

Intraoperative hemodilution involves removing one or more units of blood at the beginning of surgery. The blood removed is replaced with crystalloid or colloid solutions to restore fluid volume. The blood is stored for reinfusion during or at the end of surgery.

The units must be labeled with the patient's name, a unique identifying number, the date and time of phlebotomy, and an "autologous use only" label. Blood collected in this manner can be stored at room temperature for up to 8 hours, or at 1° to 6° C for up to 24 hours.[9]

Intraoperative Collection

During intraoperative blood collection a medical device is used to collect shed blood from the operative field. Following collection it is reinfused to the patient. The process can include collecting and directly reinfusing the blood using a device that washes, filters, and concentrates it. Washing does not remove bacteria; therefore intraoperative blood collection should not be used if the operative field has bacterial contamination (Fig. 9-2).

Units collected from a sterile operating field and processed with a device for intraoperative blood collection that washes with 0.9% saline can be stored at room temperature for up to 6 hours or at 1° to 6° C for up to 24 hours. Transfusion of blood collected intraoperatively by other means should begin within 6 hours.[9] The labeling of these units is the same as that for units collected by intraoperative hemodilution.

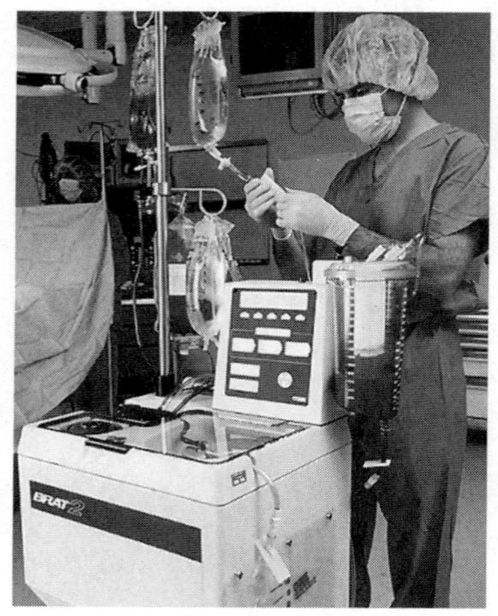

Fig. 9-2 Intraoperative cell recovery instrument.

Courtesy of COBE Cardiovascular, Arvada, Colo.

Postoperative Collection

With postoperative collection blood is collected from surgical drains followed by reinfusion with or without processing. Blood is often collected into sterile canisters. Transfusion must begin within 6 hours of initiating the collection.[9]

Directed Donations

The public's concern for the safety of blood supply led to demands from potential recipients to chose their own donors. Although no substantial evidence exists that directed donations provide safer blood than allogeneic donations, most blood centers and hospitals participate in a directed-donor program. Donor requirements and testing must meet the same criteria as donations not reserved for certain patients. The donor screening, health history, and phlebotomy are the same for directed donors as for routine blood donors. Policies regarding crossover to the general patient population, determination of the ABO type before collection, additional fees, and time for unit availability vary among institutions. The 56-day interval between donations may be waived with the medical director's approval.

Hemapheresis

Heme means "related to blood," and *apheresis* means "to remove." Hemapheresis is a category of procedures in which whole blood is removed from a donor or patient, a component is separated by mechanical means, and the remainder of the blood is returned. The following terms describe the portion that is removed:

- Leukapheresis: white blood cells are removed
- Plateletpheresis: platelets are removed
- Plasmapheresis: plasma is removed

These procedures are used with donors to collect a greater quantity of a specific component than can be obtained from single whole blood donations. The procedure in patients is used to treat various diseases (**therapeutic apheresis**), which is described in more detail in Chapter 14.

Therapeutic apheresis: removal of blood from a patient and retainment of the portion that may be contributing to a pathologic condition; remainder is returned along with a replacement fluid such as colloid or fresh frozen plasma.

Apheresis was originally performed manually. The process involved removing a unit of whole blood, centrifuging it, removing the desired component, and returning the remaining blood before removing the next unit. Currently apheresis is routinely performed with a cell separator machine (Fig. 9-3). Centrifugal force is used to separate the blood into components based on their specific gravity. The blood flows directly from the donor's arm into the centrifuge bowl, a specific component is removed, and the remainder of the blood is returned to the donor; all of this occurs within a closed system. Depending on the procedure and the equipment used, the process can vary from 30 minutes to 2 hours. The procedure can be performed by intermittent or continuous flow. An intermittent flow process involves one venipuncture; blood is removed, centrifuged, and returned in alternating steps. A continuous flow procedure necessitates a venipuncture in both arms; blood is removed from one arm, centrifuged, and returned in the other arm.

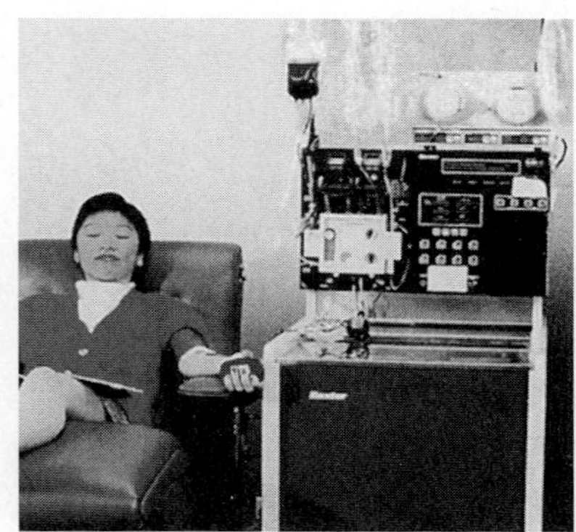

Fig. 9-3 Apheresis instrument.
Courtesy of Baxter Healthcare Corp., Deerfield, Ill.

In general the same standards that apply to whole blood donation apply to plasmapheresis, plateletpheresis, and leukapheresis donation. Frequency of donation and additional donor testing vary according to the type of apheresis performed. Plateletpheresis donors must have a platelet count of at least 150,000 per μl, and at least 48 hours must elapse between donations.[9] Donors cannot donate more than twice per week or 24 times per year. Collection of plasma by pheresis more often than once every 8 weeks necessitates that total plasma protein, IgG, and IgM levels be monitored at 4-month intervals.[10]

Therapeutic Phlebotomy

A therapeutic phlebotomy is performed to withdraw blood from a patient for medical reasons. Although the removal does not cure the diseases, it can help treat the patient's symptoms. Common indications for therapeutic phlebotomy include polycythemia, hemochromatosis, and porphyrias. Blood collected for therapeutic reasons cannot be used for allogeneic transfusion.[9]

CHAPTER SUMMARY

Careful donor selection by trained blood bank personnel is the most important element in ensuring a safe blood supply. Registration and donor identification determine whether insufficient time has elapsed for donating or if the donor was previously deferred. Donors must be informed of high-risk behavior and discouraged from donating if they have the potential of transmitting infection through the blood supply. Blood is not tested for certain diseases, such as malaria and babesiosis; therefore questions regarding exposure and travel are important for screening purposes. In addition medical history questions and a brief physical examination determine whether the donation process might adversely affect the donor. Thus the safety of the donor and the recipient is an important element of the screening process.

Confirmation of donor identity and careful bag and sample labeling must be performed before phlebotomy. Arm preparation to avoid contamination with bacteria involves a two-step disinfecting procedure. Signs of adverse donor reactions during phlebotomy, although uncommon, must be recognized and responded to quickly. Postdonation instructions to the donor regarding activities to avoid and the importance of increasing fluid intake complete the donation process.

Special donations, such as autologous, directed, apheresis, and therapeutic phlebotomy, are important donor and patient services that necessitate unique policies and procedures. The minimum requirements for allogeneic and special donation procedures, determined by the AABB and FDA, must be carefully followed. Careful donor screening, along with testing described in Chapter 10, ensures the safest possible blood supply.

CRITICAL THINKING EXERCISES

◆ *EXERCISE 9-1*

A potential donor is being questioned regarding her previous medical history, and she states that she has been in Ethiopia (a malarial area) for 1 year doing Peace Corps activities. She just returned last week. Can she donate? If not, how long must she wait?

◆ *EXERCISE 9-2*

A potential donor has the following results on a physical exam:

Hemoglobin:	14 g/dl
Temperature:	98.9° F
Weight:	150 lb
Blood pressure:	140/80
Pulse:	80 beats per minute

She states she has had aspirin for a headache that day and received hepatitis B immune globulin for a needle-stick 3 months ago. Can she donate? Is there a deferral time?

◆ *EXERCISE 9-3*

A 16-year-old female would like to donate blood for her relative. She weighs 108 lb and has finished the hepatitis-B vaccination series 2 weeks ago as a school requirement.

1. Is she an eligible donor?
2. Are exceptions made for directed donations?
3. If she were donating for herself, could she donate?
4. What are some of the issues surrounding directed donations?

◆ ***EXERCISE 9-4***

An 18-year-old male donated for the first time at a blood drive at his high school. Concerned that he may have contacted HIV, he used the CUE to keep his unit out of the blood supply. Explain the reasons why he used the CUE, and why he may have donated. Why are questions regarding HIV so important when there are tests performed to detect the virus?

◆ ***EXERCISE 9-5***

While scrubbing a donor's arm, the phlebotomist was distracted by another donor's reaction and did not use the second cleansing solution. What potential problems could this cause? Would it affect the donor or the recipient of those blood products?

STUDY QUESTIONS

For questions 1 through 10, determine the best course of action based on the information for potential whole blood allogeneic donors. Indicate whether you would:

A	=	Accept
TD	=	Temporarily defer
PD	=	Permanently defer

1. A 28-year-old female; 112 lb; hemoglobin, 12.5 g/dl; miscarried 2 weeks ago

2. A 56-year-old man; 168 lb; hematocrit, 44%; blood pressure, 180/95; took aspirin 4 hours ago for arthritis pain

3. A 35-year-old female; copper sulfate screen, blood drop sinks in 12 seconds; 115 lb; blood pressure, 118/76; pulse, 65; temperature, 37° C.

4. A high-school student; 17-year-old female; taking Accutane for acne

5. Donor center volunteer; 75-year-old male; first-time blood donor; had hepatitis 20 years ago following surgery

6. A 21-year-old male; received tattoo in the service 4 months ago

7. A 65-year-old female; has instructions from physician to donate for upcoming surgery; had syphilis and was treated 40 years ago; blood pressure, 130/80; pulse, 78; hematocrit, 37%; temperature, 99° F

8. A 38-year-old male; received rabies vaccine after a dog bite 3 months ago

9. A 19-year-old first-time donor; received human growth hormone 12 years ago

10. A 24-year-old donor with history of a positive test for hepatitis C from another blood center

11. Which is a cause for temporary deferral of a whole blood donor?
    a. influenza injection
    b. antibiotics 4 weeks ago
    c. oral polio vaccine 4 weeks ago
    d. rubella injection 2 weeks ago

12. A donor with a physician's request to donate for planned surgery in 3 weeks has a hemoglobin of 10 g/dl. She is:
    a. permitted to donate as an autologous donor
    b. deferred because of a low hemoglobin
    c. permitted to donate with the approval of the blood bank's medical director
    d. permitted to donate a smaller unit of blood

13. Plateletpheresis donors cannot donate more than:
    a. twice a week
    b. 24 times a year
    c. every 48 hours
    d. all of the above

True or False

___ 14. Viral marker tests are not required on autologous blood to be used within the collection facility.

___ 15. Autologous units may be given to other patients if they are not used for the patient who donated it.

REFERENCES

1. Food and Drug Administration: *Code of federal regulations,* 21 CFR 600-799 (revised annually), Washington, DC, 1996, Office of the Federal Register.
2. Food and Drug Administration: *Memorandum: revised recommendations for the prevention of human immunodeficiency virus (HIV) transmission by blood and blood products,* Rockville, Md, April 23, 1992, Congressional and Consumer Affairs.
3. American Association of Blood Banks: Uniform donor history questionnaire. Available at: www.aabb.org/docs/ab98-3public.htm. Accessed June 3, 1999.
4. Vengelen-Tyler V, editor: *Technical manual,* ed 13, Bethesda, Md, 1999, American Association of Blood Banks.
5. Food and Drug Administration: *Memorandum: deferral of blood and plasma donors based on medications,* Rockville, Md, July 28, 1993, Congressional and Consumer Affairs.
6. Food and Drug Administration: *Memorandum: revised guideline for the collection of platelets, pheresis,* Rockville, Md, October 7, 1988, Congressional and Consumer Affairs.
7. Food and Drug Administration: *Memorandum: precautionary measures to further reduce the possible risk of transmission of Creutzfeldt-Jakob disease by blood products,* Rockville, Md, August 8, 1995, Congressional and Consumer Affairs.
8. Food and Drug Administration: *Memorandum: clarification of FDA recommendations for donor deferral and product distribution based on the results of syphilis testing,* Rockville, Md, December 12, 1991, Congressional and Consumer Affairs.
9. Menitove JE, editor: *Standards for blood banks and transfusion services,* ed 19, Bethesda, Md, 1999, American Association of Blood Banks.
10. Food and Drug Administration: *Code of federal regulations,* 21 CFR 640.65 (revised annually), Washington DC, 1996, US Government Printing Office.

DONOR BLOOD TESTING

10

Carol J. Grant

CHAPTER OUTLINE

LEARNING OBJECTIVES

Upon completion of this chapter, the reader should be able to:

1. Describe the enzyme-linked immunosorbent assay (EIA), and differentiate among sandwich, indirect, and competitive EIA techniques.
2. Compare internal and external controls in EIA testing.
3. Compare sensitivity with specificity.
4. List the required tests performed on allogeneic and autologous donor blood.
5. List the optional tests performed on allogeneic blood donors.
6. Discuss the theory and use of the Western blot test as a confirmatory test.
7. Describe when cytomegalovirus screening is performed.
8. State the frequency of positive tests on blood donated for allogeneic transfusion.
9. Define *look-back* and the Food and Drug Administration requirements with regard to hepatitis C virus and human immunodeficiency virus testing on blood donors.

Table 10-1 Currently Required Viral Marker Tests

Virus	Test
Hepatitis	HBsAg Anti-HBc Anti-HCV ALT
HIV-1/2	Anti–HIV-1/2 HIV-1 p24 antigen
HTLV-I/II	Anti–HTLV-I/II

HBsAg, Hepatitis B surface antigen; *anti-HBc,* antibody to hepatitis B core; *ALT,* alanine aminotransferase; *anti-HCV,* antibody to hepatitis C virus; *HIV,* human immunodeficiency virus; *HTLV,* human T-cell lymphotropic viruses.

The laboratory testing of each unit of blood collected follows careful donor screening in ensuring the safety of the blood supply. Tests include ABO- and Rh-typing, antibody screening, and an ever-expanding series of tests to detect infectious diseases (Tables 10-1 and 10-2).

INFECTIOUS DISEASE TESTING

Infectious disease testing involves a variety of methodologies, but none is more important than the enzyme-linked immunosorbent assay (EIA, or ELISA).

General Enzyme-Linked Immunosorbent Assay Theory

EIA technology can be used to detect the presence of small amounts of antigen or antibody. EIA tests use a solid object such as a plastic bead in a tray, or the well of a plastic microplate, coated with antigen or antibody, depending on the test being run (Fig. 10-1). Although each test varies, the general principles of the test are the same. The **indirect EIA** procedure detects antibodies, whereas the technique used to detect antigen is **sandwich EIA. Competitive EIA** can be used to detect antigen or antibody. Fig. 10-2 illustrates the principle of these EIA techniques. Box 10-1 defines terminology commonly used in EIA testing.

Indirect EIA: enzyme-linked immunosorbent assay technique used to determine the presence or quantity of an antibody.
Sandwich EIA: enzyme-linked immunosorbent assay technique used to determine the presence or quantity of an antigen.
Competitive EIA: enzyme-linked immunosorbent assay technique used to determine the presence or quantity of an antigen or antibody. In this test a lower absorbance indicates detection of the marker.

The interpretation of the results obtained upon completion of the sandwich or indirect EIA test is summarized as follows:

- Specimens with absorbance values less than the cutoff value are considered nonreactive; further testing is not required
- Specimens with absorbance values greater than or equal to the cutoff value are defined as initially reactive
- All initially reactive tests are repeated in duplicate; if both repeat tests are negative, the sample is considered nonreactive, and the donor unit is acceptable for transfusion; if one or both of the repeat tests are positive, the sample is considered reactive, and the unit is discarded
- If a confirmatory test is available, it is routinely performed on tests that are positive after repeat testing

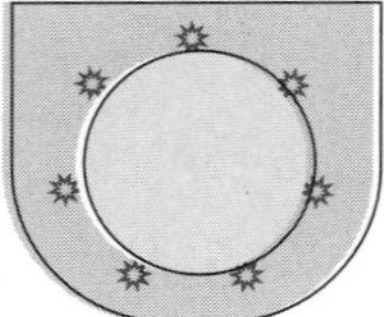
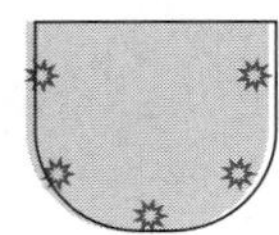

Fig. 10-1 Enzyme-linked immunosorbent assay methodologies. Enzyme-linked immunosorbent assay tests are performed either in a microplate well *(right)* or in a tray containing wells with beads *(left).* The well or the bead contains the antigen or antibody that combines with the antibody or antigen being detected (if present).

Table 10-2 Other Tests Performed on Donated Blood

TEST FOR	METHOD	COMMENTS
Syphilis	Rapid plasma reagin Hemagglutination	Confirmed by fluorescent antibody test
Cytomegalovirus	Hemagglutination Latex agglutination EIA	Not required; performed on units to be transfused to at-risk patients
Chagas' disease	EIA Hemagglutination	Testing is performed in areas endemic for *T. cruzi*
Clinically significant red blood cell antibodies	Tube: indirect AHG Gel card: Gel (e.g., ID-MTS, ReACT) Microplate	Units with antibodies must be labeled to indicate the antibody detected (except for washed or deglycerolized red blood cells or cryoprecipitate)
ABO and Rh	Tube Microplate	Results must be checked with previous donations

EIA, Enzyme-linked immunosorbent assay; *T. cruzi, Trypanosoma cruzi; AHG,* antihuman globulin.

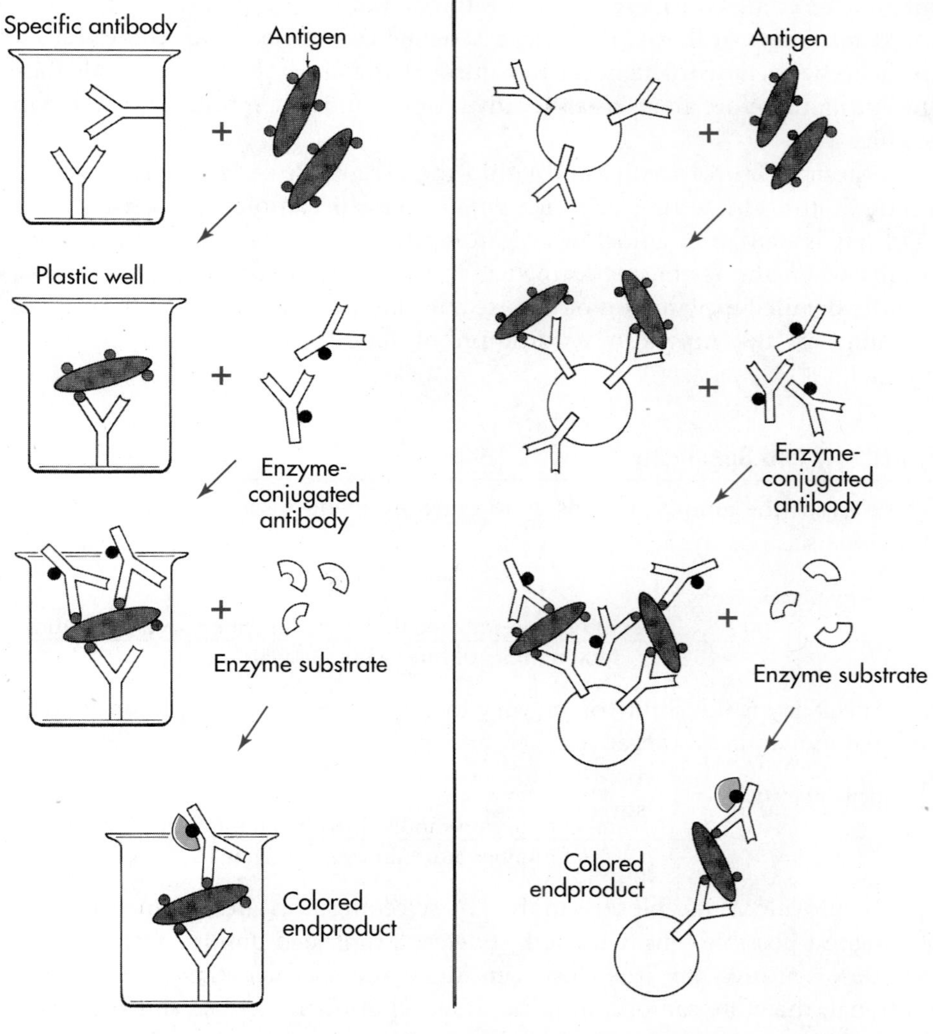

Fig. 10-2 Principle of the solid phase enzyme immunosorbent assay.
Courtesy of Baron EJ, Peterson LR, Finegold SM: *Diagnostic microbiology,* ed 9, St Louis, 1994, Mosby.

BOX 10-1

Enzyme-Linked Immunosorbent Assay Test Terms and Definitions

Internal controls: Validation materials provided with the assay kit
External controls: Reagents or materials that are not part of the test kit used for surveillance of test performance
Cutoff value: Absorbance value unique to each test run that determines a positive or negative result; calculated from the internal controls
Conjugate: Enzyme, usually horseradish peroxidase, labeled antibody or antigen
Substrate: Color developer, usually *o*-phenylenediamine

- If a sample is repeatedly reactive, whether or not the confirmatory test is positive, the blood is not used for allogeneic transfusion

Controls

Internal Controls

EIA testing is performed in donor testing facilities with "kits," which contain specific reagents for each assay, licensed by the Food and Drug Administration (FDA). Positive and negative controls are included in the EIA kit and are run on each microplate or tray of beads. The cutoff value is calculated based on the absorbance values of the controls and a "blank" or background absorbance.

External Controls

The **Clinical Laboratory Improvement Act** regulations state that a positive and a negative control must be tested with each run of patient specimens. The same rule applies to donor testing. Controls provided by a test kit

Clinical Laboratory Improvement Act: enacted to ensure that laboratory tests are consistently reliable and of high quality.

manufacturer are considered calibration material if they are used to calculate the cutoff value. If that is the case, a separate control external to the test kit needs to be included. The negative control in the kit is often used to calculate the cutoff; therefore an external negative control must be routinely included in testing.

External control results not within the acceptable stated range may "invalidate" the EIA testing and necessitate that all samples be retested. The FDA has issued strict guidelines regarding the interpretation of reactive test results when the testing performed is invalid because of external controls.[1] A more detailed explanation of the use and interpretation of external controls is found in the American Association of Blood Banks' (AABB) *Technical Manual.*[2]

Sensitivity and Specificity

Sensitivity is the ability of an assay to correctly identify samples from infected individuals as positive.

$$\text{Sensitivity percentage} = \frac{100 \times \text{Number of positive individuals detected in an infected population}}{\text{Total number of infected individuals tested}}$$

Specificity is the ability of an assay to correctly identify samples from noninfected individuals as negative.

$$\text{Specificity percentage} = \frac{100 \times \text{Number of negative individuals in a noninfected population}}{\text{Total number of noninfected individuals tested}}$$

To provide a safe blood supply, EIA screening tests are designed to have the highest possible sensitivity and to detect all infected donors. Testing is not yet 100% sensitive, but it is close. Sensitivity and specificity are inversely proportional; therefore samples from noninfected donors may occasionally give a false-positive reaction. Because of this limitation, reactive samples must be retested, and confirmatory or supplemental testing must then proceed. The frequency of repeat-reactive test results in the blood donor population appears in Table 10-3.

Table 10-3 Incidence of Repeat Reactive Rates Among Blood and Plasma Donors

Test	Repeat Reactive Rate (%)
HBsAg[3]	0.02
Anti–HIV-1/2[4]	0.09
Anti–HTLV-I/II[5]	0.34
Anti-HCV[6]	0.63
Anti-HBc[7]	1.65
HIV-1 p24[8]	0.11

HBsAg, Hepatitis B surface antigen; *anti-HIV,* antibody to human immunodeficiency virus; *anti-HTLV,* antibody to human T-cell lymphotropic viruses; *anti-HCV,* antibody to hepatitis C virus; *anti-HBc,* antibody to hepatitis B core.

HEPATITIS

Hepatitis Viruses

Hepatitis is an inflammation of the liver that can be caused by bacteria, drugs, alcohol, toxins, and several different viruses, including hepatitis A, B, C, D, and E. The hepatitis viruses are compared on Table 10-4.

Hepatitis A

Hepatitis A, also known as infectious hepatitis, is almost always transmitted by fecal contamination and oral ingestion. The hepatitis A virus (HAV) circulates in the bloodstream only during the initial phase of infection when an individual is usually too ill to donate; however, if blood is collected while the virus is circulating, it can be transmitted by transfusion. Because transfusion-transmission is extremely rare, donated blood is not tested for hepatitis A antigen or antibody.

Table 10-4 Hepatitis Viruses

	HEPATITIS A	HEPATITIS B	HEPATITIS C	HEPATITIS D	HEPATITIS E
Transmission	Enteric; oral and fecal	Parenteral; sexual; perinatal	Parenteral; sexual; perinatal	Parenteral; sexual; perinatal	Enteric; oral and fecal
Incubation	15-50 days	40-160 days	14-300 days	30-50 days	21-42 days
Classification	Picornavirus	Hepadnavirus	Flavivirus	Satellite	Calicivirus
Nucleic acid	RNA	DNA	RNA	RNA	RNA
Tested for	No	Yes	Yes	No	No

RNA, Ribonucleic acid; *DNA*, deoxyribonucleic acid.

Hepatitis B

Originally called serum hepatitis, hepatitis B was the first known hepatitis virus transmitted by blood transfusion. It can also be transmitted **parenterally,** by sexual contact, and **perinatally.**

Parenterally: by routes other than the digestive tract, including needle-stick and transfusion.

Perinatally: exposure before, during, or after the time of birth.

Hepatitis C

Posttransfusion hepatitis persisted after hepatitis B testing was implemented. With no specific virus identified, the posttransfusion hepatitis was termed non-A, non-B hepatitis, but current knowledge shows that most posttransfusion hepatitis is due to hepatitis C.[9] This virus is transmitted by the same methods as hepatitis B.

Hepatitis D

Although hepatitis D is also transmitted by blood, the presence of hepatitis B is necessary to cause disease. Blood is not screened for hepatitis D, since testing for hepatitis B is sufficient to avoid hepatitis-D transmission.

Hepatitis E

Hepatitis E is spread much the same as hepatitis A, through an oral-fecal route; therefore donated blood is not tested.

Hepatitis Tests

To prevent the transmission of hepatitis by transfusion, four tests are currently run on donor blood: hepatitis B surface antigen (HBsAg), antibody to hepatitis B core (anti-HBc), alanine aminotransferase (ALT), and antibody to hepatitis C virus (anti-HCV).

Hepatitis B Surface Antigen

Studies published in 1965 by Blumberg and associates[10] described an antigen in the blood of Australian aborigines that was later named HBsAg. Not all of the hepatitis B virus consists of intact viral particles. Excess noninfectious forms of the antigen consisting of the outer surface of the virus can be found in addition to the intact virus. Because of the large amount present, it is possible to test for the antigen directly.

The HBsAg confirmatory assay uses the principle of specific antibody neutralization to confirm the presence of HBsAg. In the neutralization procedure antibody to HBsAg is incubated with the donor's serum. If HBsAg is present in the serum, it is bound by the antibody. The neutralized HBsAg is then blocked from binding to the antibody-coated solid medium. If the neutralization causes the reaction to disappear or diminish by at least 50%, the original result is considered positive for HBsAg.[2] The neutralization principle is similar to competitive EIA.

Surrogate markers: disease markers such as antibodies or elevations in enzymes that may be used as indicators for other potential infectious diseases; often used when direct testing is not available.

Antibody to Hepatitis B Core

In 1986 anti-HBc and ALT were added as **surrogate markers.** Anti-HBc is an antibody to the inner portion or core of the hepatitis B antigen. These antibodies generally appear after HBsAg is detected, but before the beginning of hepatitis symptoms (Fig. 10-3). Anti-HBc can persist at detectable levels for many years following infection and has been demonstrated in individuals who have transmitted other types of hepatitis. No specific confirmatory test for anti-HBc exists.

Alanine Aminotransferase

ALT is an enzyme highly concentrated in the liver with relatively lower concentrations in heart and other muscle tissues. The level of ALT in the serum is elevated when the liver has been damaged because of various conditions, such as biliary tract disease, viral infections, or alcohol toxicity. An elevated result is often the first indication of liver inflammation.

Standard chemistry analyzers can be used to measure ALT levels. A common method for ALT determination is a coupled enzyme assay that determines the amount of pyruvate produced by L-alanine and α–ketoglutarate in the presence of ALT.[11] The pyruvate produced is combined with nicotinamide adenine diphosphate (NADH) in the presence of lactic dehydrogenase. The rate of disappearance of the NADH is proportional to the amount of pyruvate in the sample. The measurement is done by a spectrophotometer. Although not required by either the

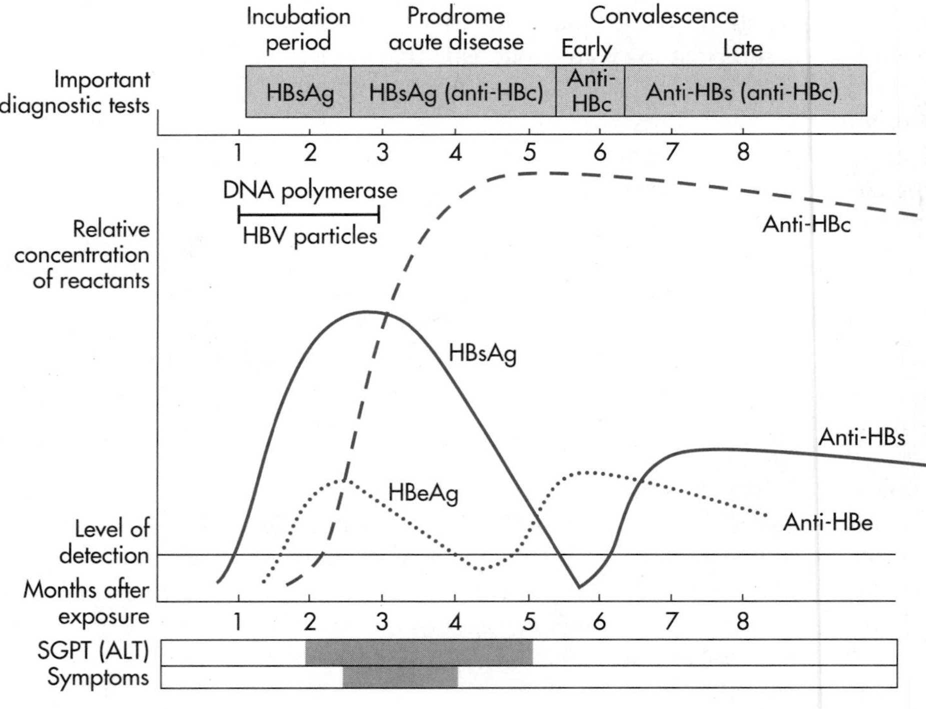

Fig. 10-3 Serologic and clinical patterns observed in hepatitis B. *HBsAg*, Hepatitis B surface antigen; *anti-HBc*, antibody to hepatitis B core; *HBV*, hepatitis B virus; *HBeAg*, hepatitis B e antigen; *anti-HBe*, antibody to hepatitis B e antigen; *ALT*, alanine aminotransferase; *SGPT*, serum glutamate pyruvate transaminase.

Courtesy of Hollinger FB, Dreesman GR. In Rose RN, Friedman H, editors: *Manual of clinical immunology*, ed 2, Washington DC, 1980, American Society for Microbiology.

FDA or AABB, many blood centers continue to perform ALT testing, since it is a requirement of some plasma fractionators in non–United States markets.

For allogeneic transfusion, blood with a level above a predetermined cutoff should not be transfused. No standard cutoff value exists; it is established at each testing facility based on local ALT values.

Antibody to Hepatitis C Virus

In 1989 the existence of hepatitis C was demonstrated, and a test was developed and implemented by 1990. After the EIA test for anti-HCV was added to routine donor blood testing, the incidence of post-transfusion hepatitis dramatically decreased.[12] Nucleic acid amplification testing (NAT), which is also referred to as genome amplification technology, recently has been introduced into blood centers for viral hepatitis C detection. Implementation of NAT by blood centers supplying plasma products for the manufacture of derivatives is required as of July 1, 1999. Polymerase chain reaction (PCR) testing and transcription-mediated amplification are two examples of testing procedures using NAT. By amplifying segments of viral nucleic acids to the level at which they can be detected, it is hoped that the "window period" for HCV and HIV will be shortened. Initial NAT screening by donor centers for HCV is being performed to gather data on the efficacy of this test for general blood donor screening. Chapter 3 describes the principle of the PCR test, and the suggested reading list provides sources of information on current NAT viral marker screening for blood donors.

A recombinant immunoblot assay (RIBA) is used as a supplemental test to determine the specificity of the antibody to HCV. If the EIA test is positive, this assay uses a nitrocellulose strip to which recombinant HCV antigens have been immobilized. During incubation the anti-HCV, if present, reacts with the bound antigen.[13] A positive test strongly correlates with infectivity and is used with the donor's clinical condition to diagnose HCV.

HUMAN RETROVIRUSES

Retroviruses contain reverse transcriptase, which allows the virus to copy its RNA onto DNA and integrate this DNA into that of the host cell. Three subfamilies of retroviruses exist: lentivirus (human immunodeficiency virus [HIV] types 1 and 2), oncornavirus or oncovirus (human T-cell lymphotropic virus [HTLV] types 1, 2, and 5), and spumavirus (no association with human disease).[14]

Three tests are currently used as a screen for retroviruses in donated blood: antibody to HIV type 1 or type 2 (anti–HIV-1/2), HIV type 1 p24 antigen (HIV-1 Ag), and antibody to HTLV types I and II (anti–HTLV-I/II).

Human Immunodeficiency Virus Types 1 and 2

HIV-1 was the first virus designated as the causative agent of acquired immunodeficiency syndrome (AIDS). The long incubation period before symptoms appear promotes the spread of the disease by sexual contact and exposure to blood products. A second type of HIV, HIV-2, was also discovered to cause AIDS. This form of the virus is more common in Africa than in the United States, and it appears to produce a less severe disease. Both forms of the virus are spread by sexual contact, perinatal, breast-feeding, and parenteral exposure to blood.

Testing for the antibody to HIV-1 has been included in donor blood testing since 1985. In 1992 anti–HIV-2 was added to the requirements for donor testing. Most donor centers use a combination test, which detects anti–HIV-1 and anti–HIV-2. Because this test detects antibody, a 22- to 25-day window exists between the time a person is infected and the time the antibody is measurable.[15]

Human Immunodeficiency Virus Type 1 p24 Antigen

In 1996 testing for the HIV antigen type 1 p24 was added to the test for anti-HIV required on all donor blood. The core protein, p24, is the major internal structural protein of HIV-1. Because this is a test for antigen instead of antibody, the time between infection and positive test results was reduced by approximately 6 to 10 days.[16] More sensitive tests using NAT is expected to further shorten the time.

Human T-Cell Lymphotropic Virus Types I and II

HTLV-I has been associated with adult T-cell leukemia (ATL), a rare neoplasm, and tropical spastic paraparesis and HTLV-I associated myelopathy, a semiprogressive neurologic disease.[17,18]

The first reported patients with HTLV-II infections showed an atypical T-cell variant of hairy cell leukemia. HTLV-II is currently assumed to be associated with large granular lymphocyte leukemia[19] and leukopenic chronic T-cell leukemia.[20] HTLV-I and HTLV-II are transmitted through cellular blood products, breast milk, sexual contact, and contaminated needles.

In 1997 the requirement to test for antibody to HTLV-II was added to the requirement to test for antibody to HTLV-I. The two are combined in one assay.

Western Blotting

The Western blot is the most common confirmatory test for both anti–HIV-1/2 and anti–HTLV-I/II. Viral antigen is separated into bands according to molecular weight by polyacrylamide gel electrophoresis in the presence of sodium dodecyl sulfate.[21] The separated bands are then transferred to nitrocellulose membrane strips by blotting. Antibodies in the test serum are then tested for reaction with the individual protein bands (antigen) on the strips. Enzyme-labeled conjugate detects the antibodies bound to the specific proteins on the strip. The pattern of distinct bands is visually compared with a strip that has been tested for reaction with a specimen containing antibodies to *all* HIV proteins (Fig. 10-4). Each licensed Western blot has specific interpretation criteria. Samples producing band patterns that do not fit the criteria for positivity are classified as indeterminate.

LOOK-BACK

Look-back: identification of persons who have received seronegative or untested blood from a donor subsequently found to be positive for HIV or HCV.

The act of identifying and notifying patients who have received seronegative or untested blood from a donor subsequently found to be positive for a viral marker is referred to as **look-back.** Look-back is required for donors with confirmed positive HIV–1/2 antibody or HIV p24 antigen results. The FDA has recently required donors with positive anti-HCV test results to also be included in look-back procedures.[22] Look-back for HCV involves the following steps:

- Identifying all donors who have tested positive for HCV since March, 1992

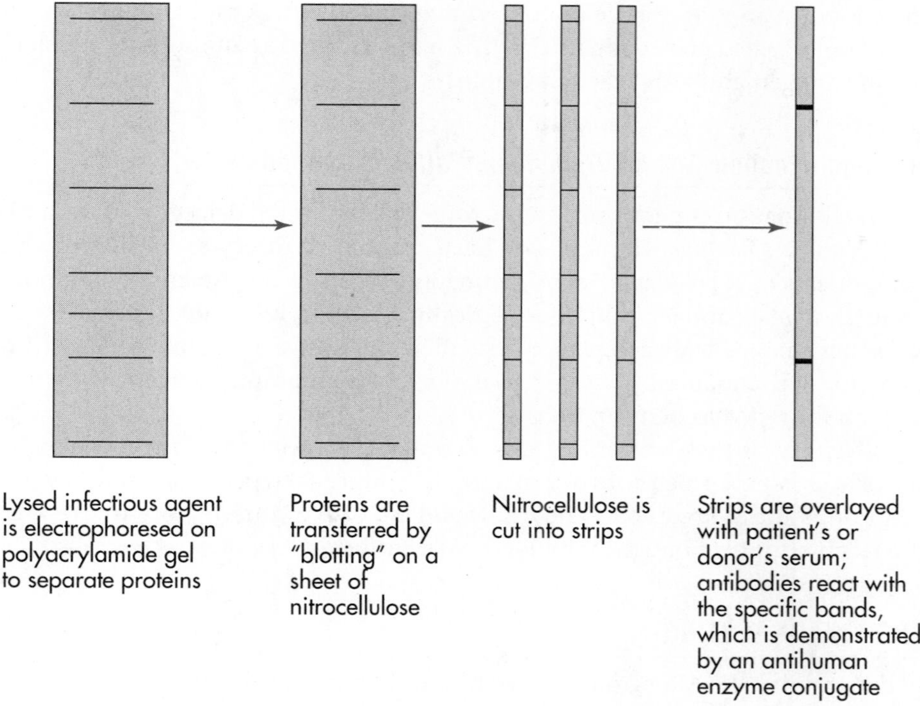

Fig. 10-4 Western blot. Interpretation: Certain band patterns that represent specific antibodies must be present for confirmation of HIV-1. If a definite band pattern does not exist, the sample is considered indeterminate.

- Identifying all blood products provided by these donors before the positive test
- Notifying facilities (hospitals, clinics, etc.) that received these products
- Tracing the product to the patient and notifying him or her of the potential exposure to HCV

Notification of the patient is the responsibility of the facility that transfused the blood.

SYPHILIS

Syphilis is a venereal disease caused by the spirochete *Treponema pallidum*. Although the most common method of transmission is direct sexual contact, at least one case of transmission has occurred through transfusion.[23] Spirochetes do not survive refrigerator temperatures, but fresh blood or platelets stored at room temperature could transmit the organisms. Donated blood can be tested by a variety of methods, including rapid plasma reagin (RPR) or hemagglutination tests.

Rapid Plasma Reagin

The RPR test is a common screening test, even though it is not specific for antibodies to *T. pallidum*. It instead detects reagin, an antibody-like substance in the blood directed against cardiolipin, a widely distributed lipoidal antigen. Cardiolipin antibodies routinely develop in individuals who have had untreated syphilis infection; however, they may also develop after the appearance of other infections. In an RPR test the donor serum is placed onto a card and mixed with cardiolipin-coated charcoal particles. The particles serve as an indicator by making the antigen-antibody reaction visible.

Hemagglutination Test for *Treponema Pallidum* Antibodies

Hemagglutination is performed in microtiter plates for the detection of the antibodies to *T. palladum*. The test uses fixed chicken erythrocytes sensitized with components of *T. pallidum*. Hemagglutination occurs in the presence of antibodies to *T. pallidum* and is read photometrically.[24] Hemagglutination tests for *T. pallidum* have gained wide acceptance since their emergence in the mid-1960s.[25] Automation has enhanced the value of the test by significantly reducing the time and labor needed to perform the assay.[26]

If either of these screening tests is reactive, a specific test for the syphilis spirochete is performed for confirmation. Fluorescent treponemal antibody absorption is the procedure of choice. Regardless of the confirmatory test results, the reactive unit is not used for allogeneic transfusion.

ABO AND Rh TESTING

In determining the ABO group the red blood cells are tested with anti-A and anti-B to detect the presence of A or B antigens. The serum or plasma is tested with A_1 and B cells to detect anti-A or anti-B. The results of the ABO testing are compared to previous ABO results if available. Discrepancies among the cell and serum testing or with previous ABO determinations must be resolved before labeling. Manual techniques are described in Chapter 4.

Routine Rh typing for donors involves testing with reagent anti-D. If the initial D antigen typing is negative, an additional test for weak D is performed. If the initial test or the test for weak D is positive, the unit is labeled as Rh positive. When tests for both D and weak D are negative, the unit is labeled as Rh negative. Manual techniques are described in Chapter 5. In donor centers ABO and Rh typing are often performed on automated equipment using microplate methods.

ANTIBODY SCREEN

The antibody screen is used to detect unexpected blood group antibodies in the donor plasma. Anti-A and anti-B are expected antibodies and are not detected by this test. The antibodies considered most important are those produced after exposure to red blood cells from transfusion or pregnancy. Although this test is required only on donors who have been transfused or pregnant, most blood centers test all donor samples rather than sort samples for testing.

The method used to perform the antibody screen should demonstrate antibodies considered clinically significant. Donor samples can be tested separately or in pools. The screening cells can be separate or pooled. Standard tube, gel technology, and microplates can be used in addition to automated techniques.

If a clinically significant antibody is present, the plasma and platelets are not used for transfusion because the antibody is present in the plasma. Red blood cell products that have not been washed or frozen or deglycerolized still have at least a minimal amount of plasma present. If used for transfusion, the antibody interpretation is required on the red blood cell label.

OPTIONAL TESTS

Cytomegalovirus

Cytomegalovirus (CMV) is a widespread infection that can be transmitted through transfusion. In the majority of individuals CMV infection is asymptomatic, but mononucleosis-like symptoms are occasionally seen. For immunosuppressed patients, including premature infants, exposure to CMV has been shown to cause motor disabilities, mental retardation, and even death.

The incidence of viral exposure and subsequent antibody formation varies with age and geographic location and ranges from 40% to 100%.[27] When selecting units to screen for CMV, younger donors have a lower incidence of positivity.

Tests to detect antibody to CMV are not required for blood donors and are usually performed only on a portion of the blood collected. Units that test negative for CMV are set aside for intrauterine transfusion or blood replacement for premature infants and immunocompromised adults.

CMV testing for antibodies can be performed by EIA, latex agglutination, or hemagglutination.

Chagas' Disease

Chagas' disease, or American trypanosomiasis, is a disease endemic in Central and South America and caused by the protozoan parasite *Trypanosoma cruzi*. Infection usually results after contact with feces of infected reduviid bugs. Transmission is also possible by transfusion.

Because cases of transfusion-transmitted Chagas' have been reported in the United States, some blood centers with many immigrants from endemic areas perform an EIA test to detect the antibodies to *T. cruzi*.

CHAPTER SUMMARY

Within the last 15 years testing performed on blood from volunteer donors has increased from one viral test to seven. These tests are also more specific and sensitive in detecting hepatitis, HIV, and HTLV diseases that could be potentially spread by transfusion. The safety of the blood supply continues to be a serious concern, however, and new testing methods and disease markers no doubt will be added in the future. NAT technology is being evaluated to supplement EIA testing for HIV and HCV detection to increase the ability to detect recently infected donors.

CRITICAL THINKING EXERCISES

◆ ***EXERCISE 10-1***

A test for the HIV-1/2 antibody contained an external control that did not fall into the range required. What is the correct procedure for this problem? Why are external controls tested?

◆ ***EXERCISE 10-2***

A sample was tested and found to be positive for the hemagglutination test for syphilis. A confirmatory test was negative, and donor history indicated no high-risk behavior. In fact the donor was 68 years old and donating an autologous unit for surgery. Can her unit be used?

◆ ***EXERCISE 10-3***

On completion of the hepatitis test using the EIA procedure, an acid is added to stop the color development of the conjugate-substrate. On this particular day, a delay caused by a power failure resulted in equipment downtime. The acid was not added until 10 minutes past the allowable time. How would a delay in the addition of the acid affect the test results?

◆ ***EXERCISE 10-4***

A donor is identified with an anti-Le^a in her serum. Can her plasma be used for transfusion or should it be discarded?

◆ ***EXERCISE 10-5***

A donor's computer record lists her as CMV-antibody negative. The most recent donation indicated that antibodies are currently present. Can she still donate? Why have her results changed? What patients require CMV-negative blood? Do alternatives exist to providing CMV antibody–negative blood?

STUDY QUESTIONS

1. Which disease has the highest potential for transmission by a transfusion?
   a. AIDS
   b. syphilis
   c. CMV
   d. hepatitis

2. Syphilis tests on donors are usually performed by which methodology or methodologies?
   a. RPR
   b. Venereal Disease Research Laboratory
   c. hemagglutination
   d. both a and b

3. HTLV-I/II is:
   a. transmissible by contaminated needles
   b. an oncornavirus
   c. found in patients with tropical spastic paraparesis
   d. associated with adult T-cell leukemia
   e. all of the above

4. The marker that demonstrates a previous exposure to hepatitis B that remains in convalescence is:
   a. anti-HCV
   b. anti-HBc
   c. anti-HAV
   d. HBsAg

5. Which of the following is the confirmatory test for a positive anti-HIV screen?
   a. Western blot
   b. RIBA
   c. PCR
   d. Southern blot

6. Which of the following requires a thorough donor history, since it is not a routinely tested disease?
   a. syphilis
   b. CMV
   c. Chagas' disease
   d. HTLV-I

7. HAV transmission through a blood transfusion is unusual because it is:
   a. transmitted enterically
   b. an acute hepatitis
   c. not infective after 2 weeks
   d. all of the above

8. A donor who is positive for HBsAg is:
   a. temporarily deferred
   b. permanently deferred
   c. deferred if the antibody to HBc is also present
   d. deferred if the ALT is elevated

9. Which of the following is a surrogate test for hepatitis that is no longer required?
   a. ALT
   b. CMV
   c. anti-HBc
   d. anti-HBsAg

10. The EIA test used to detect antibody to a virus uses which technique?
   a. indirect EIA
   b. sandwich EIA
   c. competitive EIA
   d. neutralization

REFERENCES

1. Food and Drug Administration: *Memorandum: Recommendations for the invalidation of test results when using licensed viral marker assays to screen donors*, Rockville, Md, January 3, 1994, Congressional and Consumer Affairs.
2. Vengelen-Tyler V, editor: *Technical manual*, ed 12, Bethesda, Md, 1996, American Association of Blood Banks.
3. *Auszyme®* Monoclonal, Product insert, Abbott Park, Ill, 1995, Abbott Laboratories.
4. *HIVAB™* HIV-1/HIV-2 (rDNA) EIA, Product insert, Abbott Park, Ill, 1996, Abbott Laboratories.
5. HTLV-I/HTLV-II EIA, Product insert, Abbott Park, Ill, 1997, Abbott Laboratories.
6. HCV EIA 2.0, Product insert, Abbott Park, Ill, 1995, Abbott Laboratories.
7. *Corzyme* Hepatitis B virus core antigen, Product insert, Abbott Park, Ill, 1995, Abbott Laboratories.
8. *HIVAG™-1* Monoclonal antibody to HIV-1, Product insert, Abbott Park, Ill, 1998, Abbott Laboratories.
9. Smith DM, Dodd RY, editors: *Transfusion transmitted infections*, Chicago, 1991, American Association of Clinical Pathologists.
10. Blumberg BS, Alter HJ, Visnich S: A "new" antigen in leukemia sera, *JAMA* 191:541, 1965.
11. a-gent® SGPT (ALT), Product insert, Abbott Park, Ill, 1986, Abbott Laboratories.
12. Busch MP: Let's look at human immunodeficiency virus look-back before leaping into hepatitis C virus look-back, *Transfusion* 31:655, 1991.
13. CHIRON/RIBA/HCV 3.0 Strip immunoblot assay (SIA) for the detection of anti-HCV in human serum or plasma, Product insert, Emeryville, Calif, 1995, Chiron Corporation, distributed by Ortho Diagnostic Systems.
14. Murray PR, Kobayashi GS, Pfaller MA, Rosenthal KS: *Medical microbiology*, ed 3, St Louis, 1997, Mosby.
15. Busch MP, Lee LL, Satten GA, et al: Time course of detection of viral and serologic markers preceding human immunodeficiency virus type 1 seroconversion: implications for screening of blood and tissue donors, *Transfusion* 35:91, 1995.
16. Stanley J: Blood collection and processing. In Quinley ED: *Immunohematology principles and practice*, ed 2, Philadelphia, 1998, Lippincott.
17. McFarlin DE, Blattner WA: Non-AIDS retroviral infections in humans, *Annu Rev Med* 42:97, 1991.
18. Janssen RS, Kaplan JE, Khabbaz RF, et al: HTLV-I-associated myelopathy/tropical spastic paraparesis in the United States, *Neurology* 41:1355, 1991.
19. Loughran TP Jr, Coyle T, Sherman MP, et al: Detection of human T-cell leukemia/lymphoma virus, type II, in a patient with large granular lymphocyte leukemia, *Blood* 80: 1116, 1992.
20. Sohn CC, Blayney DW, Misset JL, et al: Leukopenic chronic T cell leukemia mimicking hairy cell leukemia: association with human retroviruses, *Blood* 67:949, 1986.
21. Kuby J: *Immunology*, ed 3, New York, 1997, WH Freeman.

22. Food and Drug Administration: CBER guidelines for industry: Supplemental testing and the notification of consignees of donor test results for antibody to hepatitis C (Anti-HCV), docket number 98D-0143, March 20, 1998.
23. Chambers RW, Foley HT, Schmidt PJ: Transmission of syphilis by fresh blood components, *Transfusion* 9:32, 1969.
24. Olympus PK-TP System, Product insert, Irving, Tex, 1990, Olympus.
25. Rathlev T: Hemagglutination tests utilizing antigens from pathogenic and apathogenic *Treponema pallidum*, World Health Organization document venereal disease testing/RES 77.65, 1965.
26. Cox PM, Logan LC, Norins LC: Automated quantitative microhemagglutination assay for *Treponema pallidum* antibodies, *Appl Microbiol* 18:485, 1969.
27. Turgeon ML: *Immunology and serology in laboratory medicine*, ed 2, St Louis, MO, 1996, Mosby.

SUGGESTED READINGS

American Association of Blood Banks, Association bulletin No. 99-3, *NAT implementation*, Bethesda, Md, Feb 8, 1999, American Association of Blood Banks.

American Association of Blood Banks, Association bulletin No. 99-6, *NAT implementation–additional guidance*, Bethesda, Md, March 10, 1999, American Association of Blood Banks.

11 BLOOD COMPONENT PREPARATION AND THERAPY

Kathy D. Blaney

CHAPTER OUTLINE

Blood Collection Bag
Anticoagulant-Preservative Solutions
Storage Lesion
Types of Anticoagulant-Preservative Solutions
Additive Solutions
Rejuvenation Solutions
Blood Component Preparation
Whole Blood
Indications for Use
Red Blood Cells
Indications for Use
Leukocyte-Reduced Red Blood Cells
Frozen Red Blood Cells
Deglycerolized Red Blood Cells
Washed Red Blood Cells
Irradiated Red Blood Cells
Platelets
Indications for Use
Platelet Concentrates
Platelets, Pooled
Platelets, Pheresis
Fresh Frozen Plasma
Indications for Use
Fresh Frozen Plasma, Thawed
Solvent-Detergent–Treated Plasma
Cryoprecipitated Antihemophilic Factor
Indications for Use
Cryoprecipitated Antihemophilic Factor, Pooled
Fibrin Glue from Cryoprecipitated Antihemophilic Factor
Granulocytes, Pheresis
Indications for Use
Labeling
Storage and Transportation
Transportation of Blood Components
Administration of Blood Components

LEARNING OBJECTIVES

Upon completion of this chapter, the reader should be able to:

1. List the benefits of component separation.
2. Define *storage lesion* and the elements that change during blood storage.
3. Compare the anticoagulant and preservative solutions with regard to expiration and content.
4. Describe the steps in blood component preparation.
5. Provide a description of each blood component and its clinical use.
6. State the storage temperature and storage limits for each blood component.
7. Describe the quality control requirements for each component.
8. Understand the Food and Drug Administration's and American Association of Blood Bank's role in regulation and accreditation issues regarding blood component preparation, storage, and distribution.
9. List the labeling requirements common to all blood components.
10. Discuss the importance of monitored storage equipment for blood components and the alarm requirements.
11. Describe essential aspects of safe blood administration.

Whole blood: blood collected from a donor before separation into its components.
Components: parts of whole blood that can be separated by centrifugation; consists of red blood cells, plasma, cryoprecipitated antihemophilic factor, and platelets.
Hemotherapy: treatment of a disease or condition by the use of blood or blood derivatives.
Good manufacturing practices: methods used in, and the facilities or controls used for, the manufacture, processing, packing, or holding of a drug (including a blood product) to ensure that it meets safety, purity, and potency standards.
Closed system: collection of blood in an airtight, sterile system.
Open system: collection or exposure to air that would shorten the expiration because of potential bacterial contamination.

The separation of **whole blood** into its parts, or **components,** allows for optimal storage of each part and the ability to provide appropriate therapy for patients. Each unit of whole blood can be separated into several components that can be transfused into patients, depending on their medical requirements. The separation of blood into components maximizes a limited resource and allows for a method of transfusing patients who require a large amount of a specific blood component. Thus the availability of blood components permits patients to receive specific **hemotherapy** that is more effective and usually safer than the use of whole blood.[1]

The primary goal of facilities that prepare components is to provide a product of optimal benefit to the recipient. It is important to understand the elements involved in the preparation and handling of blood products to ensure that **good manufacturing practices** (GMPs) are followed. All processes in the collection, testing, separation, and distribution of components are highly regulated by the Food and Drug Administration (FDA), which considers blood a "drug."[2] This chapter describes the preparation, labeling, and storage of blood components. A summary of the clinical indications for each component and general administration policies are also reviewed.

BLOOD COLLECTION BAG

Blood is collected in a primary bag that contains an anticoagulant-preservative mixture. The entire blood bag, including integrally attached satellite bags and tubing, is sterile and considered a **closed system.** The airtight system becomes an **open system** once entered, and the allowable storage time is reduced because of potential bacterial contamination (Fig. 11-1).

The facility's inventory requirements and the drawing location usually determine the number of satellite bags or the "bag configuration" used for collecting blood from donors. The primary bag can have as many as four additional bags attached. Storage temperature and time constraints following collection also affect which components are to be prepared. For example, if platelets are prepared from the whole blood, the unit must be stored between 20° to 24° C, and the platelets must be separated from the whole blood within 8 hours. If platelets are not separated from the whole blood, units are stored at 1° to 6° C before component preparation.

A

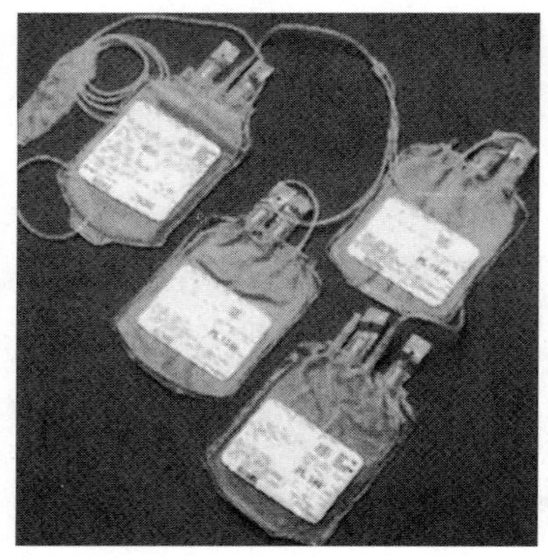

B

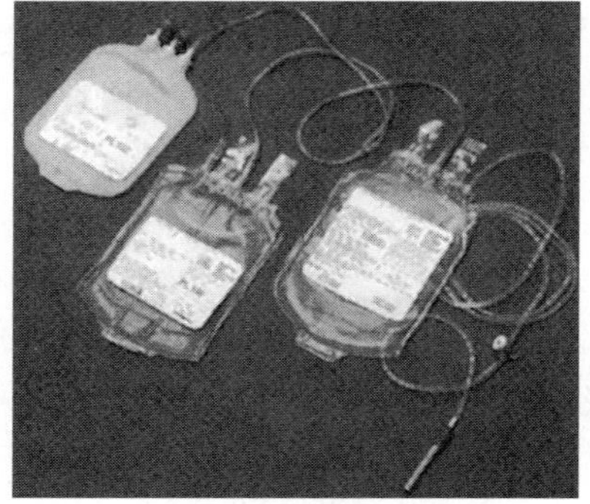

Fig. 11-1 Blood collection bags. *A*, Quad-bag system. *B*, Triple-bag system.

Courtesy of Baxter Healthcare Corp., Deerfield, Ill.

ANTICOAGULANT-PRESERVATIVE SOLUTIONS

Anticoagulant-preservative solutions work together to prevent clotting and extend the storage of red blood cells. The volume of this solution in the primary collection bag is either 63 ml or 70 ml. The standard whole blood collection volume is 450 ml ± 45 ml for blood collected in a 63 ml anticoagulant or 500 ml ± 50 ml for the larger volume bag. If collection is planned for less than 350 ml, the volume of anticoagulant-preservative solution should be reduced proportionately. This may be necessary if an autologous unit is collected from an individual weighing less than 110 pounds. Fig. 11-2 shows this calculation,[3] and Table 11-1 summarizes the function of the chemical elements in these solutions.

Storage Lesion

Biochemical changes occur when blood is stored at 1° to 6° C, which affects red blood cell viability and function. These changes are called the storage lesion. The

$$\frac{\text{Weight of patient}}{110 \text{ lb}} = \text{factor to use to reduce volumes (A)}$$

A × 70 ml = amount of anticoagulant (B)

70 − B = amount of anticoagulant to remove

A × 500 ml = amount of blood that should be withdrawn

Example: An 85-lb donor would yield a "factor" of .77 (A)
.77 × 70 = 54 ml anticoagulant should be used
70 − 54 = 16 ml should be removed
.77 × 500 = 385 ml blood should be drawn

Fig. 11-2 Calculation for adjusting anticoagulant and blood volume drawn.

Table 11-1 Anticoagulant-Preservative Composition and Purpose

CHEMICAL	PURPOSE
Dextrose	Supports ATP generation by glycolytic pathway
Adenine*	Acts as substrate for red blood cell ATP synthesis
Citrate	Prevents coagulation by chelating calcium
Sodium biphosphate	Prevents excessive drop in pH

*Only in citrate-phosphate-dextrose-adenine–1 and additive solutions.
ATP, Adenosine triphosphate.

criterion for measuring acceptable storage limit or "shelf life" is that at least 75% of the original red blood cells be in the recipient's circulation 24 hours after transfusion.[3] The purposes of the preservative solutions are to minimize the effects of the biochemical changes and to maximize the shelf life of the components. The biochemical changes that occur during storage of red blood cells are summarized in Fig. 11-3.

Glucose, adenosine triphosphate (ATP), and pH decrease as red blood cells are stored. Storage also affects the level of 2,3-diphosphoglycerate (2,3-DPG), which is important in the release of oxygen from hemoglobin. High levels of 2,3-DPG cause greater oxygen release whereas lower levels increase the affinity of hemoglobin for oxygen. In red blood cells stored in citrate-phosphate-dextrose-adenine (CPDA-1) or additive solution, 2,3-DPG levels steadily decrease to zero after 2 weeks of storage.[3] After these cells are transfused, stored cells regenerate ATP and 2,3-DPG to normal levels after about 24 hours.[4] Although the storage lesions seem significant, these changes rarely have clinical implications, with the exception of infants requiring exchange transfusions.[3]

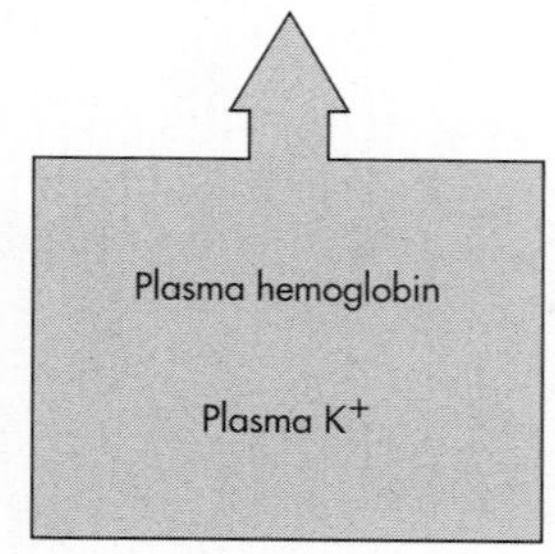

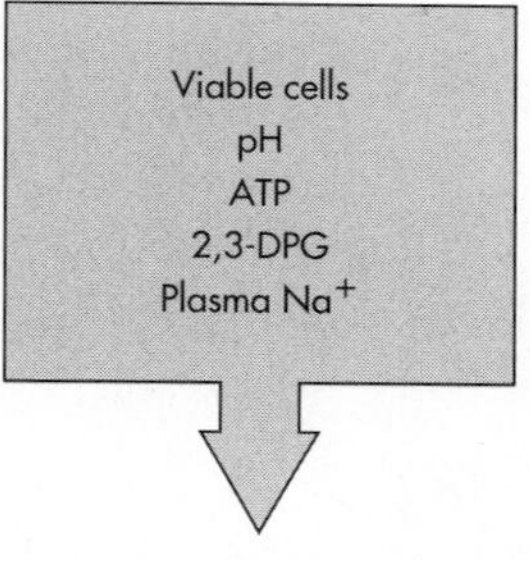

Fig. 11-3 Storage lesion: biochemical changes to stored red blood cells. *ATP,* Adenosine triphosphate; *2,3-DPG,* 2,3-diphosphoglycerate.

Types of Anticoagulant-Preservative Solutions

Anticoagulant-preservative solutions in the primary collection bag may be citrate-phosphate-dextrose (CPD), citrate-phosphate-2-dextrose (CP2D), or CPDA-1. Blood collected in CPD and CP2D is approved for storage for 21 days at 1° to 6° C, whereas blood collected in CPDA-1 can be stored for 35 days.

Additive Solutions

Additive solutions (AS-1, AS-3, or AS-5) are provided as an integral part of the collection bag system. After the whole blood is collected in CPD or CP2D and the plasma is separated from the red blood cells, the additive "pouch" of normal saline, glucose, and adenine is allowed to flow into the red blood cells to enhance red blood cell survival and function.[5] AS-1 and AS-5 solutions also contain mannitol as a red blood cell stabilizing agent. AS-3 contains additional citrate and phosphate and does not contain mannitol.[6] This 100-ml solution must be added within 72 hours of the whole blood collection. In addition to extending the storage to 42 days from collection, the additive solution reduces the red blood cell

Table 11-2 Expiration Limits for Red Blood Cells in Different Solutions

Anticoagulant preservative	Storage limit (days)
CPD	21
CP2D	21
CPDA-1	35
AS-1, AS-3, AS-5	42

CPD, Citrate-phosphate-dextrose; *CP2D,* citrate-phosphate-2-dextrose; *CPDA-1,* citrate-phosphate-dextrose-adenine; *AS,* additive solution.

viscosity and improves the flow rate during administration. Table 11-2 summarizes the expiration limits for the various anticoagulants.

Rejuvenation Solutions

Although the procedure is not routine, it may be necessary to restore 2,3-DPG and ATP levels in red blood cell units collected in CPD or CPDA-1, during storage or up to 3 days after expiration, with a solution containing pyruvate, inosine, phosphate, and adenine. This product extends the expiration date for freezing or transfusing a red blood cell unit, which may be necessary when a rare or autologous unit is involved. Washing to remove the inosine before use is required, since it may be toxic to the recipient.[7]

BLOOD COMPONENT PREPARATION

The separation of components from the original whole blood unit is performed by centrifugation. Red blood cells settle to the bottom, since they are the heaviest component, whereas the platelets and plasma components remain on top. Variables that affect the yield of the product being prepared include speed of the centrifuge (revolutions per minute, or RPM) and length of time of centrifugation.

Each centrifuge used for preparing components is calibrated for optimal time and speed for each product made. Quality control measures are performed to evaluate the products and determine whether the centrifugation parameters are set for maximum product yield. A short centrifugation time at a low RPM is usually called a "light spin," whereas a longer spin time at a higher RPM is called a "heavy spin." Steps in the preparation of red blood cells, fresh frozen plasma (FFP), platelets, and cryoprecipitated antihemophilic factor (CRYO) are outlined below. The American Association of Blood Banks (AABB) *Technical Manual* provides detailed procedures for the preparation of blood components. Fig. 11-4 illustrates component separation. Table 11-3 summarizes the storage temperatures, expiration limits, and quality control requirements for these components.

- After the whole blood unit is centrifuged at a "light spin," the platelet-rich plasma (PRP) is expressed or pushed through the attached tubing into an empty satellite bag. The red blood cells remain in the original bag. If collected in an additive system, the additive solution (AS-1, AS-3, or AS-5) is added to the red blood cells. The red blood cells are then sealed and split from the remaining bags and refrigerated at 1° to 6° C.
- The PRP unit is recentrifuged at a "heavy spin," which causes the platelets to sediment to the bottom of the bag. All but about 50 to 70 ml of plasma is removed from the platelets. The additional plasma that remains with the platelets is required to maintain a pH of 6.2 or higher during the storage period. The platelets are sealed and allowed to "rest" for a period of at least 1 hour before they are stored on a rotator that maintains continuous gentle agitation. Platelet concentrates are maintained at 20° to 24° C for a maximum of 5 days.
- The plasma that had been expressed into another empty attached bag can be frozen as FFP or used as recovered plasma for further manufacture. FFP must be frozen within 8 hours of collection and stored at or below −18° C for up to 1 year or stored at *or below* −65° C for 7 years. Recovered plasma is usually shipped to a fractionator for processing into derivatives such as albumin, immune globulin, and coagulation factor concentrates.

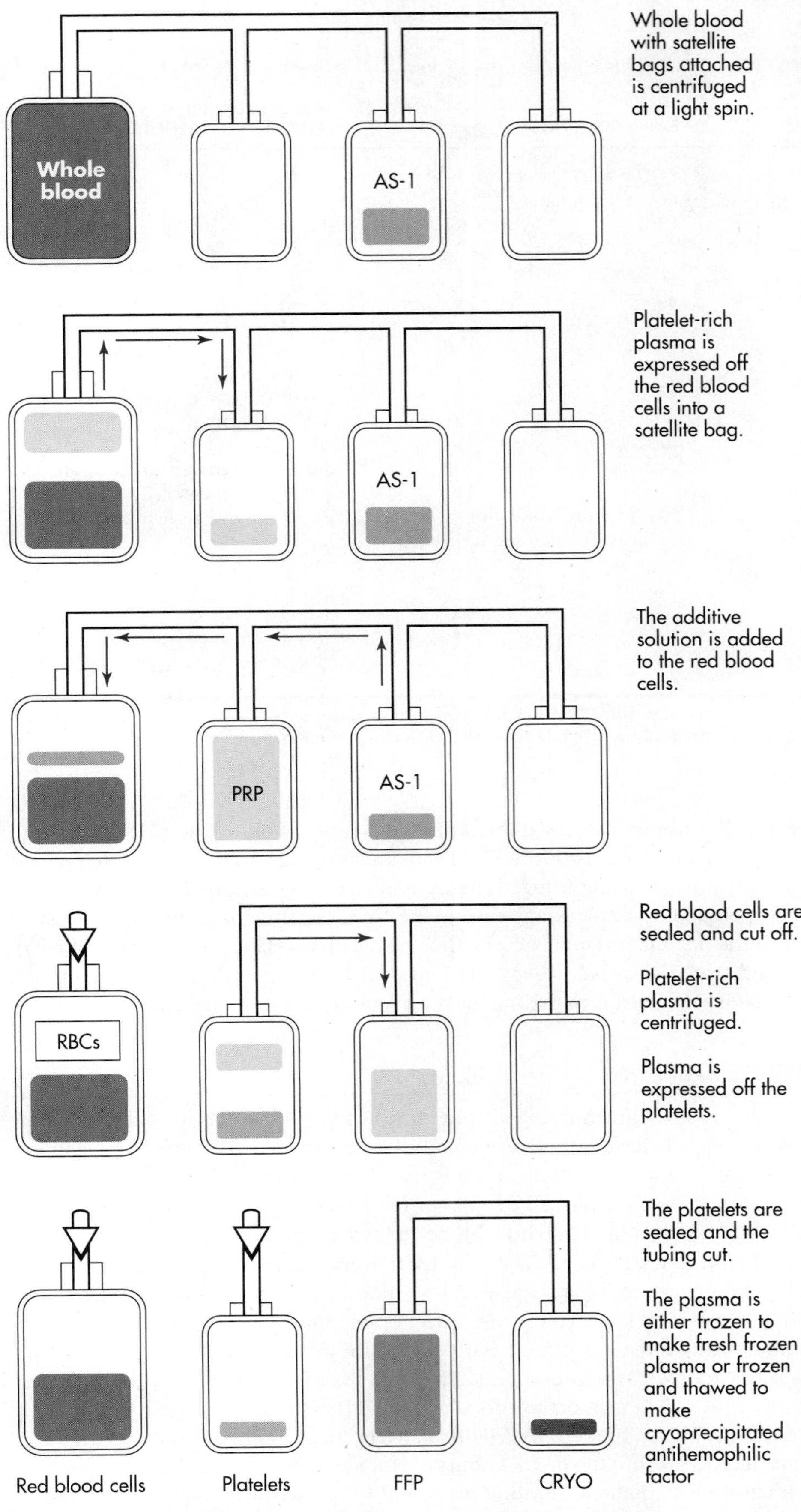

Fig. 11-4 Component separation. *AS*, Additive solution; *PRP*, platelet-rich plasma; *RBCs*, red blood cells; *FFP*, fresh frozen plasma; *CRYO*, cryoprecipitated antihemophilic factor.

Table 11-3 Storage Temperature, Expiration Limits, and Quality Control Requirements of Selected Blood Components

COMPONENT	STORAGE TEMPERATURE	EXPIRATION LIMITS	QUALITY CONTROL: MINIMUM REQUIREMENTS
Whole blood	1°-6° C Shipping: 1°-10° C	CPD, CP2D: 21 days CPDA-1: 35 days	None
RBCs	1°-6° C Shipping: 1°-10° C	CPD, CP2D: 21 days CPDA-1: 35 days AS-1, AS-3, AS-5: 42 days	Hematocrit: ≤80% in CPDA-1 units
Platelet concentrates	20°-24° C	5 days	5.5 × 10^{10} in 75% of units tested; pH: ≥6.2
FFP	≤−18° C	1 year	None
FFP	≤−65° C	7 years	None
CRYO	≤−18° C	1 year	Factor VIII: ≥80 IU and ≥150 mg fibrinogen
RBCs, frozen	≤−65° C	10 years	None
RBCs, deglycerolized or washed (open system)	1°-6° C	24 hours	80% RBC recovery; deglycerolized: visual hemoglobin check
RBCs, irradiated	1°-6° C	28 days from irradiation or original outdate, whichever is first	Irradiator QC applied 2500 cGy in center
Platelets, pooled	20°-24° C	4 hours	None
Pooled CRYO	20°-24° C	4 hours	None
FFP, thawed	1°-6° C	24 hours	None
Platelets, pheresis	20°-24° C	5 days	3 × 10^{11} in 75% of units tested
Granulocytes, pheresis	20°-24° C	24 hours	1 × 10^{10} in 75% of units tested

CPD, Citrate-phosphate-dextrose; *CP2D*, citrate-phosphate-2-dextrose; *CPDA-1*, citrate-phosphate-dextrose-adenine; *RBCs*, red blood cells; *AS*, additive solution; *FFP*, fresh frozen plasma; *CRYO*, cryoprecipitated antihemophilic factor; *QC*, quality control; *cGy*, centigray.

- If FFP is further processed into CRYO, an empty satellite bag is left attached to the FFP and frozen with it. The FFP is thawed at 1° to 6° C. A white precipitate forms and is centrifuged (heavy spin) with all but about 10 to 15 ml of the supernatant plasma expressed into the empty satellite bag. The CRYO remains in the bag that originally contained the FFP. It is relabeled as CRYO, refrozen, and stored at or below −18° C for up to 1 year from donation. The plasma that is expressed into the satellite bag is used as recovered plasma.

WHOLE BLOOD

Whole blood is the unmodified component drawn from a donor that consists of erythrocytes, leukocytes, platelets, and plasma proteins with the anticoagulant-preservative solution. Whole blood is stored in a monitored refrigerator at 1° to 6° C for 21 days if collected in CPD or for 35 days if in CPDA-1. Additive solutions cannot be added to whole blood to increase the storage period.

Before the development of the technology involved in blood component preparation, whole blood was the only blood product available. In the 1960s, when plastic replaced glass as the collection medium, separation of whole blood into its components became possible. Availability of whole blood declined and was replaced with red blood cells. Problems associated with whole blood transfusions include circulatory overload in patients who require only oxygen-carrying capacity from red blood cells. Viable platelets are lost and labile coagulation factors decrease within the first 24 hours of storage. Whole blood must also be ABO identical to the patient, limiting its flexibility in inventory management and in emergency situations. Whole blood, therefore, has a limited use in most clinical situations.

Indications for Use

Whole blood is indicated for patients who are actively bleeding and who have lost more than 25% of their blood volume and for patients undergoing an exchange transfusion.[3] Whole blood increases the hemoglobin by about 1 g/dl or the hematocrit by about 3%. Whole blood must be ABO identical and crossmatched before administration. When whole blood is not available, red blood cells administered with crystalloid solutions are usually effective in restoring both oxygen-carrying capacity and blood volume.[8] Reconstituted whole blood (red blood cells reconstituted with type AB FFP from a different donor) is usually prepared for exchange transfusions in infants.[9]

RED BLOOD CELLS

Indications for Use

Red blood cells contain hemoglobin, which transports oxygen through the bloodstream and to the tissues. Red blood cell transfusions increase the mass of circulating red blood cells in situations where tissue oxygenation may be impaired by acute or chronic blood loss, such as in hemorrhage or anemia. Conditions commonly requiring red blood cell transfusion support include (but are not limited to):

- Oncology patients undergoing chemotherapy or radiation therapy
- Trauma victims
- Patients undergoing cardiac, orthopedic, and other surgeries
- Patients with end-stage renal disease
- Premature infants
- Patients with sickle cell disease

The diseases and conditions that commonly necessitate component therapy are reviewed in Chapter 14. Transfusing 1 unit of red blood cells usually increases the hemoglobin by about 1 g/dl and increases the hematocrit by about 3% in the average 70-kg adult. Red blood cells necessitate crossmatching before issue.

Red blood cells are often modified into additional products needed for specific patient requirements. The following section summarizes the preparation, storage, and use of leukocyte-reduced, frozen and deglycerolized, washed, and irradiated red blood cells.

Leukocyte-Reduced Red Blood Cells

White blood cells remaining in red blood cell units have been implicated in adverse transfusion reactions and immunization to white blood cell antigens. A reaction caused by leukocytes can be extremely uncomfortable for a patient, causing shaking chills and a rise in temperature soon after initiating the red blood cell transfusion. In addition to the white blood cells, cytokines produced by leukocytes during red blood cell storage are also responsible for febrile reactions.[10] Removing leukocytes from red blood cells may not be cost effective for all patients; it is indicated for chronically transfused patients to prevent alloimmunization to leukocyte antigens, patients transfused outside the hospital setting, and patients

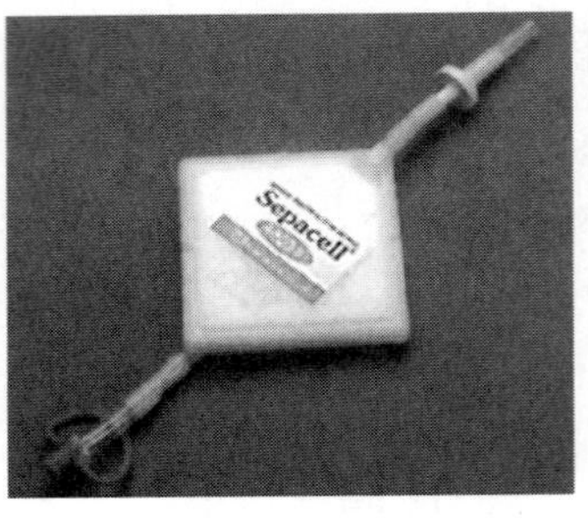

Fig. 11-5 Leukocyte reduction filter.
Courtesy of Baxter Healthcare Corp., Deerfield, Ill.

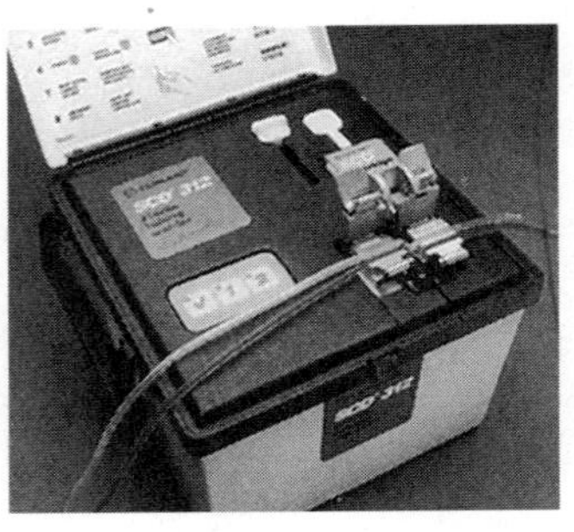

Fig. 11-6 Sterile connection device.
Courtesy of Baxter Healthcare Corp., Deerfield, Ill.

Cryoprotective: solution added to protect against cell damage that occurs at or below freezing temperatures.

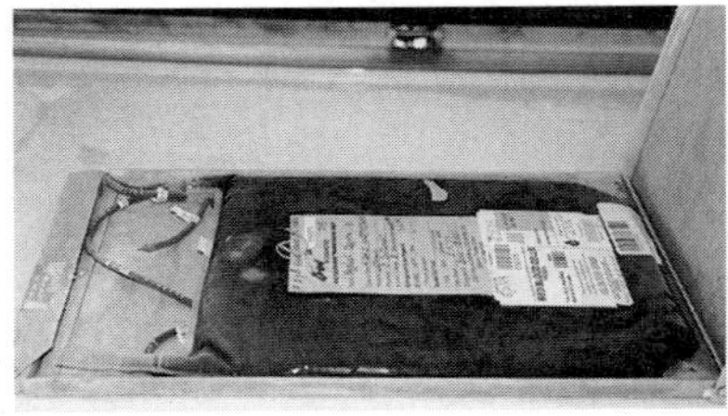

Fig. 11-7 Frozen red blood cells.
Courtesy of Central Florida Blood Bank, Inc., Orlando, Fla.

previously reactive to leukocytes.[1] Reduction in leukocytes *before* red blood cell storage is optimal, since it reduces the leukocyte fragments and cytokines that increase during storage.[10]

The standard 170-micron blood filter does not remove leukocytes. White blood cell removal is best accomplished by the use of commercially available leukocyte removal or leukoreduction filters (Fig. 11-5). Filtration can be performed by:

- Using in-line filters integral to the collection set that allows red blood cells to be filtered, since they are prepared before storage
- Sterile-connecting a leukocyte reduction filter to the red blood cells and filtering before storage; FDA-approved sterile-connecting devices allow for the attachment of tubing from filters, transfer pacts, and between units without creating an "open system" (Fig. 11-6)
- Using a bedside leukocyte reduction filter when the unit is transfused. When this filter is used, the unit's expiration changes to 24 hours, since it results in an open system.

In addition to preventing reactions, the removal of leukocytes reduces the danger of transfusion-transmitted cytomegalovirus (CMV), since this virus resides in the cytoplasm of white blood cells.[11]

According to AABB's *Standards*,[12] leukoreduced red blood cells are to be prepared with a method known to retain at least 85% of the original red blood cells and reduce the leukocyte number in the final component to less than 5×10^6 in each unit.

Frozen Red Blood Cells

Red blood cells can be frozen for long-term preservation to maintain an inventory of rare units or extend the availability of autologous units. Freezing extends the storage up to 10 years from collection when stored at or below −65° C. To prepare a red blood cell unit for freezing, glycerol is added as a **cryoprotective** agent to prevent cell dehydration and the formation of ice crystals, which causes cell lysis.[11] Glycerol is slowly added to the unit for a final glycerol concentration of 40% weight per volume.[3] The unit is transferred to a polyolefin or polyvinyl chloride bag and placed in a metal or cardboard canister to prevent breakage at low temperatures. Initial freezing temperatures should be −80° C. Units can subsequently be stored at −65° C (Fig. 11-7).[3]

Freezing can also be accomplished with a lower glycerol concentration if a liquid nitrogen freezer is used. This method is not as common for red blood cells. Glycerol concentration is approximately 20%, and the initial freezing temperature is −196° C. Maximum storage temperature is −120° C for a period of 10 years.

Deglycerolized Red Blood Cells

Frozen red blood cells are thawed, and the glycerol removed by the process of deglycerolization. After thawing in a 37° C water bath, the unit is washed in a series of saline solutions of decreasing osmolarity. Saline solutions of 12% and 1.6% followed by 0.9% normal saline are used to draw the glycerol out of the cells. This process is usually performed on an instrument called a blood cell processor, which gradually adds preset saline volumes, mixes and centrifuges the cells, and removes supernatant automatically (Fig. 11-8). Since the process of glycerolization and deglycerolization involves entering the blood unit, the system is considered "open," and the product must be transfused within 24 hours.

Washed Red Blood Cells

Washing red blood cells with normal saline may be indicated for patients who react to the small amount of plasma proteins that remain in a unit of red blood cells. Reactions can be allergic, febrile, or anaphylactic. An IgA-deficient patient with clinically significant anti-IgA requires washed red blood cells if a transfusion is necessary. Washed red blood cells may also be used in infant or intrauterine transfusions.[1] Washing is accomplished with approximately 1000 ml of 0.9% saline using the automatic blood cell processor described for deglycerolizing frozen red blood cells. Washing is associated with a loss of about 10% to 20% of the original red blood cells and is no longer considered an effective method of removing leukocytes.[3]

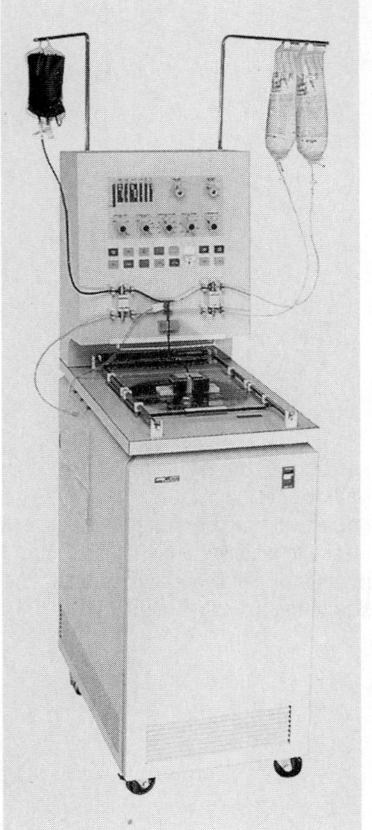

A

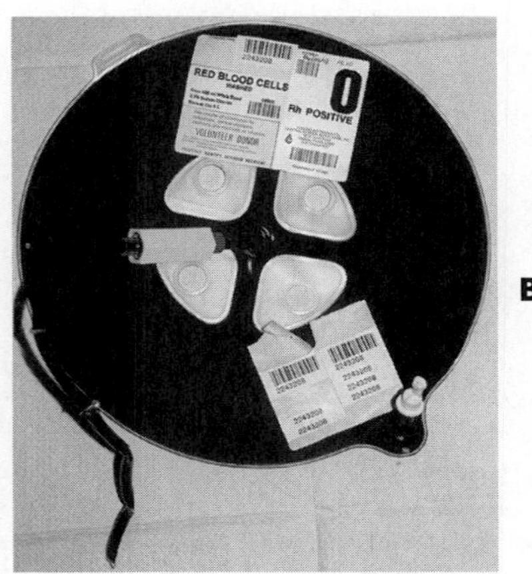

B

Fig. 11-8 Blood cell processor *(A)* and washed red blood cells *(B)*.

Courtesy of COBE Cardiovascular, Arvada, Colo.

Irradiated Red Blood Cells

Viable T cells in cellular blood components may cause transfusion-associated graft versus host disease (GVHD), which is fatal in over 90% of affected patients.[14] Factors that determine a patient's risk for transfusion-associated GVHD include whether, and to what degree, the patient is immunodeficient; the degree of similarity between donor and recipient regarding human leukocyte antigens (HLAs); and the number of transfused T cells capable of multiplication.[15] Gamma irradiation of cellular blood components prevents proliferation of T cells that cause transfusion-associated GVHD. Red blood cells that have been leukoreduced by filtration do not prevent GVHD, since some leukocytes remain in the final product. AABB's *Standards*[12] requires irradiation of cellular components (red blood cells and platelets) if the donor unit is from a blood relative of the intended recipient or the donor unit is HLA-matched for the recipient.

In addition, irradiation to prevent GVHD is suggested for:

- Patients receiving an intrauterine transfusion
- Patients suffering from immunoincompetence or immunodeficiency
- Patients who have received allogeneic marrow or peripheral blood progenitor cells
- Premature newborns
- Patients undergoing intensive chemotherapy and irradiation

The required dose of irradiation is 2500 cGy, or 25 Gy, in the middle of the canister, and the lowest dose should be 1500 cGy.[12] Periodic verification and documentation of dose delivery are required.

Irradiation induces erythrocyte membrane damage that causes red blood cell units to have a higher plasma potassium level and a decrease in ATP and 2,3-DPG levels.[16] Cell activities that are not dependent on reproduction (notably platelet activation and oxygen delivery) are not significantly affected by irradiation. The expiration date of irradiated red blood cells is changed to 28 days after irradiation if the available shelf life exceeds 28 days.[17] The irradiated cells can be given to a recipient other than the originally intended recipient.

PLATELETS

Indications for Use

Normal platelet function and adequate numbers of circulating platelets are essential for hemostasis. Their function includes:

- Maintenance of vascular integrity

- Initial arrest of bleeding by formation of platelet plug
- Stabilization of the hemostatic plug by contributing to the process of fibrin formation[18]

Platelets are transfused to control or prevent bleeding associated with critically decreased circulating platelet numbers or functionally abnormal platelets. Platelet transfusions are not usually effective or indicated for patients with destruction of circulating platelets caused by autoimmune disorders such as idiopathic thrombocytopenic purpura, or ITP. Patients requiring platelet transfusions typically include:

- Cancer patients undergoing chemotherapy or radiation therapy
- Post–bone marrow transplant recipients
- Postoperative bleeding

Since transfused platelets normally circulate with a life span of only 3 to 4 days, frequent transfusion support is often necessary for patients using platelets. Evaluation of the effectiveness of platelet transfusions is important in determining if the patient is **refractory**, or unresponsive to the platelet transfusions. The **corrected count increment**, outlined in Fig. 11-9, determines the increase in platelet count adjusted for the number of platelets infused and the size of the patient.[6] Box 11-1 lists conditions associated with refractoriness.[19] Platelets do not necessitate crossmatching before issue and should be ABO matched whenever possible. It is not necessary to delay transfusion to obtain ABO-compatible or ABO-matched platelets.[3]

Refractory: Unresponsive to platelet transfusions.
Corrected count increment: relative increase in platelet count adjusted for the number of platelets transfused and the size of the patient.

Platelet Concentrates

Platelets prepared from a unit of whole blood, as described in the Blood Component Preparation section, contain at least 5.5×10^{10} platelets per unit and, under optimal conditions, should elevate the platelet count by about 5000 μl in a recipient weighing 75 kg.[19] These platelets are also referred to as random platelets or platelet concentrates.

Platelets, Pooled

To achieve a therapeutic dose, platelets are pooled for transfusion in adults. This is accomplished by transferring the platelet concentrates into a transfer set while

$$\textbf{CCI} = \frac{\textbf{posttransfusion}\text{ platelet count} - \textbf{pretransfusion}\text{ platelet count}}{\text{Number of platelets transfused (multiples of }10^{11})} \times \textbf{BSA}$$

Example: Patient: BSA = 1.5 M^2
Precount: 2000/μl
Postcount: 29,000/μl
Platelets transfused: 4.5×10^{11}

$$\text{CCI} = \frac{29{,}000 - 2000}{4.5} \times 1.5 = 9000$$

A CCI of greater than 7500 indicates adequate platelet count increment

To calculate the BSA, a nomogram is used. The height and weight of the patient are needed to determine the BSA.

Fig. 11-9 Corrected count increment. *CCI*, Corrected count increment; *BSA*, body surface area.

BOX 11-1

Conditions Causing Platelet Refractoriness or Poor Response to Platelet Transfusions

IMMUNE
HLA alloantibodies
Platelet alloantibodies
Autoantibodies

NONIMMUNE
Splenomegaly
Medications
Sepsis
Active bleeding
Fever

being careful not to contaminate the ports. An approximate dose is 1 unit per 10 kg of patient body weight, yielding pools of 6 to 10 platelets. Since it is necessary to create an "open system" when pooling platelets, the expiration of the pooled product changes to 4 hours. The pooled platelets should be stored at 20° to 24° C with gentle agitation until transfusion.

Platelets, Pheresis

Hemapheresis is an effective method of harvesting a therapeutic dose of platelets from one individual donor (Fig. 11-10). During plateletpheresis, whole blood is collected from a donor using automated apheresis equipment, which separates whole blood into components. The platelets are retained, and the remaining elements are returned. Platelets can be collected in approximately 1 to 2 hours. The product is also referred to as "single-donor platelets." Platelet pheresis donors may donate as often as twice a week or 24 times a year with an interval of 48 hours between procedures.[12] A unit of platelets prepared by pheresis should contain a minimum of 3×10^{11} platelets, which is about the same as a pool of 5 to 8 platelets prepared from whole blood.

Hemapheresis: whole blood is removed from a donor or patient and separated into components; one or more of the components are retained, and the remainder is returned.

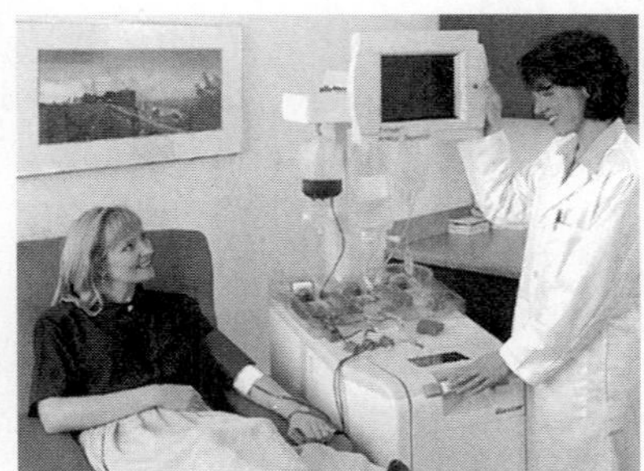

A

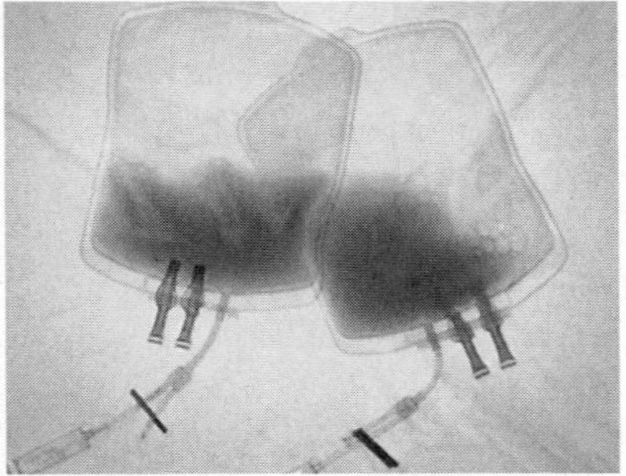

B

Fig. 11-10 ***A*, Apheresis instrument. *B*, Platelet, pheresis product.**

Courtesy of Baxter Healthcare Corp., Deerfield, Ill.

Platelets, Pheresis: Human Leukocyte Antigen–Matched

Platelets manifest Class I HLA. Class I antigens refer to the A, B, and C antigens. Platelets also demonstrate platelet antigens that may elicit an immune response from a patient receiving frequent platelet components. Patients who have developed antibodies to HLA or platelet antigens usually require platelets matched for HLA antigens or crossmatched for platelet antigens to achieve satisfactory increment.[3] The incidence of HLA antibody production causing platelet refractoriness among patients receiving repeated transfusions of cellular components is 30% to 60%.[20] Locating HLA-matched donors from previously typed HLA plateletpheresis donors requires a large donor base. Identical HLA-A,B antigen matching from unrelated donors is rare (1 in 5000 to 20,000) However, less than perfect matching may be sufficient to overcome the refractory state.

When donors are selected for HLA compatibility, the products should be irradiated to prevent GVHD.[12]

Platelets, Leukocytes Reduced

Leukocyte reduction to less than 5×10^6 can be achieved using certain apheresis devices and leukocyte reduction filters designed for bedside and prestorage filtration. The indication for leukocyte reduction is to prevent recurrent febrile nonhemolytic reactions and HLA alloimmunization for patients requiring long-term platelet support or eventual transplantation.[21] As with leukocyte reduction in red blood cell products, leukocyte removal before storage also reduces cytokines and the potential febrile reactions they cause. Leukocyte-reduced platelets are also effective in preventing CMV infection.[11]

FRESH FROZEN PLASMA

Indications for Use

The process of blood coagulation involves a series of biochemical reactions that transform circulating blood into an insoluble gel through conversion of fibrinogen to fibrin.[18] This process requires certain plasma proteins or coagulation factors as well as phospholipids and calcium. Impairment of the coagulation system can occur because of decreased synthesis of the coagulation factors or a consumption of the factors. Defects in the plasma clotting factors may be due to congenital or acquired conditions.

FFP contains all the coagulation factors, including the **labile factors** V and VIII that do not store well at temperatures below −18° C (Table 11-4). One milliliter of FFP contains approximately 1 unit of coagulation factor activity. FFP is indicated for the following[1,3,6]:

- Management of bleeding in patients who require coagulation Factors II, V, VII, X, or XI, when the concentrates are not available or are not appropriate
- Abnormal coagulation assays resulting from massive transfusion
- Patients anticoagulated with warfarin who are bleeding or require emergency surgery
- Replacement solution for therapeutic plasmapheresis for the treatment of thrombotic thrombocytopenic purpura and hemolytic uremic syndrome
- Correction or prevention of bleeding complications in patients who have severe liver disease with multiple factor deficiencies
- Patients with deficiencies of the inhibitor antithrombin III who are undergoing surgery
- Disseminated intravascular coagulation when fibrinogen level is below 100 mg/dl

Fresh Frozen Plasma, Thawed

A unit of FFP is thawed prior to administration in a 30° to 37° C waterbath for approximately 30 to 45 minutes. Units may be placed in protective overwraps to prevent contamination of the administration ports or in a device that maintains the ports above water. Waterbaths with an agitator accelerate the thawing process. FDA-approved microwaves specially designed for plasma thawing also can be used by carefully following the manufacturer's instructions. Standard microwaves should never be used, since they denature plasma proteins. After thawing, FFP is stored at 1° to 6° C and should be transfused within 24 hours from thawing.

Table 11-4 Coagulation Factors and Their Sources

FACTOR	NAME	STABILITY	SOURCE
I	Fibrinogen	S	CRYO
II	Prothrombin	S	Factor IX complex; FFP
V	Proaccelerin	L	FFP
VII	Proconvertin	S	Factor IX complex
VIII	Antihemophilic factor	L	Factor VIII concentrate; CRYO; FFP
IX	Christmas factor	S	Factor IX complex; Factor IX concentrate
X	Stuart-Prower factor	S	Factor IX complex
XI	Plasma thromboplastin antecedent	S	FFP
XII	Hageman factor/contract factor	S	FFP
XIII	Fibrin stabilizing factor	S	CRYO
vWF	von Willebrand's factor	L	Factor VIII concentrate; CRYO; FFP

S, Stable; *L*, labile; *CRYO*, cryoprecipitated antihemophilic factor; *FFP*, fresh frozen plasma.

The dose of FFP depends on the clinical situation and the underlying disease process.[1] If coagulation factor replacement is necessary, the dose is 10 to 20 ml/kg (4 to 6 units in an adult). Crossmatching is not necessary and should be ABO compatible with the patient's red blood cells.

Solvent-Detergent–Treated Plasma

Solvent-detergent–treated FFP has recently been licensed by the FDA as an alternative to FFP.[22] PLAS+SD (pooled plasma, treated with solvent-detergent) has a lower potential for transmission of infectious agents, since the manufacturing process destroys lipid-enveloped viruses (human immunodeficiency virus and hepatitis B and C). The product is manufactured by pooling thawed FFP from volunteer donors and treating it with the organic solvent tri(n-butyl)phosphate and the detergent Triton X-100. It is then realiquoted and frozen in uniform plastic containers containing 200 ml of PLAS+SD. The indications for use, handling, and storage are the same as for FFP. PLAS+SD is manufactured by V.I. Technologies, Inc., and distributed by the American Red Cross.

CRYOPRECIPITATED ANTIHEMOPHILIC FACTOR

Indications for Use

CRYO is the cold insoluble precipitate that forms when a unit of FFP is thawed between 1° and 6° C. It contains, in a concentrated form, most of the coagulation factors that are found in FFP. These factors include:

- von Willebrand's factor (vWF), which is needed for platelet adhesion to damaged endothelium
- Fibrinogen, which is cleaved into fibrin in the presence of thrombin to form a clot
- Factor VIII, a deficiency associated with hemophilia A
- Fibronectin, an opsonic glycoprotein that may help in the clearance of bloodborne particulate matter[3]

The primary clinical uses of CRYO are as a supplement for patients with deficiencies of Factor XIII and fibrinogen and as a fibrin sealant.[3] Since viral inactivated Factor VIII concentrates are currently available for patients with hemophilia A, von Willebrand's disease, and Factor VIII:C deficiency, CRYO is less commonly used for correcting or preventing bleeding in these patients. CRYO is the only concentrated fibrinogen product available and is used to treat patients with congenital or acquired fibrinogen defects. Dysfibrinogenemia, a condition in which fibrinogen is not functionally effective, is associated with severe liver disease.[3]

Quality control of CRYO must demonstrate 150 mg of fibrinogen and 80 international units of Factor VII per unit tested.[12] In facilities that pool CRYO before freezing, the final unit must have 150 mg of fibrinogen and 80 international units of Factor VIII times the number in the pool.

Cryoprecipitated Antihemophilic Factor, Pooled

CRYO is pooled into a transfer bag to achieve a therapeutic dose. The frozen units first must be thawed in a 30° to 37° C waterbath for up to 15 minutes using overwraps to prevent contamination of the ports or by using a device that keeps the ports above water. The contents of bags can be rinsed with 10 to 15 ml of 0.9%

$$\text{No. of Factor VIII units} = \frac{\text{plasma volume} \times (\text{desired level \%} - \text{initial level \%})}{80\ \text{U/bag}}$$

Example: Plasma volume (PV, ml): 40 ml/kg × body weight (kg)
Quantity of Factor VIII coagulant activity: stated on bottle
Factor VIII in CRYO: 80 U/bag

Patient: 70 kg
Initial Factor VIII level: 2 units/dl: 2% activity
Desired Factor VIII level: 50 units/dl: 50% activity

$$\text{No. of Factor VIII units} = \frac{2800 \times (.50 - .02)}{80} = 16.8\ \text{bags of CRYO}$$

Fig. 11-11 Calculating the dose of Factor VIII. *CRYO,* Cryoprecipitated antihemophilic factor.

sodium chloride while pooling. Pooled CRYO must be administered within 4 hours of first entry and should be stored at room temperature until transfusion. Dosage varies with the patient's condition, weight, and level of the factor requiring replacement. This formula is shown in Fig. 11-11.[6] If large volumes of CRYO are to be administered, ABO-compatible units should be selected. CRYO does not necessitate crossmatching. Coagulation factor levels and other laboratory studies are performed to determine the effectiveness and the need for repeat doses.

CRYO can also be pooled after separation from FFP at the collection facility. The number of the units in the pool is indicated on the label. The same storage temperature and outdate apply.

Fibrin Glue from Cryoprecipitated Antihemophilic Factor

CRYO is also used to prepare a topical hemostatic solution useful in controlling bleeding during surgery and a variety of procedures, including aortic surgery, patch grafts, cerebrospinal fluid leaks, cosmetic surgery, and nasal narrowing surgery.[23] Additional applications include controlling bleeding during tooth extraction and minor surgical procedures for patients with von Willebrand's disease, hemophilia, and thrombasthenia.[24] One to two units of CRYO are mixed with thrombin and applied to the bleeding surface by layering, mixing, or spraying on the surgical field. Fibrinogen is converted to fibrin by the action of thrombin, which forms a clot to stop bleeding.

GRANULOCYTES, PHERESIS

Indications for Use

Three major types of leukocytes are found in blood: lymphocytes, granulocytes, and monocytes. Granulocytes are further subdivided into neutrophils, eosinophils, and basophils by their appearance and function. Neutrophils are the most numerous leukocytes in the blood and are involved in phagocytosis of bacteria and fungi. Adequate numbers of neutrophils are essential in responding to infection.

The use of granulocyte transfusions is rare and limited to a small number of patients. Better success with granulocyte transfusions has been observed in the treatment of septic infants.[25] The reason for the decreased use of granulocytes is due to:

- ◆ More effective antibiotics
- ◆ Recombinant growth factor that stimulates the bone marrow to produce leukocytes
- ◆ Adverse reactions associated with granulocyte transfusions

Granulocytes are limited to patients with the following conditions:

- ◆ Neutropenia (generally less than 0.5×10^9/L or 500/μl)
- ◆ Documented infections, especially gram-negative bacteria and fungi
- ◆ Lack of response to antibiotics

Granulocytes are prepared by hemapheresis. This product contains leukocytes and platelets as well as 20 to 50 ml of red blood cells. The number of granulocytes in each product equals or is greater than 1.0×10^{10}. Granulocytes deteriorate rapidly on storage and should be administered within 24 hours of collection. They are maintained at 20° to 24° C without agitation until transfused. A standard blood filter should be used, but not one that removes leukocytes. A crossmatch is usually required before transfusion because of red blood cell contamination above 2 ml.[12] Granulocyte support is usually continued until the granulocyte count increases and the infection is cured. Since patients undergoing this therapy are severely immunosuppressed, irradiation of the product to prevent GVHD is important.

LABELING

The labeling of whole blood and components is required to conform with the most recent version of the U.S. Industry Consensus Standard for the Uniform Labeling of Blood and Blood Components.[12] Currently, labeling must conform with the 1985 Uniform Labeling Guideline by the FDA and Title 21 of the Code of Federal Regulations (CFR), section 606.121, which is revised annually. A move toward the **ISBT-128** standard is being made that would standardize blood component labels internationally. Because of the overwhelming impact and large scope of this change, the original proposed deadline of 1998 has been delayed. A summary of current label requirements is included in Fig. 11-12.

ISBT-128: International Society of Blood Transfusion recommendations regarding the uniform labeling of blood products for international bar code recognition by computers.

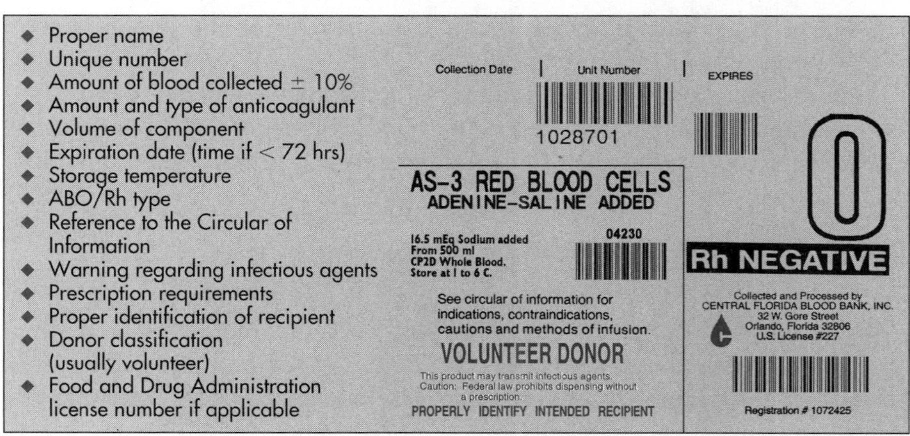

Fig. 11-12 Label requirements.

Courtesy of Central Florida Blood Bank, Inc., Orlando, Fla.

Labels on units are intended to provide sufficient information regarding the product without creating confusion. Standardization with regard to label placement, readability of bar codes by various computer systems, and product names is essential to prevent errors in transfusion and shipping. Required labels must be placed on the bag and cannot be substituted with tie tags (except for autologous blood labels). In addition to the standard label, specific requirements for other products follow:

- Irradiated components must have the name of the facility performing the irradiation
- Pooled components must include the final volume, unique number assigned to the pool, and name of the facility preparing the pooled component
- Autologous units must be labeled "For Autologous Use Only"

A facility receiving a unit of blood from another institution can place its own number on the unit; however, no more than two unique numeric or alphanumeric identification numbers should be visible on a blood component container. The original number must never be removed, since it may be necessary to remove numbers assigned by intermediary facilities.

The *Circular of Information* is referenced on the label as an important extension to component labels. This clear, concise guideline provides a description of each component, indications and contraindications for use, and information on dosage, administration, storage, side effects, and hazards. It is frequently updated and contains recent FDA guidelines.

STORAGE AND TRANSPORTATION

Proper storage of blood components is important to maintain product potency and prevent bacterial growth. FDA and AABB guidelines define procedures for the calibration and maintenance of equipment designed for product storage, storage temperature limits, and monitoring parameters. Specifically all refrigerators, freezers, and platelet incubators used for storing blood components must have the following:

- Recording devices to monitor the temperature at least every 4 hours
- Audible alarms to ensure a response 24 hours a day and an alarm set to signal the undesirable temperature *before* it is reached
- Alarm checks, performed on a regular basis
- Emergency procedures for power failure and alarm activation
- Emergency power backup systems; continuous power source for alarms
- Use of calibrated thermometers checked against referenced thermometers
- Written procedures for all of the above

Appropriate storage temperatures for blood components are listed in Table 11-3. During storage blood should be examined for evidence of hemolysis, abnormal coloring, or clots, any of which may indicate bacterial contamination.

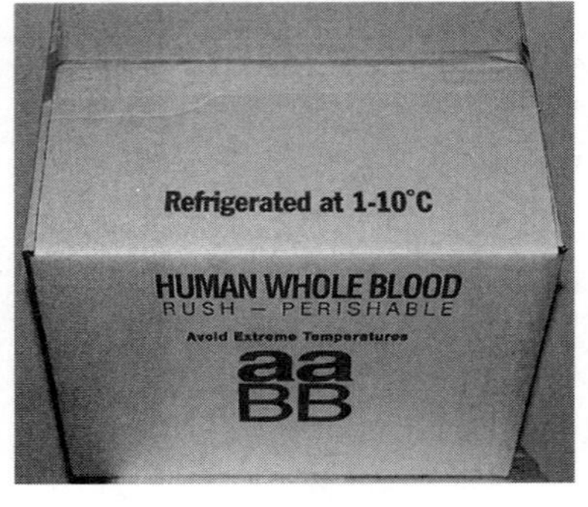

Fig. 11-13 Blood container for transporting blood products.
Courtesy of Central Florida Blood Bank, Inc., Orlando, Fla.

Transportation of Blood Components

Whole blood or red blood cells that are packaged for shipping must be maintained between 1° and 10° C. Plastic bags of wet ice placed on top of the units can maintain appropriate temperatures for 24 hours if properly packed. Containers used for shipping must be validated periodically to ensure their effectiveness for shipping at wide ranges of outdoor temperatures (Fig. 11-13).

Frozen units are shipped on dry ice. Since frozen products are brittle, they must be wrapped carefully. As dry ice evaporates, extra space allows the units to move about in the box and potentially break. Platelets must be maintained as close as possible to 20° to 24° C during shipping. Discontinuation of the agitation of platelets during transportation should not exceed 24 hours.[12]

On receipt of a shipment of blood components, the temperature and appearance of the units must be observed and recorded. Container closure and attached segments should also be inspected (Box 11-2). Units that are received out of the designated temperature range must be evaluated for their suitability for transfusion. The shipping facility should be notified if the product is unacceptable. Questionable units should be quarantined until a responsible person determines the disposition.[3] Shipping records, including details of problems and the outcomes, must be maintained.

Units that are issued to an unmonitored area, such as a patient's room, are usually not accepted back into inventory unless a time limit (usually 30 minutes) is set or the units have been transported in an insulated cooler or container. Only 1 unit is typically issued at a time unless the transfusion requirement is urgent.

Appropriate training of staff involved in the shipping and transportation of blood and blood components, in both the hospital and blood center setting, is essential for the maintenance of quality products. Policies and procedures for all aspects of component packaging, inspection, record keeping, and monitoring must be understood and followed carefully.

BOX 11-2

Checklist for Receiving Blood

- Temperature acceptable for component
- Appearance:
  Clots
  Discoloration
  Hemolysis
- Container closure
- Attached segments intact: red blood cells
- Expiration date/time
- Shipping list correct
- Intact labels

ADMINISTRATION OF BLOOD COMPONENTS

This section summarizes important aspects of blood administration that pertain to the components described earlier. A more detailed discussion can be found in the *Technical Manual* and the *Physician's Handbook on Blood Transfusion Therapy*, both published by the AABB. Although laboratory personnel have limited involvement in blood administration, an understanding of the critical elements improves the communication between health care workers and therefore the safety of the transfusion. Box 11-3 lists these elements.

Requirements of safe blood administration include the following:

- *Positive identification* of the patient and blood sample is critical to avoid transfusion reactions that may be fatal.
- A *system to avoid and detect clerical errors* also contributes to avoiding serious reactions. Strict adherence to policies regarding identification numbers and mislabeled tubes should be followed.
- *Direct observation* of the patient should occur during the first 15 minutes after infusion begins and every 30 minutes thereafter. Prompt intervention of a transfusion reaction is important in reducing its severity.
- *Only normal saline* (0.9% USP) should be administered with blood components. Hypotonic solutions such as 5% dextrose cause hemolysis in vitro. Ringer's lactate, which contains calcium, can initiate in vitro coagulation by reversing the action of citrate. The additions of medications to blood can cause hemolysis and mask adverse reactions.
- *Use of filters*: A 170-micron standard filter must be used with all blood components. Leukoreduction filters, which can be substituted to prevent febrile reactions and HLA alloimmunization, are specific for platelets and red blood cells and cannot be interchanged.
- *Time limits*: Blood should be infused within 4 hours because of the risk of bacterial growth. If the patient's condition requires blood infusion to extend past

BOX 11-3

Checklist for Blood Administration

- Positive identification:
  Tubes
  Patient
  Unit
- Only normal saline (0.9% USP)
- 170-micron standard filter
- Appropriate Leukopoor filter
- Observe patient: first 15 minutes, every 30 minutes thereafter
- Time: no more than 4 hours
- Correct documentation

4 hours, the unit should be divided and kept in the blood bank refrigerator until needed.

- *Documentation and record keeping* are essential. The patient's medical record must include the following information with regard to a transfusion:
  - Donor unit number or pool number
  - Date and time of transfusion
  - Pretransfusion and posttransfusion vital signs
  - Amount transfused
  - Identification of the transfusionist
  - Whether a transfusion reaction occurred[12]

Adverse transfusion reactions can occur, regardless of how carefully the component was prepared, tested, crossmatched, and administered. The reporting of a reaction that occurs during or following administration is an important procedure that must be followed without deviation. Good communication between the transfusing personnel and the laboratory in the event of a reaction expedites its resolution and prevents further complications. Adverse consequences of transfusions are thoroughly discussed in Chapter 12.

CHAPTER SUMMARY

A summary of blood components and their indications for use, and ABO and Rh compatibility for the selection of both plasma products and red blood cells, is shown below. Important concepts in the preparation and transfusion of blood components are listed as follows:

1. The ability to separate a unit of whole blood maximizes the use of a limited resource and provides a product of optimal therapeutic value to the patient.
2. The separation of a unit of whole blood into its parts is performed by centrifugation. Each product has an optimal storage temperature and expiration limit.
3. Adherence to the FDA's good manufacturing practices is required to ensure proper procedures are followed and accurate records are maintained during the manufacturing, labeling, storage, and distribution of blood components.
4. Product potency is monitored by periodic quality control. These standards are part of the FDA and AABB requirements.
5. Additional product preparation may be necessary, including HLA matching, leukocyte reduction, and irradiation, to prevent or reduce the risk of complications related to certain patient diseases or conditions.
6. The proper dispensing and administration of all blood products is important in transfusion safety. Patient and unit identification is a critical step in this process.

SUMMARY OF BLOOD COMPONENT THERAPY

Component	Approximate Volume	Indications
Whole blood	500 ml	Increases oxygen-carrying capacity and plasma volume
Red blood cells	250 ml	Increase oxygen-carrying capacity: anemia, trauma, and surgery
Platelets	50 ml	Bleeding caused by thrombocytopenia or thrombocytopathy

SUMMARY OF BLOOD COMPONENT THERAPY—CONT'D

Platelets, pheresis	300 ml	Bleeding caused by thrombocytopenia or thrombocytopathy
Fresh frozen plasma	200 ml	Replace stable and labile coagulation factors
Cryoprecipitated antihemophilic factor	10-15 ml	Treatment of Factor VII, XIII, and von Willebrand's deficiencies
Granulocytes	600 ml	Increase granulocytes in severe sepsis
Leukocyte reduced products		Avoid febrile nonhemolytic reactions and prevent human leukocyte antigen alloimmunization
Red blood cells, washed	200 ml	Reduce plasma proteins to avoid allergic and anaphylactic reactions
Red blood cells, frozen	200 ml	Rare blood and autologous storage

ABO/Rh COMPATIBILITY: PLASMA AND RED BLOOD CELLS

Plasma

	Donor					
Recipient	**A**	**B**	**O**	**AB**	**Rh+**	**Rh−**
A						
B						
O						
AB						
Rh+						
Rh−						

Red Blood Cells

	Donor					
Recipient	**A**	**B**	**O**	**AB**	**Rh+**	**Rh−**
A						
B						
O						
AB						
Rh+						
Rh−						

◊ CRITICAL THINKING EXERCISES

◆ *EXERCISE 11-1*

Is it possible to prepare CRYO and FFP from the same blood unit? Explain your answer.

◆ *EXERCISE 11-2*

A nonbleeding adult of average height and weight with chronic anemia is transfused with 2 units of red blood cells. The pretransfusion hemoglobin is 7.0 g/dl. What is the expected posttransfusion hemoglobin? If the hemoglobin does not increase as expected, list potential reasons.

◆ *EXERCISE 11-3*

A severely immunosuppressed adult patient has been transfused with a pool of 10 units of platelets, pooled. The pretransfusion platelet count was 6000 μl. What is the expected platelet count 1 hour from transfusion? If the platelet count does not increase as expected, what are some potential causes?

◆ ***EXERCISE 11-4***

A unit of blood is released for a patient on the oncology floor. Fifteen minutes later the nurse calls the blood bank and reports that the patient has a visitor and doesn't want the transfusion until later that day. The nurse would like to hold the unit in the refrigerator on the floor since she is too busy to return it right now. How do you respond?

◆ ***EXERCISE 11-5***

A 60-kg hemophilic patient is going to have a small tumor removed. The physician requests enough CRYO to maintain the patient at 50% activity for surgery. The patient is currently at 15%. Determine how many units need to be pooled for surgery.

◆ ***EXERCISE 11-6***

1. A 70-lb child is scheduled for orthopedic surgery in 3 weeks. The physician requested that 2 units of autologous red blood cells be drawn before surgery. Determine the amount to be drawn and the anticoagulant adjustment for drawing from this child.
2. On the day of surgery, the patient becomes ill and surgery is postponed. Because of the tight operating room schedule, the surgery cannot take place for 2 months. Do the units need to be discarded and redrawn? Do any options exist?
3. The patient's older sister would like to be a donor for this patient. She meets the regular blood donor criteria and donates as a directed donor 1 week before the new surgery date. What needs to be performed before this unit can be made available to her sister? Will the expiration date change? If her sister does not use the unit during surgery, can it be returned to regular inventory?

◆ ***EXERCISE 11-7***

1. A nurse is completing her shift in 1 hour and needs to start a transfusion and give the same patient an intravenous medication before she leaves. To expedite the process she opts to give both through the Y-set she has prepared for the blood administration. She is not sure if this is allowed, so she calls the blood bank before she picks up the blood. What should she be advised to do?
2. The nurse is in a hurry to start this transfusion and realizes that the intravenous solution she attached to the blood administration set is 2% dextrose instead of 0.9% saline. Can she proceed with this transfusion, or should she wait for 0.9% saline? Why?

STUDY QUESTIONS

For questions 1 through 7 match the clinical condition to the component that would have the best therapeutic value. Components may be used more than once.

Patient Problem	Component
1. von Willebrand's disease	a. FFP
2. Hemophilia A	b. CRYO
3. Thrombocytopenia	c. Red blood cells, washed
4. Refractory platelet response	d. Granulocytes
5. Newborn exchange transfusion	e. Platelets
6. Sickle cell disease	f. Platelets, HLA matched
7. IgA-deficient patient with anti-IgA	g. Red blood cells

8. The average content of fibrinogen in 1 unit of CRYO is:
   a. 100 to 150 mg
   b. 200 to 250 mg
   c. 700 to 750 mg
   d. 750 to 1000 mg

9. Acute loss of 10% of blood volume usually necessitates:
   a. replacement with red blood cells
   b. replacement with whole blood
   c. replacement with colloid solutions
   d. no replacement

For questions 10 through 17 match the correct expiration times on the right with the appropriate blood component on the left. Expiration times can be used more than once.

Component	Expiration Times
10. Red blood cells, AS-1	a. 35 days
11. Red blood cells, washed	b. 28 days
12. Red blood cells, irradiated	c. 3 days
13. Red blood cells, CPDA-1	d. 24 hours
14. Red blood cells, rejuvenated	e. 42 days
15. Red blood cells, frozen	f. 10 years
16. Red blood cells, open system	g. 21 days
17. Red blood cells, CPD	h. 1 year

18. Eight units of platelets were pooled. The new expiration is:
    a. 2 hours
    b. 4 hours
    c. 6 hours
    d. 24 hours

19. In preparing platelets from a unit of whole blood, the correct order of centrifugation is:
    a. hard spin followed by a hard spin
    b. light spin followed by a light spin
    c. hard spin followed by a light spin
    d. light spin followed by a hard spin

20. Red blood cells that have been frozen are stored at:
    a. −65° C for 5 years
    b. −85° C for 10 years
    c. −65° C for 10 years
    d. −80° C for 10 years

21. Platelets, pheresis must contain a minimum of how many platelets to be acceptable?
    a. 5.5×10^{10}
    b. 3.3×10^{11}
    c. 5.0×10^{11}
    d. 3.0×10^{11}

22. Sterile connecting devices are used to:
    a. filter leukocytes from whole blood
    b. deglycerolize frozen red blood cells
    c. weld tubing to maintain sterility
    d. connect platelets for pooling

23. Temperature limits for shipping red blood cells are:
    a. 1° to 6° C
    b. 1° to 10° C
    c. 2° to 8° C
    d. 20° to 24° C

REFERENCES

1. Lane T: *Blood transfusion therapy, a physician's handbook*, ed 5, Bethesda, Md, 1996, American Association of Blood Banks.
2. Quinley ED, Caglioti TA: *GMP fundamentals*, Raritan, NJ, 1994, Ortho Diagnostics.
3. Vengelen-Tyler V, editor: *Technical manual*, ed 12, Bethesda, Md, 1996, American Association of Blood Banks.
4. Beutler E, Wood L: The in vivo regeneration of red cell 2,3 diphosphoglyceric acid (DPG) after transfusion of stored blood, *J Lab Clin Med* 74:300, 1969.
5. Beutler E: Preservation of liquid red cells. In Rossi EC, Simon TL, Moss GS, Gould SA, editors: *Principles of transfusion medicine*, ed 2, Baltimore, Md, 1995, Williams & Wilkins.
6. American Association of Blood Banks/America's Blood Centers/American Red Cross: *Circular of information for the use of human blood and blood components*, April 1997.
7. *Rejuvesol*, Product insert, Braintree, Mass., 1993, Cytosol Laboratories.
8. Shackford SR, Virgilio R, Peters RM: Whole blood versus packed-cell transfusion: a physiologic comparison, *Ann Surg* 193:337, 1981.
9. Levy GJ, Strauss RG, Hume H, et al: National survey of neonatal transfusion practices. I. red blood cell therapy, *Pediatrics* 91:523, 1993.
10. Heaton A: Introduction: timing of leukodepletion of blood products, *Semin Hematol* 28:1,1991.
11. Bowden RA, Slichter SJ, Sayers M, et al: A comparison of filtered leukocyte-reduced and cytomegalovirus (CMV) seronegative blood products for the prevention of transfusion-associated CMV infection after marrow transplant, *Blood* 86:3598,1995.
12. Menitove JE, editor: *Standards for blood banks and transfusion services*, ed 18, Bethesda, Md, 1997, American Association of Blood Banks.
13. Meryman HT: Principles of cryopreservation and the current role of frozen red blood cells in blood banking and clinical medicine. In Glassman AB, Umlas J: *Cryopreservation of tissue and solid organs for transplantation*, Arlington, Va, 1983, American Association of Blood Banks.
14. Shivdasani RA, Anderson KC: Graft-versus-host disease. In Petz LD, Swisher SN, Kleinman S, et al, editors: *Clinical practice of transfusion medicine*, ed 3, New York, 1996, Churchill Livingstone.
15. Sazama K, Holland P: Transfusion induced graft-versus-host disease. In Garratty G, editor: *Immunobiology of transfusion medicine*, New York, 1994, Marcel Dekker.
16. Baldwin M, Jefferies L, editors: *Irradiation of blood components*, Bethesda, Md, 1992, American Association of Blood Banks.
17. Food and Drug Administration: *Memorandum: Recommendations regarding license amendments and procedures for gamma irradiation of blood products*, Rockville, Md, July 22, 1993, Congressional and Consumer Affairs.
18. Harmening DM: Introduction to hemostasis: an overview of hemostatic mechanism, platelet structure and function, and extrinsic and intrinsic functions. In Harmening DM, editor: *Clinical hematology and fundamentals of hemostasis*, ed 2, Philadelphia, 1992, FA Davis.
19. Slichter SJ: Mechanisms and management of platelet refractoriness. In Nance SJ, editor: *Transfusion medicine in the 1990's*, Arlington, Va, 1990, American Association of Blood Banks.
20. Heyman MR, Schiffer CA: Platelet transfusion to patients receiving chemotherapy. In Rossi EC, Simon TL, Moss GS, editors: *Principles of transfusion medicine*, Baltimore, 1991, Williams & Wilkins.
21. Slichter SJ: Platelet transfusion therapy, *Hematol Oncol Clin North Am* 4:291, 1990.
22. American Red Cross: *Red Cross announces launch of first virus-inactivated blood component: new advance offers increased protection of the US plasma blood supply*, April 10, 1998. Available at: www.redcross.org/news/inthenews/98/4-10-98. Accessed Sept. 13, 1998.
23. Bulova S: New literature review: surgical transfusion practice. In *The compendium: a collection of short topic presentations*, Bethesda, Md, 1997, American Association of Blood Banks.
24. Martinowitz U, Schulman S, Horoszowski H, Heim M: Role of fibrin sealants in surgical procedures on patients with hemostatic disorders, *Clin Orthop* 328:65, 1996, and related research.
25. Strauss RG: Granulocyte transfusions. In Rossi EC, Simon TL, Moss GS, Gould SA, editors: *Principles of transfusion medicine*, ed 2, New York, 1996, Churchill Livingstone.

Clinical Considerations in Immunohematology

V

12 ADVERSE COMPLICATIONS OF TRANSFUSIONS

Paula R. Howard

CHAPTER OUTLINE

LEARNING OBJECTIVES

Upon completion of this chapter, the reader should be able to:

1. Categorize the adverse complications of transfusion.
2. Describe the immunobiology of in vivo red blood cell destruction and discuss factors that influence the severity of the clinical features.
3. Distinguish the features characteristic of an acute and delayed immune-mediated hemolytic transfusion reaction.
4. Discuss the mechanisms that may effect non-immune-mediated red blood cell destruction.
5. Describe the major features of the following immune-mediated nonhemolytic transfusion reactions: febrile, urticarial, anaphylactic, transfusion-related acute lung injury, and transfusion-associated graft versus host disease.
6. Discuss the mechanism and clinical features of the bacterial contamination of blood products.
7. Describe the clinical features of a transfusion reaction caused by circulatory overload.
8. Describe the mechanisms of transfusion hemosiderosis, citrate toxicity, and posttransfusion purpura in relation to the adverse complications of transfusions.
9. List the responsibilities of medical personnel performing the transfusion in the event of an adverse reaction.
10. Identify steps taken in the transfusion service on receipt of a patient sample postreaction.
11. Identify other testing that may be required in the investigation of transfusion reactions and the rationale for selecting these tests.
12. Describe the documentation required for a transfusion service in the investigation of a transfusion reaction.

The primary objective of the blood banking community is the provision of a safe and adequate blood supply. Blood banks and transfusion services strive to provide blood products for the recipient's optimal hematologic benefit. Many systems and procedures have been designed to reduce the risk of adverse complications of blood transfusions. Transfusion safety measures incorporated at all steps of the blood collection, donor unit processing, and transfusion protocols. This chapter provides an overview of the proposed mechanisms, risks, and preventive measures associated with complications of blood transfusion.

OVERVIEW OF COMPLICATIONS IN TRANSFUSION

Transfusion reaction: any unfavorable response by a patient to the infusion of blood or blood products.

The term **transfusion reaction** is defined as any unfavorable response by a patient to the infusion of blood or blood products.[1] Millions of donor units are collected and transfused to patients. Within this frame of reference, the relative risks of a complication to transfusion are varied. Urticarial reactions, the most common complication of transfusion, have been reported at 10,000 to 20,000 incidents per million units transfused; febrile reactions followed with 5,000 to 10,000 incidents per million units transfused.[2] In comparison, ABO-related fatal acute hemolytic reactions occurred with 1.7 incidents per 1 million units transfused.[3]

Adverse complications of transfusion may be classified into several categories:

- *Hemolytic versus nonhemolytic* – Hemolytic reactions result in the destruction of red blood cells and may proceed to the point where free hemoglobin is liberated. These reactions may be due to either an immune process or some sort of physical or chemical damage to the transfused red blood cells. Nonhemolytic reactions, such as febrile and allergic reactions, do not involve the destruction of red blood cells.
- *Acute versus delayed* – In acute reactions onset is rapid and occurs within hours of the transfusion. In delayed reactions onset of reaction occurs days or even weeks after the transfusion.
- *Immune-mediated versus non-immune-mediated* – Immune-mediated reactions occur as a result of antigen-antibody interactions. These reactions may involve antibodies with specificities toward antigens of the red blood cells, white blood cells (human leukocyte antigen [HLA] and granulocytes), or platelets. The activation of complement may be involved along with the generation of identifiable cytokines.
- *Infectious versus noninfectious* – Bacterial, viral, and parasitic blood-borne agents have been linked to complications of transfusion.

The acute and delayed adverse effects of blood transfusions are summarized in Boxes 12-1 and 12-2 by categories.

BOX 12-1

Acute Adverse Complications of Blood Transfusion

IMMUNE-MEDIATED
Hemolytic
Febrile nonhemolytic
Urticarial
Anaphylactic
Transfusion-related acute lung injury

NON-IMMUNE-MEDIATED
Bacterial contamination
Physical red blood cell damage
Citrate toxicity
Circulatory overload

BOX 12-2

Delayed Adverse Complications of Blood Transfusion

IMMUNE-MEDIATED
Hemolytic
Transfusion-associated graft versus host disease
Posttransfusion purpura

NON-IMMUNE-MEDIATED
Disease transmission
Transfusion hemosiderosis

IN VIVO RED BLOOD CELL DESTRUCTION

The clinical sequelae of a hemolytic transfusion reaction (HTR) were documented more than 70 years ago in the literature. Since these first reports much research has been performed to discern the underlying mechanisms of these events. The clinical signs and symptoms of HTRs have not been completely elucidated to date. An HTR may be the manifestation of the clinical consequences of the immune destruction of transfused red blood cells that results in intravascular or extravascular hemolysis or a combination of both. In addition, an HTR may stem from a nonimmune etiology. Thermal damage, mechanical damage, osmotic destruction, and bacterial contamination are several factors that may also generate a hemolytic episode in the transfusion recipient.

The clinical presentation of an immune-mediated HTR encompasses many clinical signs, ranging in severity from fever to death. The severe clinical consequences of HTR include hypotension progressing to irreversible shock, disseminated intravascular coagulation, and renal failure (Fig. 12-1). Acute HTR commonly manifests an intravascular hemolysis accompanied by hemoglobinemia and hemoglobinuria. In contrast to an acute HTR, a delayed HTR is less severe and often misdiagnosed. The clinical variability of these HTRs can be explained in terms of the pathophysiologic mechanisms involved. A multitude of simultaneous clinical events contributes to the degree of severity resulting from the in vivo destruction of red blood cells.[4,5] Events of great significance in an immune-mediated HTR include:

- Antibody binding to red blood cells
- Activation of complement
- Activation of mononuclear phagocytes and cytokines
- Activation of coagulation
- Renal failure

Antibody Binding to Red Blood Cells

The first event in an immune-mediated HTR is the interaction of red blood cell antibodies with respective red blood cell antigens. This antigen-antibody complex formation initiates the clinical sequence of events associated with HTR. Characteristics of both the red blood cell alloantibody and corresponding antigen are major determinants for the course and severity of an HTR.[4]

Properties of the Antibodies

1. Immunoglobulin (Ig) class, whether IgM or IgG, influences the course of the reaction.
   - IgM molecules readily activate the classical pathway of complement leading to the potential of intravascular hemolysis (destruction of the transfused red blood cells within the vascular component). Intravascular hemolysis releases free hemoglobin and **red blood cell stroma** into the plasma. ABO antibodies have been implicated with intravascular hemolysis in the

Red blood cell stroma: red blood cell membrane that remains following hemolysis.

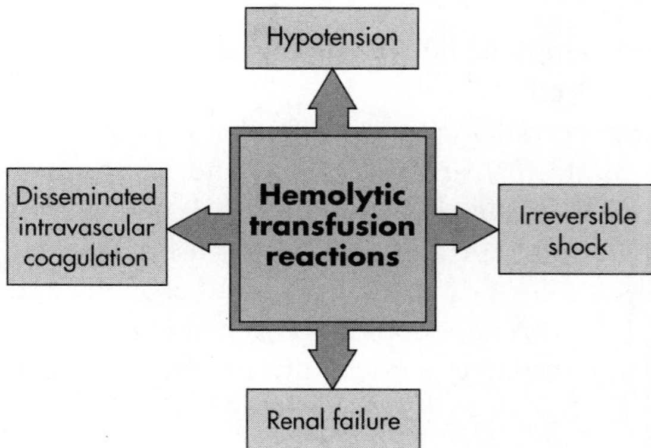

Fig. 12-1 Clinical consequences of hemolytic transfusion reactions.

transfusion recipient. Almost all ABO system antibodies are capable of binding to antigen-positive red blood cells at 37° C. In addition, both IgM and IgG forms of the ABO antibodies are capable of the activation of complement.
- IgG molecules less commonly activate the complement pathway but can interact with Fc receptors of mononuclear phagocytes, effecting phagocytosis and cellular activation.

2. The concentration or titer of the red blood cell alloantibody also influences the extent and severity of HTR. Higher concentrations of circulating antibody in a transfusion recipient are more likely to produce severe clinical manifestations. For example, ABO antibodies are often of high titer and **avidity** in individuals never exposed to foreign red blood cells.

Avidity: sum total of the strength of binding of two molecules (e.g., antigen and antibody).

Properties of the Antigens

The density (number of antigens per red blood cell) and distribution of the targeted red blood cell antigens also influence the severity of an HTR. Scattered surface antigens bind fewer antibody molecules per red blood cell and are less likely to initiate severe hemolytic episodes. In contrast, antigens that are clustered together on the red blood cell surface increase the chances for the activation of the classical pathway of complement.

Other Effects of Immune Complexes

In addition to the activation of complement, antigen-antibody complexes may contribute in alternate pathways of the pathophysiology of a transfusion reaction. **Bradykinin,** a potent vasodilator and one of the plasma **kinins,** is generated as a sequela of immune complex formation. The physiologic consequences produce vasodilation and hypotension. In addition, antigen-antibody complex formation plays a role in the release of **norepinephrine,** which contributes to the vasoconstriction observed in the kidneys and lungs.[1]

Bradykinin: potent vasodilator of the kinin family.
Kinins: group of proteins associated with contraction of smooth muscle, vascular permeability, and vasodilation.
Norepinephrine: hormone that increases blood pressure by vasoconstriction.

Activation of Complement

In an HTR, complement functions in three capacities, including opsonization, anaphylatoxin generation, and red blood cell lysis.[4] Activated in HTR through the classical pathway, complement necessitates the presence of either IgM or IgG antibodies to begin the activation of C1q. The process proceeds to the cleavage of C3 and the binding of C3b to the red blood cell membrane. Complement activation may further proceed to the assembly of the membrane attack complex and the hemolysis of cells.

As a consequence of the activation of complement, the following events are noted:

- Opsonization occurs because the membrane-bound complement products are cleared by mononuclear phagocytic cells.
- Anaphylatoxins, potent inducers of inflammation, are liberated into the plasma. These products act on mast cells, smooth muscle, and neutrophils. C5a acts on smooth muscle to effect contraction with an overall net effect of vascular dilation and bronchospasm.[3] C3a and C5a also cause vasoactive amine (**serotonin** and **histamine**) release by mast cells and basophils and effect degranulation of neutrophils. The net effect of the systemic release of serotonin and histamine is increased vascular permeability. An overall state of hypotension is created.

Serotonin: potent vasoconstrictor liberated by platelets.
Histamine: compound that causes constriction of bronchial smooth muscle, dilation of capillaries, and decrease in blood pressure.

- The final pathway in complement activation assembles the membrane attack complex with the end result of red blood cell lysis. The liberated hemoglobin is bound by plasma **haptoglobin**. When the hemoglobin-binding capacity of plasma haptoglobin is exceeded, hemoglobinemia and hemoglobinuria are detectable.

Haptoglobin: plasma protein with sole function of binding free hemoglobin and carrying the molecule to the hepatocytes for further catabolism.

Activation of Mononuclear Phagocytes and Cytokines

Red blood cells sensitized with either immunoglobulin or complement are removed from the circulation by the mononuclear phagocyte system. The macrophages, located in the spleen, are probably most active in this mechanism, although the Kupffer cells of the liver also participate.

These mononuclear phagocytes also generate cytokines that mediate the systemic effects often associated with HTRs. The term *cytokines* refers to protein hormones involved in cell-to-cell communication. The combined effects of these cytokines include fever, hypotension, activation of T cells and B cells, and activation of endothelial cells to express procoagulant activity.[5,6]

Activation of Coagulation

Antigen-antibody–complement complexes may initiate the coagulation and fibrinolytic systems. Disseminated intravascular coagulation (DIC) is often associated with an acute HTR. The cardinal signs of DIC include the consumption of clotting factors (particularly fibrinogen, Factor V, and Factor VIII) and platelets with resulting diffuse, uncontrolled microvascular bleeding. The microvascular thrombi promote tissue **ischemia** and release of tissue factor, further encouraging the activation of more thrombin. Hemostatic profiles of patients in DIC demonstrate low platelet counts and decreased fibrinogen levels with the presence of fibrin degradation products.

Ischemia: decreased supply of oxygenated blood to an organ or body part.

Renal Failure

Renal failure caused by a severe HTR is a multifactorial event and most prominent in an untreated acute HTR. Contributing factors to the renal failure include systemic hypotension, reactive renal vasoconstriction, and deposition of intravascular thrombi whose cumulative effects compromise the renal cortical blood supply.[1] The release of norepinephrine in a physiologic reaction to the hypotension and shock produces the vasoconstriction observed in the kidneys and lungs. The developing renal ischemia may be transient or advance to acute tubular necrosis and renal loss.

ACUTE AND DELAYED IMMUNE-MEDIATED HEMOLYTIC TRANSFUSION REACTIONS

As outlined in the previous section, an HTR in a transfusion recipient may produce serious clinical consequences. Acute HTRs are characterized by many clinical signs, a rapid onset, and the potential for serious clinical complications in transfusion recipients. These reactions are usually associated with the transfusion of ABO-incompatible red blood cells. In contrast delayed HTRs are usually less severe in scope with no major clinical complications. The significant distinctions between acute and delayed immune-mediated hemolytic transfusion reactions are summarized in Table 12-1.

Table 12-1 Summary of Acute versus Delayed Hemolytic Transfusion Reactions

	ACUTE	DELAYED
Clinical signs/symptoms	◆ Fever, chills, flushing, pain at site of infusion, tachycardia, tachypnea, lower back pain, hemoglobinemia, hemoglobinuria, hypotension ◆ Dramatic and severe; rapid onset	◆ 5 to 7 days posttransfusion ◆ Fever (with or without chills) ◆ Unexplainable decrease in hemoglobin and hematocrit ◆ Occasional mild jaundice
Major complications	◆ DIC, renal failure, irreversible shock, death	◆ No major complications ◆ Less severe reaction
Causes	◆ Ag-Ab interaction causes rapid activation of large amounts of complement ◆ Major side ABO incompatibility (group A, B, or AB donor unit to group O recipient) ◆ Other antibodies: anti-Vel, anti-PP_1P^k	◆ Patient previous primary immune response but has a low concentration of alloantibody; anamnestic response on reexposure to red blood cell antigen ◆ Alloantibody not demonstrable by conventional antibody detection techniques ◆ Alloantibodies to Rh, Duffy, and Kidd antigens are commonly seen
Incidence	◆ 1:25,000 transfusions[4] ◆ Human error in patient and specimen identification	◆ 1:2,500 transfusions[4]
Clinical laboratory tests	◆ ↑ Plasma free hemoglobin ◆ ↑ Serum bilirubin (6 hr posttransfusion) ◆ ↓ Haptoglobin ◆ Hemoglobinuria ◆ DAT: positive or negative	◆ DAT: positive ◆ Posttransfusion antibody screen: positive ◆ ↓ Hemoglobin/hematocrit
Management	◆ Treat hypotension and DIC ◆ Maintain adequate renal blood flow ◆ Dialysis if renal failure	◆ Provide antigen-negative donor units ◆ No additional treatment necessary
Prevention	◆ Design and implement systems to avoid errors of mislabeled samples and patient identification ◆ Design and implement systems to decrease chances of technical error	◆ Check patient records

DIC, Disseminated intravascular coagulation; *Ag-Ab*, antigen-antibody; ↑, increased levels; ↓, decreased levels; *DAT*, direct antiglobulin test.

NON-IMMUNE-MEDIATED MECHANISMS OF RED BLOOD CELL DESTRUCTION

For a transfusion reaction in a patient experiencing hemoglobinemia and hemoglobinuria, the initial focus investigates the possibility of an immune-related response. When alloantibodies are not implicated, an investigation into the nonimmunologic mechanisms of red blood cell destruction should be initiated. This process necessitates examination of the segments or remaining blood from the unit in question with careful questioning of personnel regarding the transfusion process itself. If a hemolyzed donor unit is accidentally transfused, the recipient receives free hemoglobin and red blood cell stroma. The red blood cell stroma may stimulate complement activation and a procoagulant state.

Examples of the causes from non-immune-mediated red blood cell hemolysis include:

◆ Exposure of red blood cells to extreme temperatures (greater than 50° C or less than 0° C)

Exposure to extreme temperatures may produce hemolysis of red blood cells. The use of malfunctioning or unregulated blood warming devices or warming during refrigerated storage may lead to hemolyzed units. Red blood cells stored frozen without additive cryoprotectants induce the hemolysis of the units.

- Improper deglycerolization of a red blood cell unit on thawing
  A simple test to prevent this complication of transfusion is to observe the supernatant of a red blood cell suspension for evidence of hemolysis after the deglycerolization has been completed.
- Mechanical destruction of red blood cells
  Small-bore needles, mechanical valves, excessive pressure, and blood salvage equipment have been linked with nonimmune hemolysis of red blood cells.
- Incompatible solutions
  The only solution that may be added to a donor unit is physiologic saline. Blood mixed with nonphysiologic solutions such as half-strength saline, 5% dextrose in 0.18% saline, Ringer's lactate, and medications may effect osmotic rupture of the red blood cells.
- Transfusion of bacterially contaminated blood products
- Intrinsic red blood cell defect attributable to a clinical condition
  Certain clinical disease states may be responsible for hemolysis unrelated to the transfusion. These clinical conditions include sickle cell disease, thermal burns, glucose-6-phosphate dehydrogenase deficiency, and paroxysmal nocturnal hemoglobinuria.

IMMUNE-MEDIATED NONHEMOLYTIC TRANSFUSION REACTIONS

In addition to the adverse effects of immune-mediated hemolytic transfusion reactions, adverse effects that involve the immune system without producing a hemolytic state may predispose the transfusion recipient to complications. These reactions involve antibodies to HLA, granulocyte, or platelet antigens or may be hypersensitive in origin. These transfusion complications encompass the scope of mild reactions such as an urticarial consequence to the potentially fatal consequences of transfusion-associated graft versus host disease (TA-GVHD). For clarity of presentation, these reactions are summarized and presented in Tables 12-2 to 12-5.

Febrile Nonhemolytic Transfusion Reactions

The febrile nonhemolytic transfusion reaction is a commonly observed adverse effect of transfusion. Because its presenting clinical features are analogous to an acute HTR, a careful investigation is necessary to rule out this untoward consequence (Table 12-2).

Allergic Transfusion Reactions

Allergic reactions to transfusion range in clinical severity from minor urticarial effects to fulminant anaphylactic shock and death. The etiology of these reactions is derived from soluble allergens present in donor plasma. These reactions are more commonly associated with the transfusion of blood products containing a plasma component (Table 12-3).

Transfusion-Related Acute Lung Injury

Transfusion-related acute lung injury (TRALI), also referred to as transfusion-related noncardiogenic pulmonary edema, is a rare adverse complication of transfusion with an estimated risk of 50 to 100 cases per million units transfused.[2]

Table 12-2 Summary of Febrile Nonhemolytic Transfusion Reactions

Clinical signs/ symptoms	◆ Fever: Temperature 1 °C or more above baseline within 8 to 24 hours of transfusion[1] ◆ Chills may accompany fever ◆ Some recipients experience associated nausea, vomiting, headache, and back pain
Major complications	◆ Usually not life threatening for the recipient ◆ Important to differentiate from acute hemolytic reaction or bacterial contamination
Causes	◆ Recipient HLA antibodies to antigens on donor lymphocytes, monocytes, and granulocytes are responsible for most false-negative HTRs ◆ Cytokines released by white blood cells during blood product storage
Incidence	◆ Commonly occur in patients with histories of multiple pregnancies and transfusions; multiple prior exposures to white blood cell and platelet antigens ◆ More common in women ◆ 1:200 donor units transfused[7] ◆ Complicate upwards of 20% of platelet transfusions
Clinical laboratory tests	◆ DAT: negative ◆ No visible hemolysis
Management	◆ Antipyretics: acetaminophen
Prevention	◆ White blood cell reduction of blood products ◆ Reduction in the number of WBCs to less than 5×10^6 prevents most febrile reactions

HLA, Human leukocyte antigen; *DAT*, direct antiglobulin test.

Table 12-3 Summary of Allergic Transfusion Reactions

	URTICARIAL	ANAPHYLACTIC
Clinical signs/symptoms	◆ Wheals, hives, erythema, itching ◆ Occur within 15 to 20 minutes of transfusion	◆ Rapid onset and severe, after small volume is transfused ◆ Wheezing, coughing, dyspnea, bronchospasm, respiratory distress, vascular instability ◆ No fever
Major complications	◆ None	◆ Shock, loss of consciousness ◆ Death
Causes	◆ Recipient antibodies to foreign plasma proteins or other substances such as drugs or food consumed by blood donor	◆ Associated with genetic IgA deficiency in recipient ◆ Possesses IgG, complement-binding anti-IgA antibodies
Incidence	◆ 1% to 3% of recipients of blood products containing plasma[8]	◆ Rare ◆ 1:20,000 to 1:50,000 transfusions[1]
Clinical laboratory tests	◆ DAT: negative ◆ No visible hemolysis	◆ DAT: negative ◆ No visible hemolysis
Management	◆ Transfusion interrupted and antihistamine administered	◆ Transfusion terminated ◆ Epinephrine administered ◆ Oxygen administered and open airways maintained
Prevention	◆ Prophylactic premedication with antihistamine if patient history reveals repetitive allergic reactions ◆ May necessitate washed cellular products	◆ Plasma-containing products from IgA-deficient donors ◆ Washed red blood cell and platelet products

DAT, Direct antiglobulin test.

Table 12-4 Summary of Transfusion-Related Acute Lung Injury

Clinical signs/ symptoms	◆ Marked respiratory distress ◆ Fever, hypotension, chills, cyanosis ◆ Nonproductive cough ◆ Rapid onset
Major complications	◆ Severe and dramatic presentation ◆ Outcome sometimes fatal
Causes	◆ Pathophysiology poorly understood ◆ Interaction of granulocytes and HLA-specific donor antibodies (several reports of patient with the antibodies), complement activation, and promotion of the aggregation of granulocytes that leads to blockage of the pulmonary microvasculature ◆ Capillary damage, vascular leakage, pulmonary edema
Incidence	◆ 1:10,000 transfusions[1]
Clinical laboratory tests	◆ DAT: negative ◆ No visible hemolysis
Management	◆ Respiratory support ◆ Administration of steroids
Prevention	◆ Donor screening for white blood cell antibodies would eliminate these reactions; the practicality of such screening is questionable.

HLA, Human leukocyte antigen; *DAT*, direct antiglobulin test.

Table 12-5 Summary of Transfusion-Associated Graft versus Host Disease

Clinical signs/symptoms	◆ Onset 3 to 30 days posttransfusion ◆ Fever, erythematous maculopapular rash, abnormal liver function ◆ Nausea, vomiting, jaundice, abdominal pain, diarrhea
Major complications	◆ Sepsis and hemorrhage ◆ 90% mortality rate
Cause	◆ Transfused immunocompetent T-lymphocytes mount an immunologic response against the recipient
Incidence	◆ Rare
Clinical laboratory tests	◆ Confirmation by HLA typing to demonstrate a disparity between donor lymphocytes and recipient tissues
Management	◆ Unresponsive to medical intervention
Prevention	◆ Irradiation of blood products before transfusion in at-risk recipients ◆ HLA-matched platelets ◆ Gamma irradiation (25 Gray) to prevent blast transformation of the donor lymphocytes ◆ Excellent candidates for irradiated blood products include bone marrow or stem cell transplant patients, premature and term infants, fetuses requiring intrauterine transfusions, and recipients with hematologic malignancies or donor units from blood relatives.

HLA, Human leukocyte antigen.

The clinical acute respiratory distress occurs within 2 to 4 hours of transfusion (Table 12-4).

Transfusion-Associated Graft versus Host Disease

TA-GVHD is a rare but highly lethal complication of transfusion that carries a 90% mortality rate.[6] This immune reaction is mediated by immunocompetent donor lymphocytes in cellular blood components. Following the transfusion of donor lymphocytes to a recipient who is immunologically incompetent, the donor lymphocytes engraft and mount an immune response against the host tissues. Since the host is unable to destroy the transfused cells, the donor lymphocytes proliferate and respond to unshared histocompatibility antigens in the host. Recipients at high risk for developing TA-GVHD include the following: recipients with congenital or acquired immunodeficiencies, fetuses and infants less than 4 months old, and recipients of nonirradiated donor units from a blood relative (Table 12-5).

BACTERIAL CONTAMINATION OF BLOOD PRODUCTS

This serious and potentially fatal adverse complication of transfusion is the consequence of bacterial proliferation in donor units during storage. The major sources of the bacterial contamination include a transient bacteremia in an asymptomatic donor or improper cleansing of the donor's skin during blood collection. Bacterial endotoxins, generated during the storage period, exert a dramatic clinical picture on transfusion of the contaminated blood product. Transfusion recipients may experience shock rapidly. One or two fatalities per year are attributed to transfusion of contaminated blood.[8]

The introduction of plastic collection bags and closed systems has considerably decreased the probability of bacterial contamination. Care during the donor phlebotomy process is necessary to prevent entry of bacteria from the donor's skin into the collection system. Despite care in phlebotomy techniques several reports demonstrate that 2% of donor units become contaminated during the process.[9] Any contaminating bacteria in the donor unit that are unable to survive at 4°C die after several days of storage. However, those organisms capable of growth at 4°C find an ideal environment for their perpetuation. Bacteria such as *Pseudomonas fluorescens, P. putida, Yersinia enterocolitica, Escherichia freundii,* and *Enterobacter cloacae* can thrive under these conditions and promote transfusion reactions. Gram-positive saprophytes such as *Staphylococcus epidermidis* and *Bacillus cereus* are more commonly implicated in platelet contamination.

The clinical symptoms of bacterial contamination mimic HTRs. In addition, the number of infused organisms influences the symptomatic presentation and the clinical outcome. Treatment of the reaction must be initiated before confirmation of the etiology to prevent a fatal outcome. Broad-spectrum antibiotic therapy is provided to the recipient. Blood cultures from the patient and the blood bag are obtained. It is not mandated at this time to include screening studies for bacterial contamination of blood products. Visual checks of all donor units are performed at the time of issue by transfusion service personnel. The individual inspecting the donor unit should be alert for any visible discoloration, clots, cloudiness, or hemolysis. Careful attention to the cleansing of the phlebotomy site in the collection process also aids in the prevention of this category of transfusion complications.

CIRCULATORY OVERLOAD

Circulatory overload, as a category of adverse complications of transfusion, occurs when a patient's cardiopulmonary system exceeds its volume capacity. This complication of transfusion is considered if dyspnea, severe headache, peripheral edema, or other signs of congestive heart failure occur during or shortly after transfusion. Patients with compromised cardiac and pulmonary status poorly tolerate rapid elevations in total blood volume and are more susceptible to circulatory overload. Since this type of reaction may lead to fatality, prompt aggressive treatment with oxygen therapy and diuretic medications is imperative to prevent further complications.

Transfusion candidates susceptible to circulatory overload should receive red blood cell units and not whole blood. The units should also be administered at a slow rate in aliquoted small volumes. The transfusion period should proceed over 4 to 6 hours. Infusions of large volumes of plasma should be avoided.

DISEASE TRANSMISSION

A detailed discussion of disease transmission in transfusion is covered in Chapter 10 of this text. For the purposes of this chapter, viral and nonviral transfusion-transmitted diseases are listed in Box 12-3.

BOX 12-3

Summary of Transfusion-Transmitted Diseases

VIRAL
HIV-1, HIV-2
Hepatitis A (rare), B, C
HTLV-I, HTLV-II
Cytomegalovirus (CMV)
Epstein-Barr virus
Human parvovirus B19

NONVIRAL
Bacterial
Syphilis
Malaria
Chagas' disease *(Trypanosoma cruzi)*
Babesiosis
Leishmaniasis
Creutzfeldt-Jakob disease

HIV, Human immunodeficiency virus; *HTLV*, human T-cell lymphotropic virus.

MISCELLANEOUS ADVERSE CONSEQUENCES OF TRANSFUSION

Transfusion Hemosiderosis

Hemosiderosis is a condition that results from the accumulation of excess iron in macrophages in various tissues. Iron overload is a potential complication in patients undergoing long-term transfusions, such as those suffering from **thalassemia** with persistent hemolysis. In transfusion hemosiderosis, iron intake (250 mg/unit) exceeds the daily iron excretion (1 mg/day) with the subsequent deposition of excess iron in the liver, heart, and kidney. When patients have received more than 100 transfusions, iron deposition may interfere with the function of the liver, heart, or endocrine glands.

Thalassemia: inherited disorder causing anemia because of a defective production rate of either alpha- or beta-hemoglobin polypeptide.

Citrate Toxicity

The transfusion of large quantities of citrated blood in a relatively short time frame introduces the risk of citrate toxicity for the transfusion recipient. Citrate, present in the formulation of the anticoagulants used in the blood collection process, binds ionized calcium. Excess citrate may be toxic to patients receiving large volumes in massive transfusion situations or in patients with impaired liver function for the metabolism of the citrate. Injections of calcium chloride or calcium gluconate negate the toxic effects.

Posttransfusion Purpura

Posttransfusion purpura (PTP) occurs rarely in a multiparous female population. In this disorder the patient's platelet count plummets a week after the transfusion of blood or blood products containing platelets. Generalized purpura and an increased probability of bleeding episodes follow. This complication is an anamnestic response to a previous sensitization with the high-incidence platelet antigen Pl^{A1}, or HPA-la (98% frequency). Antigen-negative individuals are at risk of developing PTP. Women, who phenotype as Pl^{A1}-negative, are sensitized through multiple pregnancies and respond with the immune production of anti-Pl^{A1}. This platelet-specific alloantibody destroys not only the transfused Pl^{A1} platelets but also the patient's Pl^{A1}-negative platelets. The mechanism for the concomitant destruction of the autologous platelets with transfused platelets remains indeterminate. Treatment of PTP includes plasmapheresis, exchange transfusion, and the use of intravenous IgG.[10]

EVALUATION OF A TRANSFUSION REACTION

Role of the Medical Personnel Performing the Transfusion

Protocols for the initiation of a transfusion necessitate that the medical personnel serving as the transfusionist carefully check all the identifying information and document informed patient consent before the infusion of the blood product. This information is documented in the transfusion record with the date and time of the start of the transfusion. In addition to verifying identification the transfusionist records the patient's pretransfusion vital signs, including temperature, blood pressure, pulse, and respiration rate. The transfusionist should remain with the patient for the first few minutes of the infusion to detect any indications of acute hemolysis, anaphylaxis, or bacterial contamination. After the first 15-minute period the patient should be observed and the vital signs recorded. Clinical personnel should continue to observe the patient periodically throughout the transfusion and up to 1 hour after completion.

If an adverse reaction is suspected, the following procedure is performed[6]:

- The transfusion should be stopped; reidentification of the patient and the transfused component is initiated.
- The transfusion service and the patient's physician are notified immediately of the suspected reaction.
- An intravenous line is maintained (for administration with blood) with normal saline or a solution, approved by the Food and Drug Administration (FDA).
- The physician evaluates the patient to determine any clinical intervention and potential medical management.
- If signs and symptoms of possible acute HTR, anaphylaxis, TRALI, transfusion-induced sepsis, or other serious complications exist, a postreaction blood sample is sent to the transfusion service for evaluation. A properly labeled and carefully collected sample is forwarded to the transfusion service with the transfusion container, the administration set, the attached intravenous solutions, and all related forms and labels. In some cases the first voided post-reaction urine is collected for possible evaluation.[6]
- If the presenting clinical signs and symptoms are indicative of urticarial or circulatory overload, the transfusion service does not need to evaluate any post-reaction blood and urine samples.

Role of the Clinical Laboratory

Any suspected transfusion reaction becomes a high priority in the transfusion service. On receipt of the postreaction clinical materials, the transfusion service personnel perform the following three steps (Fig. 12-2)[6]:

- Check for any errors in identification

  Patient sample and blood component are checked for any errors relating to identification. If such an error is discovered, notification is provided to the medical personnel handling the transfusion reaction. All records are double-checked to determine whether another potential transfusion recipient is at risk because of this error. The source of the error is evaluated in light of the overall transfusion process to determine where the system failed.
- Visual check for hemolysis

  Because red blood cells immediately release free hemoglobin into the plasma during intravascular hemolysis, the postreaction sample is evaluated for any

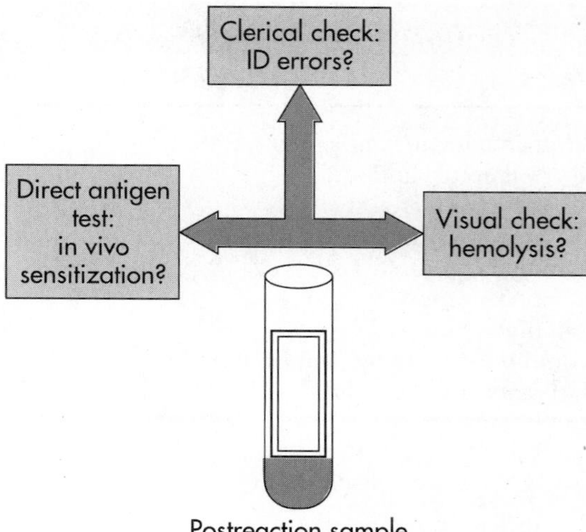

Fig. 12-2 Laboratory investigation of a transfusion reaction.

evidence of hemolysis or **icterus** and is compared to the pretransfusion sample, if available in the laboratory. Any pinkish or reddish discoloration suggests the presence of free hemoglobin. If a transfusion has occurred over a 3- to 4-hour period, icterus may be noted as the degradation of free hemoglobin to bilirubin progresses. Bilirubin levels usually peak at 5 to 7 hours following a hemolytic event.

Icterus: pertaining to or resembling jaundice.

- Direct antiglobulin test
  To check for a serologic incompatibility, a DAT is performed on a postreaction sample, preferably an ethylenediaminetetraacetic acid, or EDTA, sample. If the postreaction sample is positive, a recipient alloantibody has sensitized the transfused red blood cells and is eliciting the immune clearance of the transfused red blood cells. A positive DAT from a transfusion reaction appears as mixed field with the transfused red blood cells demonstrating agglutination and the autologous red blood cells remaining unagglutinated. If the transfused red blood cells have experienced a rapid clearance, the DAT may be negative or microscopically positive at the time of sample collection. The comparison of the postreaction sample to the DAT performed on the pretransfusion sample is helpful in evaluating the transfusion reaction.

Additional Laboratory Testing in a Transfusion Reaction

Depending on the results of the aforementioned testing, further laboratory testing may be performed (Table 12-6). The extent of the additional testing is in part at the discretion of the physician in charge of the transfusion service and preestablished policies for the investigation of a transfusion reaction. Additional laboratory testing that may follow the initial investigation includes any combination of the following analyses[6]:

- Parallel testing of pretransfusion and posttransfusion patient samples for ABO and Rh typing along with a reconfirmation of the ABO and Rh typing of the donor unit
- Any discrepancies of typing confirm an error in sample or patient identification; if an error in the patient's sample has occurred, an investigation of another potential clerical error affecting another patient should be initiated
- Parallel testing of pretransfusion and posttransfusion patient samples for antibody detection

Table 12-6 Additional Testing in a Transfusion Reaction Investigation

TEST	REASON
ABO/Rh typing	Errors in patient/sample identification
Antibody screen	Newly detected antibodies
Crossmatch	Serologic compatibility
Hemoglobin/hematocrit	Therapeutic effectiveness
Haptoglobin	Hemolytic process
Bilirubin	Hemolytic process
Urine hemoglobin	Hemolytic process
Inspection of donor unit	Nonimmune hemolysis or bacterial contamination
Gram stain and blood culture	Bacterial contamination

The use of additional enhancement techniques in the antibody screen may be helpful in the detection of a weakly reactive antibody. Polyethylene glycol or enzyme techniques may provide additional information in the workup. If a new antibody is detected, antibody identification procedures are performed. A previously undetected antibody, now evident in the posttransfusion sample, is indicative of a possible anamnestic immune response following the recent transfusion exposure. The donor unit transfused to the recipient is checked for the presence of the antigen.

- Repetition of crossmatch using pretransfusion and posttransfusion patient samples
  The recommended crossmatch procedure includes both the immediate spin and antiglobulin crossmatch phases.[5]
- Frequent checks of hematologic status
  Hemoglobin and hematocrit values are evaluated following transfusion for expected therapeutic elevations of 1 g/dl hemoglobin and 3% hematocrit for each red cell unit transfused.
- Perform analysis of haptoglobin levels on both the pretransfusion and posttransfusion patient samples
  Haptoglobin is a plasma protein with the sole function of binding free hemoglobin and carrying the molecule to hepatocytes for further catabolism. During a hemolytic process, haptoglobin levels fall in plasma because haptoglobin-hemoglobin complexes are formed. Normally 50 to 200 mg/dl of plasma haptoglobin is available for binding. Estimates show that as little as 1 to 2 ml of intravascular red blood cell destruction can deplete the normal circulating haptoglobin levels.[11]
- Examination of urine for hemoglobin in the postreaction urine sample
  Free hemoglobin, released during intravascular red blood cell destruction, is excreted into the urine after exceeding the plasma haptoglobin-binding capacity.
- Examination of returned donor unit and administration tubing for abnormal appearance or hemolysis
  If bacterial sepsis is suspected, the donor unit may be Gram stained and cultured.
- Other postreaction testing may include bilirubin, IgA levels, and HLA and granulocyte antibody detection

RECORDS OF TRANSFUSION COMPLICATIONS

Records of patients who experience an adverse reaction to a transfusion remain indefinitely in the transfusion service.[6] Cases of transfusion-transmitted disease and bacterial contamination must also be reported to the blood collection facility. These records serve as a determinant in the prevention of future reactions. For example, a patient with a history of a previous clinically relevant alloantibody, currently not demonstrable in the antibody screen test, would require a transfusion with antigen-negative donor units.

Fatalities attributable to transfusion must be reported within 24 hours to the director of the FDA's Office of Compliance, Center for Biologics Evaluation and Research, followed by a written report within 7 days.[12] The formal report includes medical and laboratory documentation and, if an autopsy was performed, an autopsy report.

CHAPTER SUMMARY

The major adverse complications of transfusion are summarized below.

SUMMARY OF ADVERSE COMPLICATIONS OF TRANSFUSION

ADVERSE EFFECT	CAUSE
Immune-mediated	
Acute hemolytic	ABO incompatibilities
Delayed hemolytic	Primary or secondary alloimmunization
Febrile	Recipient white blood cell antibodies
Urticarial	Plasma allergen
Anaphylactic	Anti-IgA in IgA-deficient recipient
TRALI	Donor WBC antibodies
TA-GVHD	Immunocompetent donor lymphocytes in immunocompromised recipient
Non-immune-mediated	
Hemolytic	Mechanical or chemical trauma to unit
Circulatory overload	Hypervolemia
Bacterial contamination	Donor septicemia/contamination during phlebotomy

TRALI, Transfusion-related acute lung injury; *TA-GVHD,* transfusion-associated graft versus host disease.

CRITICAL THINKING EXERCISES

◆ ***EXERCISE 12-1***

An inexperienced nurse in a home health facility calls the transfusion service to report a transfusion reaction. The transfusion recipient is complaining of shortness of breath and chills. The nurse is seeking advice on the appropriate action steps.

1. What advice should be provided to the customer?
2. What documentation should be returned to the transfusion service?
3. What immediate procedures should be performed on the transfusion investigation at the transfusion service?

◆ ***EXERCISE 12-2***

Seven days after the transfusion of 15 red blood cell units, a patient experiences a 5 g/dl drop in hemoglobin and is mildly jaundiced. No evidence of bleeding is identified.

1. What tests would provide evidence for a delayed transfusion reaction?
2. What is the rationale for the test selection?

◆ ***EXERCISE 12-3***

A 55-year-old man was admitted to the emergency room following a motor vehicle accident. The patient is hemorrhaging from a lacerated spleen and requires emergency surgery. Pretransfusion testing determined that the patient was group A Rh negative with a negative antibody screen. Crossmatches on donor red blood cell units were compatible by the immediate spin crossmatch. During surgery the patient receives 6 units of group A Rh-negative red blood cells and 4 units of group A Rh-positive frozen plasma. Three days later, during the first 15 minutes of a subsequent red blood cell transfusion using a blood-warming device, the patient developed fever and chills.

1. Based on the information cited above, propose three possible explanations that could account for the etiology of the transfusion reaction.
2. Determine a strategy for the evaluation of the transfusion reaction to rule in or rule out any possible mechanism.

STUDY QUESTIONS

1. A patient experiences chills and fever, nausea, flushing, and lower back pain following the infusion of 350 ml of blood. To rule out a transfusion reaction because of acute hemolysis, one should immediately:
   a. perform a DAT and observe serum on posttransfusion sample
   b. measure serum haptoglobin on prereaction and postreaction samples
   c. repeat crossmatches on prereaction and postreaction samples
   d. Gram stain and culture the unit

2. Dyspnea, severe headache, and peripheral edema occurring soon after transfusion are indicative of which type of transfusion reaction?
   a. hemolytic
   b. febrile
   c. circulatory overload
   d. anaphylactic

3. What is a common cause of a febrile nonhemolytic transfusion reaction?
   a. recipient is allergic to the donor's plasma proteins
   b. donor unit is cold
   c. donor unit has a positive DAT
   d. recipient has antibodies to the donor's HLAs

4. What plasma protein functions to bind hemoglobin following intravascular hemolysis?
   a. albumin
   b. haptoglobin
   c. transferrin
   d. C-reactive protein

5. Which of the following adverse complications of transfusion is prevented by irradiation?
   a. circulatory overload
   b. hyperkalemia
   c. iron overload
   d. TA-GVHD

6. Which of the following characteristics describes a clinical finding of delayed HTRs?
   a. hives and wheals
   b. hemosiderosis
   c. positive antibody screen postreaction sample
   d. ABO incompatibility between donor unit and recipient

7. What blood group system's antibodies are commonly associated with delayed HTRs?
   a. high titer, low avidity
   b. ABO
   c. MNS
   d. Kidd

8. A patient has experienced two febrile reactions following red blood cell transfusion. What is the preferred blood component if future transfusions are necessary?
   a. leukocyte-reduced red blood cells
   b. irradiated red blood cells
   c. CMV-negative red blood cells
   d. group O Rh-negative red blood cells

9. Which of the following patient histories might suggest future transfusions with saline-washed red blood cells?
   a. history of multiple red blood cell alloantibodies
   b. history of previous DIC
   c. history of multiple urticarial reactions
   d. history of transfusion-associated sepsis

10. What is the cause of transfusion-induced hemosiderosis?
   a. excess citrate
   b. Pl^{A1} antigen
   c. iron overload
   d. circulatory overload

11. What laboratory test is useful to detect clerical errors of sample identification in a transfusion reaction investigation?
   a. ABO and Rh typing
   b. antibody screen
   c. crossmatch
   d. DAT

12. What microorganism grows well at 4° C and may result in a transfusion-transmitted sepsis?
   a. *Staphylococcus aureus*
   b. *Yersinia enterocolitica*
   c. *Staphylococcus epidermidis*
   d. *Bacillus cereus*

13. What is the expected therapeutic effect in the recipient's hematocrit following the transfusion of 1 unit of red blood cells?
   a. increase of 0.5%
   b. increase of 1%
   c. increase of 2%
   d. increase of 3%

14. Anaphylactic reactions to transfusion are usually caused by:
   a. anti-IgA in an IgA-deficient recipient
   b. anti-IgG in an IgA-deficient recipient
   c. IgA deficiency
   d. IgG deficiency

15. A precipitous fall in a recipient's platelet count following a transfusion is associated with:
    a. circulatory overload
    b. PTP
    c. citrate toxicity
    d. Factor VIII deficiency

REFERENCES

1. Issitt PD, Anstee DJ: *Applied blood group serology,* ed 4, Durham, NC, 1998, Montgomery Scientific Publications.
2. AuBuchon JP, Kruskall MS: Transfusion safety: realigning efforts with risks, *Transfusion* 37:1211, 1997.
3. Linden JV, Paul B, Dressler KP: A report of 104 transfusion errors in New York State, *Transfusion* 32:601, 1992.
4. Davenport R: Immunobiology of hemolytic transfusion reactions. In *Transfusion reactions: refresher and update,* Bethesda, Md, 1996, American Association of Blood Banks.
5. Davenport RD: The role of cytokines in hemolytic transfusion reactions, *Immunol Invest* 24:319, 1995.
6. Vengelen-Tyler V: *Technical manual,* ed 12, Bethesda, Md, 1996, American Association of Blood Banks.
7. Walker RH: Special report: transfusion risks, *Am J Clin Pathol* 88:374, 1987.
8. Jeter EK, Spivey MA: *Introduction to transfusion medicine: a case study approach,* Bethesda, Md, 1996, American Association of Blood Banks.
9. Mollison PL, Engelfriet CP, Contreras M: *Blood transfusion in clinical medicine,* ed 9, Oxford, 1993, Blackwell Scientific Publications.
10. Harmening DH: *Clinical hematology and fundamentals of hemostasis,* ed 3, Philadelphia, 1997, FA Davis.
11. Burtis CA, Ashwood ER, Tietz N: *Textbook of clinical chemistry,* ed 2, Philadelphia, 1994, WB Saunders.
12. Food and Drug Administration: *Code of federal regulations,* 21 CFR 606.170, Washington, DC, 1996, US Government Printing Office.

SUGGESTED READINGS

Harmening D, editor: *Modern blood banking and transfusion practices,* ed 4, Philadelphia, 1999, FA Davis.

Issitt PD, Anstee DJ: *Applied blood group serology,* ed 4, Durham, NC, 1998, Montgomery Scientific Publications.

HEMOLYTIC DISEASE OF THE NEWBORN

13

Barbara V. Anderson

CHAPTER OUTLINE

Etiology of Hemolytic Disease of the Newborn
Overview of Hemolytic Disease of the Newborn
Rh Hemolytic Disease of the Newborn
ABO Hemolytic Disease of the Newborn
Alloantibodies Causing Hemolytic Disease of the Newborn Other Than Anti-D
Prediction of Hemolytic Disease of the Newborn
Maternal History
Antibody Titration
Amniocentesis
Percutaneous Umbilical Blood Sampling
Postpartum Testing
Postpartum Testing of Infants Born to D-Negative Mothers
Postpartum Testing of Infants with Suspected Hemolytic Disease of the Newborn
Prevention of Hemolytic Disease of the Newborn
Antepartum Administration
Postpartum Administration
Treatment of Hemolytic Disease of the Newborn
In Utero Treatment
Postpartum Treatment

LEARNING OBJECTIVES

Upon completion of this chapter, the reader should be able to:

1. Discuss the etiology of hemolytic disease of the newborn.
2. Discuss the metabolism of bilirubin in the fetus versus bilirubin in the newborn.
3. State what tests are included in an initial prenatal workup.
4. List examples of antibodies that are not clinically significant in terms of hemolytic disease of the newborn.
5. Explain the primary value of performing antibody titration and state what results are considered significant.
6. Explain the value of amniocentesis or percutaneous umbilical cord sampling in predicting hemolytic disease of the newborn.
7. Discuss the two main reasons cord blood is tested.
8. List the tests routinely performed on cord blood cells when hemolytic disease of the newborn is suspected, and discuss possible sources of error when performing each test.
9. Compare and contrast the clinical and laboratory findings in ABO hemolytic disease of the newborn versus Rh hemolytic disease of the newborn.
10. Discuss the composition, dosage, eligibility criteria, timing, and principle of Rh immune globulin.
11. Explain the principle, interpretation, and significance of a positive rosette test for fetomaternal hemorrhage.
12. Explain the principle, interpretation, and significance of the Kleihauer-Betke acid elution.
13. Evaluate laboratory test results and indicate if a patient is an Rh immune globulin candidate.
14. Compare and contrast intrauterine transfusion versus exchange transfusion.
15. List the special considerations that must be met when selecting blood for exchange transfusion, and explain the purpose of each requirement.
16. Evaluate maternal and cord blood cell test results and indicate if child has hemolytic disease of the newborn.

Erythroblastosis fetalis: hemolytic disease of the newborn.

Hemolytic disease of the newborn (HDN), also known as **erythroblastosis fetalis,** is a disorder of the fetus or newborn in which fetal red blood cells are destroyed by maternal IgG antibodies. These antibodies, directed against fetal antigens, cross the placenta, sensitize fetal red blood cells, and shorten red blood cell survival. This premature red blood cell destruction results in disease varying from mild anemia to death in utero. The transfusion service plays a critical role in the prediction, diagnosis, treatment, and, most important, the prevention of this potentially life-threatening disease.

ETIOLOGY OF HEMOLYTIC DISEASE OF THE NEWBORN

Fetomaternal hemorrhage: escape of fetal cells into the maternal circulation, usually occurring at the time of delivery.

During pregnancy the placenta functions as the site of oxygen, nutrient, and waste exchange. In addition, the placenta serves as a barrier between maternal and fetal circulations. This barrier limits the number of fetal red blood cells entering the maternal circulation during pregnancy and thus reduces the chances of antibody production during pregnancy. ABO incompatibility between mother and child can also provide additional protection against immunization. Intravascular hemolysis of ABO-incompatible fetal red blood cells by maternal anti-A or anti-B reduces exposure to fetal cells carrying foreign antigens. However, at the time of delivery when the placenta is separated from the uterus, a significant number of fetal red blood cells escape into the maternal circulation (known as **fetomaternal hemorrhage** [FMH]). In addition to delivery, immunization can result from fetal red blood cell exposure following amniocentesis, spontaneous or induced abortion, chorionic villus sampling, ectopic pregnancy, or abdominal trauma. Foreign antigens on the fetal red blood cells can stimulate an active immune response in the mother, which results in the production of IgG antibodies.

In a subsequent pregnancy the IgG antibodies cross the placental barrier by an active transport mechanism. The antibodies bind to the fetal antigens, which results in red blood cell destruction by macrophages in the fetal liver and spleen. Hemoglobin liberated from the damaged red blood cells is metabolized to indirect bilirubin. The indirect bilirubin is transported across the placenta, conjugated by the maternal liver, and harmlessly excreted by the mother (Fig. 13-1). However, as red blood cell destruction continues, the fetus becomes increasingly anemic. Fetal liver and spleen enlarge as erythropoiesis increases in an effort to compensate for the red blood cell destruction. Immature red blood cells (erythroblasts) are released into the fetal circulation (which explains the term *erythroblastosis fetalis*). If this condition is left untreated, cardiac failure can occur accompanied by hydrops fetalis, or edema and fluid accumulation in fetal peritoneal and pleural cavities. Thus the greatest threat to the fetus is cardiac failure resulting from uncompensated anemia.

Following delivery the infant faces a different challenge. Red blood cell destruction continues with the release of indirect bilirubin. In utero the indirect bilirubin is conjugated in the maternal liver and excreted. However, the newborn liver is deficient in glucuronyl transferase (the liver enzyme needed to conjugated indirect bilirubin). As the indirect bilirubin is released, it binds to albumin and circulates harmlessly. However, when the binding capacity of the albumin is exceeded, the indirect bilirubin binds to tissues, which results in jaundice. In particular, it may bind with tissues of the central nervous system (CNS) and cause

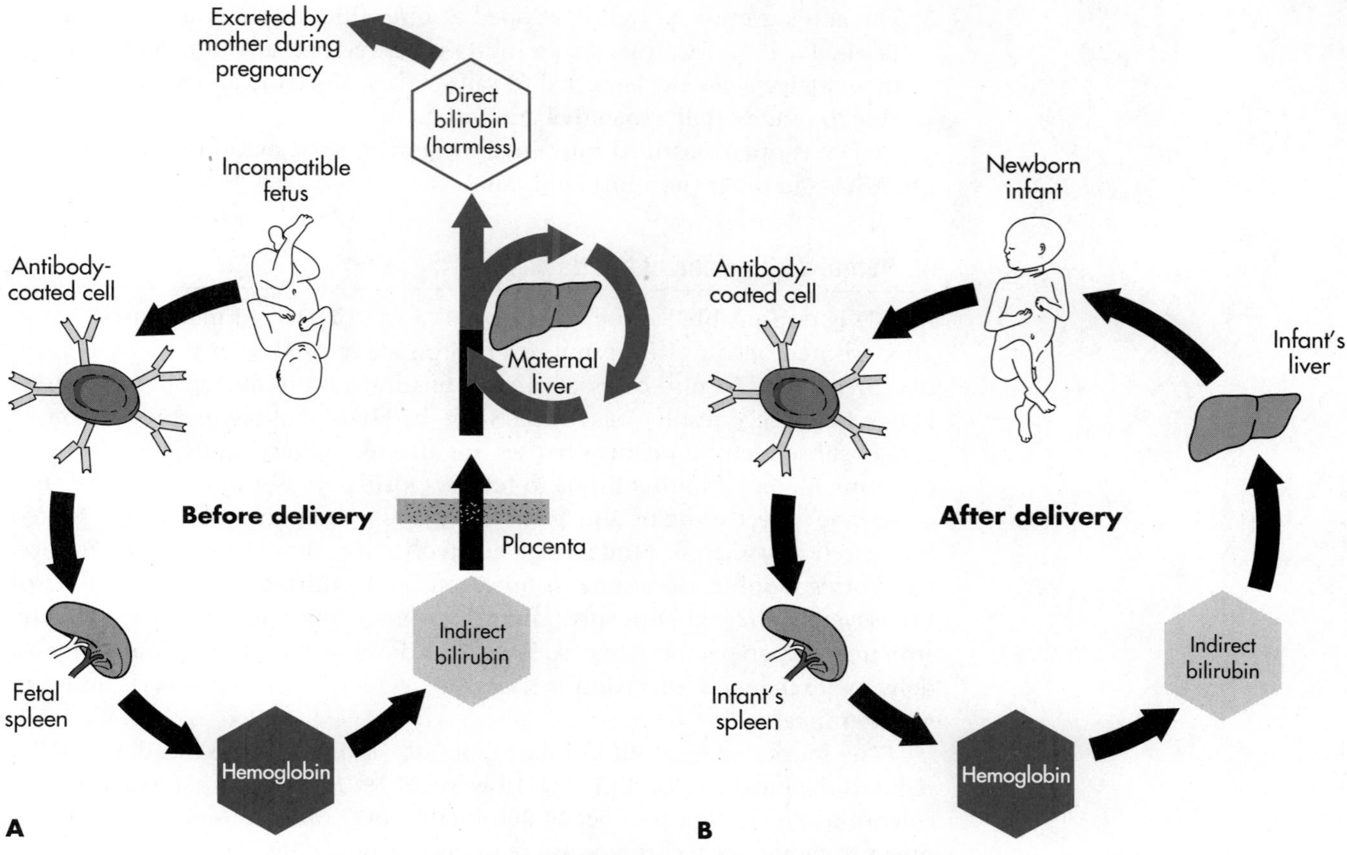

Fig. 13-1 Metabolism of bilirubin. ***A,*** Before delivery, fetal bilirubin produced by the breakdown of sensitized red blood cells in the fetal spleen is safely metabolized by the maternal liver. ***B,*** After delivery, the newborn's liver does not produce glucuronyl transferase and cannot convert bilirubin to an excretable form. As a result, it collects in tissues and causes brain damage.

From Ortho Diagnostics: *Blood group antigens and antibodies as applied to hemolytic disease of the newborn*, Raritan, NJ, 1968, Ortho Diagnostics.

permanent brain damage (kernicterus), resulting in deafness, mental retardation, or death (Fig. 13-1).

OVERVIEW OF HEMOLYTIC DISEASE OF THE NEWBORN

Three important factors must be present for HDN to occur:

1. The mother must lack the antigen and, following exposure to the antigen from previous pregnancies or transfusions, produce an antibody of the IgG class. IgG is the only immunoglobulin capable of crossing the placental barrier. This active transport across the placenta is determined by the fragment, crystallizable, or Fc, portion of the immunoglobulin molecule.[1]
2. The fetus must possess the antigen. The gene for the antigen is inherited from the father. If the father is known to be homozygous for the gene, 100% of the children inherit the gene and therefore are at risk for HDN. If the father is known to be heterozygous, only 50% of the children inherit the gene and are at risk.

3. The antigen must be well developed at birth. Blood group antigens such as Lewis, P_1, I, and Cartwright are not well developed at birth. Antibodies to these antigens are not expected to cause HDN, since the antigen is not available to bind with the maternal antibody.

HDN is often classified into three categories based on antibody specificity: Rh, ABO, and other (non-Rh) antibodies.

Rh Hemolytic Disease of the Newborn

Anti-D is responsible for the most severe cases of HDN. In most cases D-negative women become alloimmunized (produce anti-D) after the first D-positive pregnancy. In rare cases alloimmunization occurs during the first pregnancy but rarely results in clinical signs of HDN. Following production of anti-D subsequent D-positive fetuses are affected to varying degrees. In some cases the maternal anti-D binds to fetal D-positive red blood cells and causes a positive direct antiglobulin test (DAT) and minimal, if any, signs of red blood cell destruction. Moderately affected infants develop signs of jaundice, and corresponding elevations in bilirubin levels, during the first few days of life. Severely affected D-positive infants, experiencing rapid red blood cell destruction, experience anemia in utero and develop jaundice within hours of delivery. Exchange transfusion is necessary to reduce bilirubin levels and prevent kernicterus.

The introduction of Rh immune globulin (RhIG) in 1968 has dramatically reduced the incidence of Rh HDN. However, a 1991 study still estimated the incidence of Rh HDN at 10.6 per 10,000 total births.[2] HDN caused by anti-D continues to be the most common cause of death from HDN.

ABO Hemolytic Disease of the Newborn

Red blood cell destruction by ABO antibodies is more common than by anti-D. Fortunately, most cases are subclinical and do not necessitate treatment. Some infants may experience mildly elevated bilirubin levels and some degree of jaundice within the first few days of life. Based on the number of infants who develop jaundice, Mollison estimates that HDN caused by ABO incompatibility occurs in 1 in 150 births.[1] These cases can usually be treated with **phototherapy.** Possible explanations for the mild red blood cell destruction, despite high levels of maternal antibody, include the following:

Phototherapy: treatment of elevated bilirubin or other conditions with light rays.

- Presence of A or B substances in the fetal tissues and secretions that bind or neutralize ABO antibodies, which reduces the amount of ABO antibody available to destroy fetal red blood cells
- Poor development of ABO antigens on fetal or infant red blood cells
- Reduced number of A and B antigen sites on fetal or infant red blood cells

This also explains why the DAT is only weakly positive in most cases of ABO HDN.

ABO HDN occurs most frequently in group A or B babies born to group O mothers. This may be due to the increased incidence of IgG ABO antibodies in group O individuals compared to other ABO groups. Unlike Rh HDN, ABO incompatibility often affects the first pregnancy because of the presence of non–red blood cell–stimulated ABO antibodies. Table 13-1 compares the clinical and laboratory findings in ABO and Rh HDN.

Table 13-1 Comparison of ABO and Rh Hemolytic Disease of the Newborn (HDN)

	NORMAL INFANT	ABO HDN	Rh HDN
CLINICAL FINDINGS			
Jaundice	Physiologic	None to mild	Mild to severe
Hepatosplenomegaly	No	No	Mild to severe
Edema	No	No	Mild to severe
SEROLOGIC RESULTS			
ABO group	Any ABO group	Mother group O Newborn A or B	Any ABO group
Rh type	Any Rh type	Any Rh type	Mother D-negative Newborn D-positive
Direct antiglobulin test	Negative	Negative or weakly positive	Positive
Antibody	None	Anti-A, anti-B, anti-A,B	Anti-D
HEMATOLOGY RESULTS			
Hemoglobin	16 to 28 g/dl	Mild: >13 g/dl	Mild: >13 g/dl Moderate: 8 to 13 g/dl Severe: <8 g/dl
Reticulocyte count	2% to 6%	Mild increase	Greatly increased
Blood smear			
Morphology	Normal	Spherocytes	Macrocytes Hypochromia
NRBC/100 WBCs	10 to 20	Mild increase	Greatly increased
CHEMISTRY RESULTS			
Bilirubin	1 to 3 mg/dl	Mild increase	Often >20 mg/dl
VALUE OF PRENATAL TESTING		None	Useful
OCCURRENCE IN FIRST PREGNANCY		Often	Rare

NRBC, Nucleated red blood cell; *WBCs*, white blood cells.

Alloantibodies Causing Hemolytic Disease of the Newborn Other Than Anti-D

Any IgG antibody is capable of causing HDN if the fetal red blood cells possess the antigen and the antigen is well developed at birth. Other Rh-system antibodies are known to cause HDN alone or in combination with anti-D. Anti-c is the second most common cause of HDN, followed by anti-K.

PREDICTION OF HEMOLYTIC DISEASE OF THE NEWBORN

Prenatal testing serves two purposes:

- To identify D-negative women who are candidates for RhIG (see the section on Prevention of Hemolytic Disease of the Newborn)
- To identify women with antibodies capable of causing HDN, which helps assess potential risk to the fetus

Prenatal testing should be performed as early as possible in the pregnancy and should include ABO and Rh typing, including a test for weak D, and antibody screen for unexpected alloantibodies. If the antibody screen is positive, antibody identification should be performed. Women with clinically significant antibodies require careful management to monitor risk to the fetus. Box 13-1 outlines laboratory testing for prediction of HDN.

Maternal History

An accurate obstetric history is essential in predicting the course of a sensitized pregnancy. For a woman with a history of a hydropic infant because of anti-D, a greater than 90% chance exists that a subsequent D-positive fetus also will be hydropic.[3] Thus a history of a previously affected infant can be useful in predicting the prognosis for future pregnancies.

Antibody Titration

Antibody titration commonly has been used to predict the severity of HDN. However, the titer is of limited value because it predicts the severity of HDN in only 62% of fetuses.[4] Antibody titration can be helpful, however, in decisions regarding the performance and timing of invasive procedures such as amniocentesis, chorionic villus sampling, or percutaneous umbilical cord sampling (PUBS). The antibody titer should be determined as early as possible in the pregnancy and the specimen frozen for future testing. Testing should be repeated at 16 and 22 weeks and repeated at 1- to 4-week intervals thereafter. A titer rising by twofold or greater is generally accepted as an indication for further monitoring. To ensure the significance of a rising titer, successive titrations must be performed using the same methods and test cells. In addition, testing previously frozen samples in parallel with the current specimen ensures that any change in the titer is not the result of technical variables. Some institutions have established an anti-D titer of 16 as the critical value indicating the need for additional monitoring. Critical titers for antibodies other than anti-D have not been established.

Amniocentesis

Amniocentesis: process of withdrawal of amniotic fluid by aspiration for the purpose of analysis.

One measure of red blood cell destruction and the severity of HDN is the level of bilirubin pigment found in amniotic fluid. Amniotic fluid is obtained by **amniocentesis,** or the insertion of a needle through the mother's abdominal wall and

BOX 13-1 ***Laboratory Testing for Prediction of Hemolytic Disease of the Newborn***

INITIAL VISIT

- ABO and Rh test performed (including test for weak D)
- Test for unexpected IgG antibodies
- If antibody screen is positive, perform antibody identification
- Antibody titration for clinically significant antibodies performed to establish baseline

FOLLOW-UP VISITS

- Repeat ABO and Rh testing is not necessary unless for transfusion purposes
- Repeat antibody identification is not necessary
- Selected cell panel should be run to exclude other clinically significant antibodies
- Perform repeat antibody titration and consider amniocentesis

uterus and extraction of fluid from the amniotic sac. The aspirated fluid is scanned spectrophotometrically from 350 to 700 nm. The change in optical density (ΔOD) above the baseline at 450 nm is a measure of the bilirubin pigments (Fig. 13-2). The ΔOD is plotted on the **Liley graph** according to gestational age (Fig. 13-3). This graph defines three zones to estimate the severity of HDN; the upper zone correlates with severe HDN and fetal death, the lower zone indicates a mildly affected or unaffected fetus, and the midzone correlates with moderate disease and necessitates repeat testing to establish a trend.

Liley graph: graph used to predict severity of HDN during pregnancy by evaluation of the amniotic fluid.

Based on amniotic fluid analysis, three alternatives exist: allow the pregnancy to continue to term, perform intrauterine transfusion (see the section on Treatment of Hemolytic Disease of the Newborn), or induce early labor. If labor is induced, fetal lung maturity must be determined to avoid **respiratory distress syndrome.** Fetal lung maturity can be determined by calculating the **lecithin/sphingomyelin** (L/S) **ratio** using thin-layer chromatography or by an agglutination test that detects phosphatidylglycerol. Lecithin and phosphatidylglycerol are biochemical components of surfactant, a mixture of phospholipids that allows the exchange of gases in the lungs. An L/S ratio of greater than 2:1 is generally considered evidence of lung maturity.

Respiratory distress syndrome: inability to maintain stable pulmonary alveolar structures, caused by low levels of surfactant, lecithin, and other pulmonary lipids in premature infants.

Lecithin/sphingomyelin ratio: ratio of lecithin to sphingomyelin that indicates lung maturity.

Percutaneous Umbilical Blood Sampling

PUBS, also known as cordocentesis, is a useful technique both diagnostically and therapeutically. Using an ultrasound-guided needle, the umbilical vein is

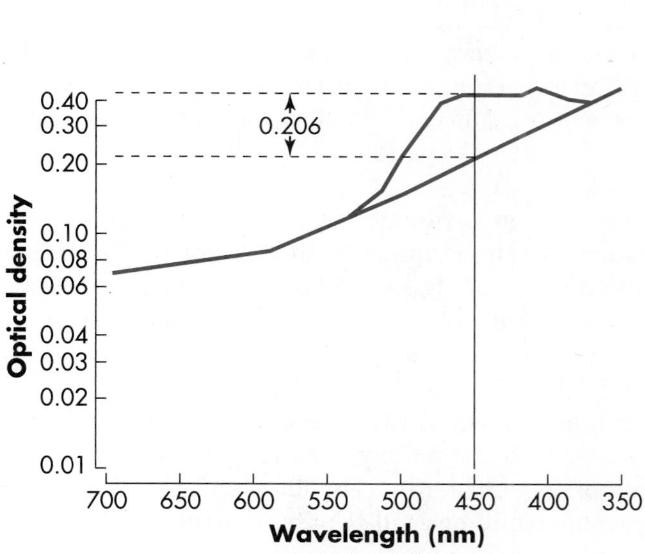

Fig. 13-2 Spectrophotometric analysis of amniotic fluid. Plot taken at 35 weeks of the optical density reading of amniotic fluid from a woman immunized to the D antigen. The difference between the baseline optical density at the 450-nm wavelength and the reading of the amniotic fluid is measured. The result in this case is 0.206, which is plotted on a Liley graph to determine the correct course of treatment according to the period of gestation.

From Mollison PL, Engelfriet CP, Contreras M: *Blood transfusion in clinical medicine*, ed 9, London, 1993, Blackwell Scientific.

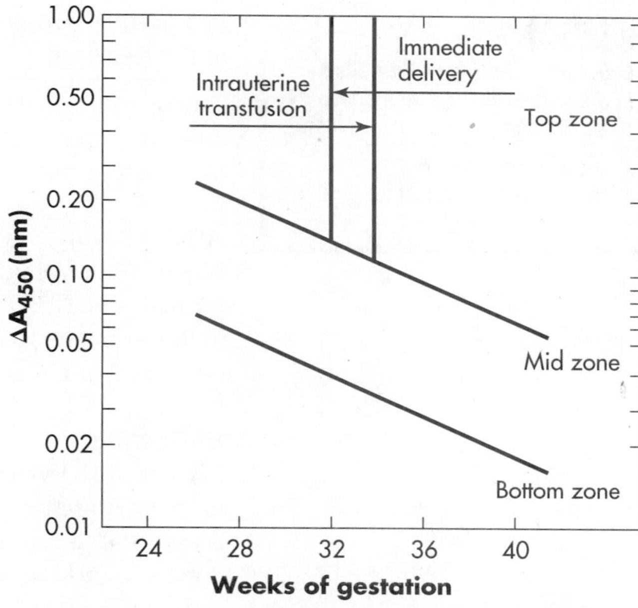

Fig. 13-3 Liley graph. Liley graph for evaluating data from spectrophotometric analysis of amniotic fluid. The optical density at 450 (Δ450) and weeks of gestation are plotted to estimate the severity of HDN. A reading of 0.206 at 35 weeks correlates with severe HDN, which may necessitate immediate delivery.

From Liley AW: Liquor amnii analysis in the management of the pregnancy complicated by rhesus sensitization, *Am J Obstet Gynecol* 82:1359, 1961.

punctured near the point of placental insertion. A fetal blood sample is aspirated, which can be used to directly measure hematologic (hemoglobin/hematocrit) or biochemical (bilirubin) variables. Before testing, the specimen must be determined to be from the fetus and not the mother by measuring fetal hemoglobin or performing red blood cell phenotyping. The fetal mortality rate associated with this technique is reported to be between 1% and 2%.[4] In cases of severe HDN, PUBS also can be used for direct intravascular transfusion to the fetus (see the section on Treatment of Hemolytic Disease of the Newborn).

POSTPARTUM TESTING

It is desirable to collect a sample of cord blood from every newborn. The specimen should be properly labeled and stored for up to 7 days where it can remain available for testing if the mother is D negative or if the newborn develops signs or symptoms of HDN. Cord blood should be washed several times before testing to avoid false-positive test results because of contamination with Wharton's jelly.

Postpartum Testing of Infants Born to D-Negative Mothers

All infants born to D-negative mothers should be tested for the D antigen, including a test for weak D. D-negative mothers whose infants are found to be D positive (including weak D positive) are candidates for RhIG therapy (see the section on Prevention of Hemolytic Disease of the Newborn).

BOX 13-2

Laboratory Testing of Cord Blood in Suspected Hemolytic Disease of the Newborn

- ABO (forward-type only)
- Rh type (including test for weak D)
- Direct antiglobulin test

Postpartum Testing of Infants with Suspected Hemolytic Disease of the Newborn

A diagnosis of HDN is based on medical history, physical examination of the newborn, and results of laboratory testing on both mother and child. Box 13-2 lists the tests that should be performed on cord blood in cases of suspected HDN.

ABO Testing

When ABO typing is carried out on newborns, only the forward type is performed, since ABO antibodies are not yet produced. In addition, it is important to follow manufacturer's directions carefully, since ABO antigens may not be fully developed and may give weaker results than those expected in an adult.

Rh Testing

In cases of HDN the DAT may be positive, which can lead to false positive or false negative Rh-testing results. To ensure the validity of an Rh-positive test result, it is essential to include appropriate Rh controls. False Rh-negative results may be due to a blocking phenomenon, requiring gentle elution to resolve.

Direct Antiglobulin Test

The DAT must be performed carefully, since the result may be weak, especially in cases of ABO HDN. In cases of a positive DAT, performing an elution is optional if antibody identification tests were performed on the mother at the time of admission.[5] If a maternal sample is unavailable, testing the eluate may be useful to confirm HDN.

If the maternal antibody screen is negative and the DAT is positive, ABO HDN should be suspected. ABO HDN can be confirmed by performing either a heat or freeze-thaw elution. The eluate should be tested against A_1, B, and O cells using an antiglobulin technique. Positive results with A_1 and/or B cells and negative results with the O cells is indicative and/or ABO HDN. If the eluate is negative with all cells, an antibody to a low-frequency antigen should be suspected and the maternal serum tested against the paternal cells.

Intrauterine Transfusions

ABO, Rh, and direct antiglobulin tests should be interpreted with extreme caution in newborns who have received intrauterine transfusions. Since group O D-negative blood is used for intrauterine transfusions, cord blood test results may be misleading. Depending on the number of transfusions, the infant may type as group O D-negative or give weak mixed-field reactions with ABO and Rh antisera. The DAT likewise may be falsely negative or only weakly positive.

PREVENTION OF HEMOLYTIC DISEASE OF THE NEWBORN

As can be seen from the previous discussions, the production of IgG antibodies (particularly anti-D) can have life-threatening consequences for the fetus. Once a woman is alloimmunized and produces antibodies, the condition cannot be reversed. Therefore the transfusion service must ensure that alloimmunization in women of childbearing age is prevented whenever possible. Fortunately RhIG is available and prevents alloimmunization in D-negative mothers exposed to D-positive red blood cells. RhIG was developed during the early 1960s and licensed for administration in 1968. Since its introduction there has been a dramatic decrease in the incidence of Rh HDN. Before the use of RhIG, 13% of D-negative women became sensitized following pregnancy. The routine postpartum administration of RhIG reduced the probability of immunization to 1% to 2%. The addition of antepartum administration at 28 weeks has further reduced the risk of immunization to less than 0.1%.[3]

RhIG is a concentrate of IgG anti-D prepared from pools of human plasma. The product is given intramuscularly to nonsensitized D-negative women at 28 weeks of gestation (antepartum) and again within 72 hours of delivery (postpartum) of an D-positive infant. RhIG suppresses the immune response following exposure to D-positive fetal red blood cells and prevents the mother from producing anti-D. The mechanism of antibody production suppression is not clearly understood, but it may involve interference of antigen presentation.[1] The product has been purified and has little or no risk of viral transmission.[3] Recently an intravenous preparation has been licensed for suppression of Rh immunization and treatment of non-splenectomized patients with immune thrombocytopenic purpura.[6]

Antepartum Administration

A full 300-μg dose of RhIG provides protection for up to 15 ml of D-positive red blood cells (approximately 30 ml of fetal whole blood). A 300-μg dose of RhIG should be given routinely to unsensitized D-negative mothers at 28 weeks of gestation and after amniocentesis, abortions, termination of ectopic pregnancy, chorionic villus sampling, PUBS, intrauterine transfusions, or abdominal trauma. For events with the potential for red blood cell exposure (FMH) before 12 weeks of gestation, when the fetal blood volume is less than 2.5 ml, a 50-μg dose can be used. As mentioned previously all women should have an ABO and Rh type and test for unexpected alloantibodies as early as possible in the pregnancy. The

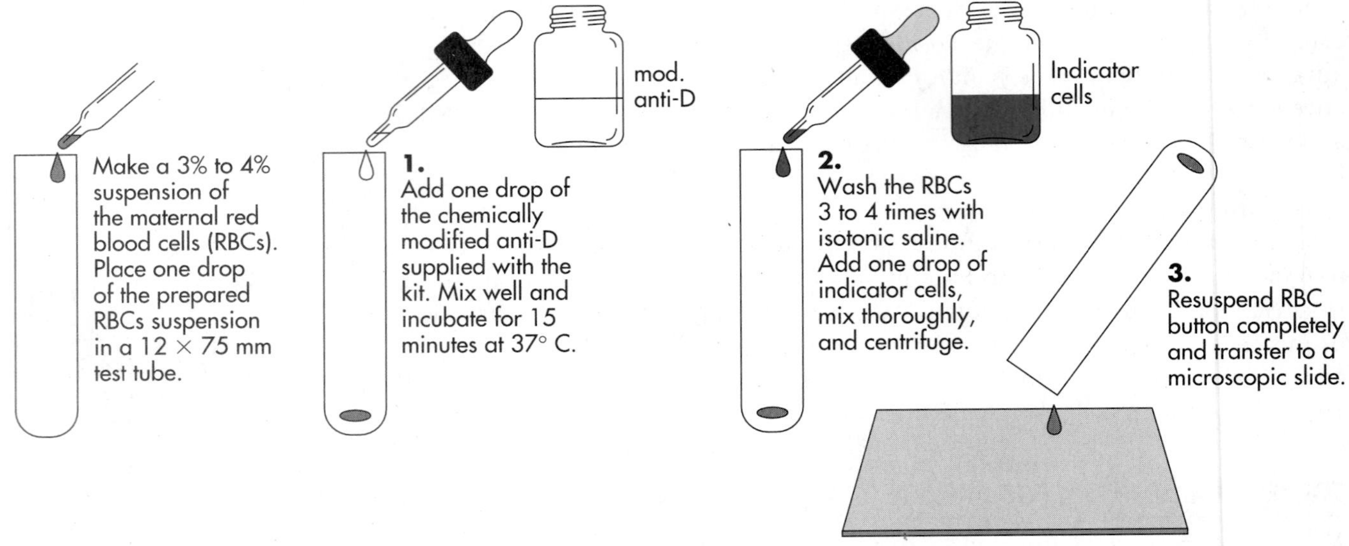

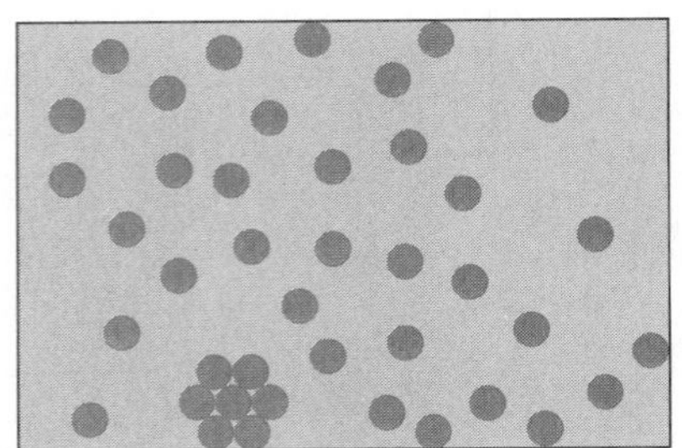

4.
Examine microscopically for mixed-field agglutination.

Feto-Maternal Hemorrhage:
< 1 rosette per 3 lpf: one dose of RhIG
> 1 rosette per 3 lpf: quantitate bleed

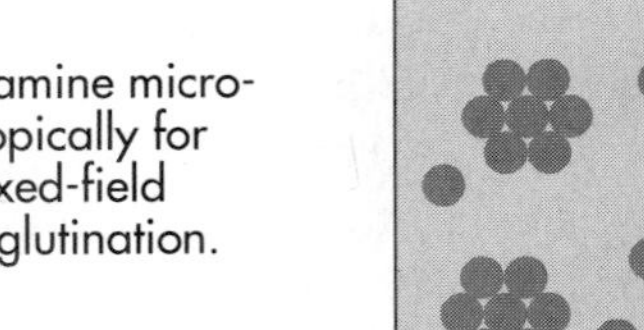

Uniform agglutination pattern: test for weak D(D^u) positive

Note:
It has been reported* that this procedure may be used to type cord bloods for the weak D(D^u) phenotype when the cord blood has a positive direct antiglobulin test because of coating by ABO antibodies. Perform test as described, using cord blood specimen in place of maternal specimen.

This procedure is not mentioned in the package insert for the Gamma Test Kit, since FDA approval has not been obtained for this use.

Fig. 13-4 Rosette test for detection of fetomaternal hemorrhage.
RhIG, Rh immune globulin; *lpf,* low power field.
Courtesy of Gamma Biologicals, Houston, Tex.
*Werch J, Todd C, Moulds M: D^u phenotyping by the rosette technique when the direct antiglobulin test is positive, *Immunohematology* 6:44, 1990.

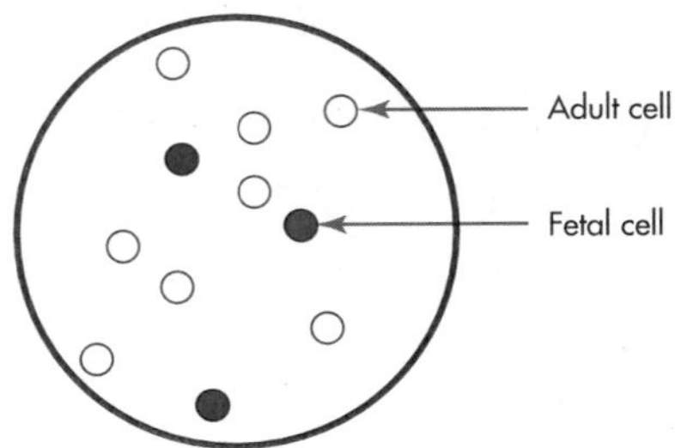

Fig. 13-5 Acid elution test for determination of hemoglobulin F. Following staining, fetal cells appear dark pink and adult cells are lighter. The fetal hemoglobin resists acid elution and remains intact, whereas the adult cells lose the hemoglobin and do not take up the stain.

antibody screen should be repeated at 26 to 28 weeks for all D-negative women. If the antibody screen remains negative for anti-D, RhIG should be administered. Other alloantibodies (anti-K, anti- E, etc.) should *not* prevent a woman from receiving RhIG.

Postpartum Administration

Cord blood from all infants born to D-negative women should be tested for the D (including weak-D) antigen. Nonimmunized (no anti-D) D-negative women who deliver a D-positive (including weak-D) infant should receive a full dose of RhIG within 72 hours of delivery. If the delivering hospital has a verified record of a negative antibody screen during the current pregnancy, the screen does not need to be repeated before administration of postpartum RhIG.[7] In those cases, when the antibody screen is repeated at delivery, results must be interpreted with caution. A weak anti-D often may be detected because of the antenatal administration of RhIG. If a check of the patient's history reveals administration of RhIG at 28 weeks, a full postpartum dose of RhIG still should be administered.

Screening for Fetomaternal Hemorrhage

If during delivery a woman experiences an FMH exceeding 30 ml of D-positive fetal red blood cells, it is essential that she receive more than one dose of RhIG. All postpartum RhIG candidates should have a postpartum specimen tested for significant FMH.[3] Currently the most frequently used method to screen for FMH is the rosette test (Fig. 13-4). In this method a suspension of the maternal cells (containing D-negative maternal red blood cells and a small number of D-positive fetal red blood cells) is incubated with anti-D. During incubation the anti-D binds to the D-positive fetal red blood cells. The suspension is washed thoroughly, and D-positive indicator cells are added, which bind to the anti-D and form a rosette around the D-positive fetal cells. A blood smear is prepared from the suspension and examined microscopically for the number of rosettes. Appropriate positive and negative controls should be run concurrently to ensure valid test results. A positive test (results vary depending on the method and reagents used) indicates a significant FMH and the potential need for more than one dose of RhIG. Since the rosette assay is only a screening test, a method to quantify the number of fetal red blood cells should be performed.

Quantifying Fetomaternal Hemorrhage

The Kleihauer-Betke acid elution is the method used most frequently to quantify the number of fetal cells in the maternal circulation. This method is based on the fact that fetal hemoglobin is resistant to acid elution and adult hemoglobin is not. A blood smear is prepared from a postpartum maternal sample and exposed to an acid buffer. Hemoglobin from adult cells leaches into the buffer and leaves only stroma, whereas the fetal cells retain their hemoglobin. Smears are washed, stained, and examined under oil immersion. Adult cells appear as "ghosts," and fetal cells appear pink (Fig. 13-5). Results are reported as the percentage of fetal cells (number of fetal cells divided by total cells counted). The volume (in milliliters of whole blood) of the FMH is equal to the percentage of fetal cells multiplied by 50. Since a full dose of RhIG protects against 30 ml of whole blood, the volume of the FMH is divided by 30 to determine the number of doses of RhIG. For example:

Results of Kleihauer-Betke: 16 fetal cells/1000 cells counted = 1.6%
Volume of FMH: 1.6 × 50 = 80 ml of Rh-positive fetal blood
Required doses of RhIG: 80/30 = 2.7 doses

Since the accuracy and precision of this method are poor, a safety margin should be provided to ensure adequate protection. If the number to the right of the decimal point is less than 5, round down and add one dose of RhIG. If the number to the right of the decimal is greater than or equal to 5, round up and add one dose of RhIG. In the example above, the final dose would be 4. Box 13-3 outlines this calculation.

BOX 13-3 ***Quantification of Fetomaternal Hemorrhage to Calculate Dose of Rh Immune Globulin (RhIG)***

STEP 1
Estimate the volume of fetal blood in maternal circulation:
Percentage of cells counted × 50 = fetal blood (ml)

STEP 2
Divide ml of fetal blood by 30, since each 300-μg dose of RhIG protects against a 30-ml whole blood bleed

STEP 3
Round the calculated dose up if ≥5 following decimal point or down if <5
Add one vial of RhIG to calculated dose to provide a safety margin

BOX 13-4 ***Laboratory Testing for Prevention of Hemolytic Disease of the Newborn Because of Anti-D***

INITIAL VISIT
ABO and Rh (including test for weak D)
Test for unexpected IgG antibodies
If antibody screen is positive, perform antibody identification:
- Anti-D identified: Not an RhIG candidate
- Anti-D not identified: Candidate for RhIG at 28 weeks
- Consider antibody titration for clinically significant antibodies

FOLLOW-UP VISIT
Repeat ABO and Rh are not necessary unless for transfusion purposes
Rh-positive: Repeat antibody screen not necessary
Rh-negative: Repeat antibody screen
- Antibody screen negative: Give RhIG at 26 to 28 weeks
- Antibody screen positive because of anti-D: No RhIG, possible HDN
- Antibody screen positive because of something other than anti-D: Give RhIG at 26 to 28 weeks

AT DELIVERY
Repeat testing not necessary unless for transfusion purposes
D negative with history of alloanti-D: Suspect HDN; test cord blood; no RhIG
D negative with no history of alloanti-D: Candidate for RhIG; test cord blood
- Cord blood: Rh-negative; no RhIG
- Cord blood: Rh-positive; screen for FMH and calculate dose of RhIG

RhIG, Rh immune globulin; *HDN,* hemolytic disease of the newborn; *FMH,* fetomaternal hemorrhage.

Appropriate laboratory testing procedures to prevent HDN because of anti-D are addressed in the American Association of Blood Banks' Bulletin No. 98-2.[7] See Box 13-4 for a summary of procedures.

TREATMENT OF HEMOLYTIC DISEASE OF THE NEWBORN

In Utero Treatment

Intrauterine transfusions are given to correct anemia in utero and prevent potential heart failure. Intrauterine transfusions historically have been administered by the intraperitoneal route. In an intraperitoneal transfusion, a needle is inserted into the mother's abdomen and into the peritoneal cavity of the fetus. The red blood cells are infused into the peritoneal cavity and absorbed into the fetal circulation through the lymphatics. Drawbacks of this procedure include the inability to perform the procedure before 25 weeks and variable absorption of red blood cells (particularly in hydropic fetuses). More recently PUBS has been used to provide direct intravascular transfusion into the umbilical vein. Benefits of this procedure include the ability to obtain a hematocrit before transfusion (to more accurately determine the amount of blood to be transfused) and the ability to perform the procedure as early as 17 weeks.

Blood for intrauterine transfusion should be group O, D-negative red blood cells less than 7 days old, irradiated, cytomegalovirus (CMV) negative, and hemoglobin S negative. Red blood cells with a hematocrit of 75% to 80% are used to avoid volume overload. Group O D-negative is used because the ABO and Rh of the fetus are usually not known and to avoid destruction by the maternal anti-D. Fresh blood is necessary to ensure longer viability, higher 2,3-diphosphoglycerate (for release of oxygen to the tissues), and lower potassium (to avoid cardiac arrhythmias). Irradiation is necessary to prevent graft versus host disease in the fetus. Donor cells are crossmatched using the maternal serum.

Postpartum Treatment

Phototherapy

Phototherapy is performed as an initial treatment for hyperbilirubinemia. Exposure of newborns to fluorescent blue light in the 420- to 475-nm range can successfully treat physiologic jaundice and mild cases of HDN, particularly ABO HDN. Bilirubin, when exposed to light, undergoes photoisomerization to form photobilirubin. These isomers of bilirubin are carried by the plasma to the liver and excreted in the bile without the need for conjugation. Cases of hyperbilirubinemia that fail to respond to phototherapy require exchange transfusion.

Exchange Transfusion

As mentioned previously, newborns suffering from HDN are at risk from anemia and hyperbilirubinemia. If left untreated elevated levels of indirect bilirubin can result in damage to the CNS. Exchange transfusion, the indicated treatment of severe HDN, successfully treats both of the above problems. Exchange transfusion:

- Corrects anemia without expanding blood volume
- Removes a sensitized newborn's red blood cells and replaces them with normal fresh donor cells
- Reduces the level of bilirubin and prevents kernicterus
- Reduces the level of maternal antibody

Many variables enter into the decision to perform exchange transfusion. A bilirubin level of 18 to 20 mg/dl historically has been used as the level at which kernicterus is a serious risk and exchange transfusion is necessary. However, complications such as low birth weight, sepsis, acidosis, or signs of CNS deterioration can affect the threshold level and indicate the need for exchange at levels well below 20 mg/dl. For these reasons premature infants may require exchange transfusions at lower bilirubin levels and more often than do full-term infants. Many physicians consider the rate of rise in the bilirubin level to be a better predictor of the need for exchange transfusion.[3]

Selection of Blood and Compatibility Testing for Exchange Transfusion

Before the initial exchange transfusion, infant cells must be tested to determine the ABO group and Rh type. Repeat ABO and Rh typing is not necessary for the remainder of the infant's hospital admission.[8] Serum or plasma from the infant or the mother may be used for the antibody screen. Maternal serum is used most commonly, since it is readily available and has a high concentration of antibodies. Since the antibody screen is positive, the red blood cells to be transfused must lack the antigen corresponding to the maternal antibody and be crossmatch compatible by the antiglobulin technique. If maternal serum is not available, the newborn's serum or an eluate from the newborn's red blood cells can be used for antibody detection and compatibility testing.

Many institutions simplify the procedure of selecting blood for exchange transfusion by using group O, Rh-negative red blood cells for all exchange transfusions, but this is not always necessary. If the mother and infant are ABO identical, group-specific red blood cells can be used. When a non–group O infant receives A or B cells, the infant's serum must be tested against A_1 and B cells using the indirect antiglobulin technique. If anti-A or anti-B is detected, group O cells must be used for transfusion.

Fresh frozen plasma (FFP) is used to reconstitute the red blood cells to a hematocrit between 40% to 50%.[3] The plasma must be ABO compatible (or group AB) with the red blood cells. The FFP restores albumin and coagulation factors. Additional requirements for CMV-negative blood and irradiation are commonly made because of the immunocompromised status of newborns. Hemoglobin S–negative blood should be provided to avoid any possibility of intravascular sickling.[3] Box 13-5 summarizes the criteria to consider when selecting blood for exchange.

BOX 13-5 ***Selection of Blood for Exchange Transfusion***

- Group O (or ABO-compatible) D-negative blood
- Fresh (less than 7 days old) red blood cells resuspended in AB fresh frozen plasma
- CMV-negative blood
- Irradiated blood
- Hemoglobin S–negative blood
- Blood lacks antigen corresponding to maternal antibody
- Compatible crossmatch with maternal serum

CHAPTER SUMMARY

HDN occurs when maternal IgG antibodies destroy fetal red blood cells. These IgG antibodies are most commonly produced following exposure to fetal red blood cells in a prior pregnancy. Fetal cells, carrying antigens inherited from the father, stimulate the mother to produce IgG antibodies. In a subsequent pregnancy, these IgG antibodies, which are capable of crossing the placenta, destroy the fetal red blood cells. In utero, this destruction can cause severe anemia, which can result in heart failure and possibly death. After delivery, red blood cell destruction continues with the release of indirect bilirubin. The fetal liver, which is deficient in the enzyme glucuronyl transferase, is unable to conjugate the indirect bilirubin. The resulting hyperbilirubinemia causes jaundice and possible damage to the CNS (kernicterus).

ABO HDN is the most common type of HDN and occurs most commonly in group O mothers who deliver A or B babies. Unlike other types of HDN, ABO HDN can occur in the first pregnancy, since it is caused by non–red blood cell–stimulated antibodies. Laboratory findings in ABO HDN include negative or weakly positive DAT, spherocytes on the blood smear, and mildly elevated bilirubin levels. ABO HDN is usually mild and can be successfully treated with phototherapy.

Rh HDN, because of anti-D, is the most severe type of HDN. It occurs in D-negative women with anti-D who deliver D-positive babies. Laboratory findings in Rh HDN include strongly positive DAT and varying degrees of anemia and bilirubinemia. Aggressive treatment may be necessary depending on the clinical symptoms and laboratory results.

Any IgG antibody can cause HDN if the child inherits the gene from the father and the red blood cell antigen is well developed on the fetal red blood cells. Anti-c and anti-K are most frequently reported after anti-D.

A number of invasive and noninvasive methods are available to help predict HDN. Titration of the maternal antibody can be helpful in deciding when to perform invasive procedures. A titer of 1:16 is often considered a critical value and indicates the need for amniocentesis or PUBS. Spectrophotometric analysis of the amniotic fluid and use of the Liley graph can aid in predicting the severity of HDN. Hemoglobin, reticulocyte count, DAT, and blood typing performed on fetal blood obtained by PUBS provide the most accurate assessments of HDN severity.

A cord blood sample should be collected from all infants born to D-negative women to determine whether the mother should receive postpartum RhIG. RhIG is a concentrate of IgG anti-D given to Rh-negative women to prevent the production of anti-D. In cases of suspected HDN, ABO/Rh typing and the DAT should be performed. Hemoglobin and bilirubin should also be closely monitored. Depending on the severity of HDN, treatment can begin in utero or after delivery. In the most severe cases (Liley upper zone), PUBS can be used for direct intravascular transfusion to the fetus. After delivery, exchange transfusion is used to correct anemia, remove sensitized red blood cells, and reduce levels of maternal antibody and bilirubin. Blood for exchange and intrauterine transfusion should be fresh (less than 7 days old), irradiated, CMV negative, hemoglobin S negative, and negative for the antigen corresponding to the maternal antibody. Group O, D-negative red blood cells resuspended in AB plasma are used most often.

Rh HDN is the only preventable type of HDN. A 300-μg dose is given at 28 weeks' gestation and again within 72 hours of delivery of a D-positive infant. This protects the mother against 30 ml of fetal D-positive blood. RhIG should always be administered after potential exposure to fetal red blood cells, including abortion, ectopic pregnancy, amniocentesis, PUBS, or abdominal trauma. If the exposure occurs before 12 weeks' gestation, a 50-μg dose of RhIG is available. Candidates for postpartum RhIG must be tested for significant FMH. The rosette assay is used to identify women who have had an FMH of greater than 30 ml and therefore need more than one dose of RhIG. The Kleihauer-Betke acid elution method can be used to quantify the FMH and calculate the number of doses of RhIG to be given.

CRITICAL THINKING EXERCISES

◆ ***EXERCISE 13-1***

R.T. was seen by her ob-gyn for her initial visit at 9 weeks of gestation. This is her first pregnancy.

1. What tests should be run for her initial prenatal workup?

◆ ***Additional Testing***

Results of prenatal testing indicate R.T. is group A D negative with a negative antibody screen.

2. Does R.T. need any additional laboratory testing during her pregnancy? If so, when should the testing be performed, what tests are needed, and why?

◆ ***Additional Testing***

R.T. was seen again by her ob-gyn at 28 weeks. Her antibody screen is repeated and found to be negative. Based on these test results, she received a 300-μg dose of RhIG. Twelve weeks later, R.T. delivered a healthy 6 lb, 4 oz boy.

3. What testing, if any, needs to be performed at the time of delivery?

◆ ***Additional Testing***

Results of the cord blood from R.T.'s baby indicate group A, D positive with a negative DAT.

4. Is R.T. a candidate for postpartum RhIG?
5. What additional test needs to be performed on R.T. before the RhIG is given, and what special specimen requirements need to be considered for this test?

◆ ***EXERCISE 13-2***

J.M. is seen at the outpatient clinic for her first prenatal visit at 15 weeks of gestation. Obstetrical history indicates one ectopic pregnancy (no RhIG given) and one full-term pregnancy (RhIG given). The last child required phototherapy. Results of prenatal testing indicate group O Rh negative with a positive antibody screen.

1. What additional testing needs to be performed?

◆ ***Additional Testing***

An antibody panel identifies anti-D with a titer of 1:16 using anti-IgG. A titer performed at 20 weeks shows the following results:

(Repeat of titer at 15 weeks:	1:16)
Titer at 20 weeks:	1:64

2. What is the purpose of performing antibody titration?

◆ ***Additional Testing***

Amniocentesis performed at 24 weeks shows a ΔOD of 0.10.

3. Using the Liley graph, what outcome might be expected for this pregnancy given this result and the patient history?

◆ ***Additional Testing***

J.M. continues to be closely monitored by amniocentesis throughout her pregnancy. She delivered a 4 lb, 10 oz girl at 37 weeks. Results of cord blood testing indicated: group A D positive with a 3+ DAT; hemoglobin of 13 g/dl; and bilirubin of 4.2 mg/dl.

4. Does this baby have HDN? If so, what is the cause? Use laboratory data to support your conclusions.

◆ ***Additional Testing***

The following evening, J.M.'s baby has a bilirubin of 17.4 mg/dl, and an exchange transfusion is requested.

5. What testing needs to be performed, and what type blood should be selected?

◆ ***EXERCISE 13-3***

B.W. was seen by her ob-gyn at 10 weeks of gestation with her first pregnancy. Results of her prenatal workup indicate she is group O D negative with a negative antibody screen. Repeat testing at 28 weeks continues to indicate a negative antibody screen, and she is given 300 μg of RhIG. The pregnancy proceeds normally, and she delivers a 7 lb, 2 oz boy at 39 weeks of gestation. Results of the cord blood testing indicated: group A D positive with a weakly positive DAT; hemoglobulin of 17.3 g/dl; and bilirubin of 0.6 mg/dl.

1. Does this baby have HDN? If so, what is the most probable cause? Use laboratory data to support your conclusions.
2. What test could be performed to confirm your suspicions?

◆ ***Additional Testing***

A freeze-thaw elution is performed. The eluate is tested against A_1, B, and O cells at 37° C using anti-IgG.

	A_1	B	O
Eluate	1+	1+	negative

3. What do these results indicate?
4. What type of treatment most likely would be recommended for this infant?
5. Is B.W. a candidate for postpartum RhIG? If so, are any additional tests necessary?

◆ ***Additional Testing***

A rosette assay performed on B.W. gives a positive result.

6. What test needs to be performed and why?

◆ ***Additional Testing***

A Kleihauer-Betke stain is performed on B.W.'s postpartum specimen to quantify the amount of the FMH. Nineteen fetal cells were counted in a total of 1000 cells.

7. How many doses of RhIG should B.W. receive?

◆ ***EXERCISE 13-4***

M.K., a 26-year-old mother of two, is admitted to labor and delivery. No prenatal records are available. Results of a type and screen follow:

Anti-A	Anti-B	Anti-D	Rh Control	Weak D	Weak D Control	A_1 Cells	B Cells	Screen Cell I	Screen Cell II	Interpretation
Neg	4+	Neg	Neg	Neg	Neg	4+	Neg	w	w	B neg

Neg, Negative; *w,* weak.

An antibody identification is performed, and anti-D is identified. Since no prenatal records are available, a cord blood is requested. The cord blood results follow:

Anti-A	Anti-B	Anti-D	Rh Control	DAT	Interpretation
Neg	Neg	3+	Neg	Neg	O pos

DAT, Direct antiglobulin test; *neg,* negative; *pos,* positive.

Based on the above results, is M.K. a candidate for postpartum RhIG? Discuss how you would proceed.

STUDY QUESTIONS

1. Objectives for performing an exchange transfusion include all of the following EXCEPT to:
   a. decrease the level of maternal antibody
   b. reduce the level of indirect bilirubin
   c. provide platelets to prevent disseminated intravascular coagulation
   d. provide compatible red blood cells to correct anemia

2. The greatest danger to the *fetus* affected by HDN is:
   a. kernicterus c. hyperbilirubinemia
   b. anemia d. low L/S ratio

3. A 300-μg dose of RhIG covers a maximum FMH of how many milliliters of whole blood?
   a. 10 c. 30
   b. 15 d. 50

4. RhIG should be administered within how many hours of delivery?
   a. 6 c. 72
   b. 48 d. 96

5. An oftentimes-fatal condition characterized by general edema that results from anemia is:
   a. kernicterus c. erythroblastosis fetalis
   b. DIC d. hydrops fetalis

6. HDN occurs when:
   a. maternal antigens react with fetal antibodies
   b. fetal antibodies react with maternal antibodies
   c. maternal antibodies react with fetal antigens
   d. fetal antigens react with maternal antigens

7. The greatest danger to the newborn affected by HDN is:
   a. kernicterus
   b. anemia
   c. conjugated bilirubin
   d. low L/S ratio

8. Which of the following women should receive postpartum RhIG?

	Mother's ABO/Rh	Mother's antibody screen	Newborn
a.	group A, D negative	negative	group O, D positive
b.	group O, D negative	negative	group A, D negative
c.	group A, D positive	negative	group B, D negative
d.	group B, D negative	anti-D	group B, D positive

9. Which of the following antibodies carries no risk of HDN?
   a. anti-Le^a
   b. anti-C
   c. anti-K
   d. anti-S

10. Which of the following is NOT characteristic of ABO HDN?
    a. may occur in first pregnancy
    b. usually treated with phototherapy
    c. strongly positive DAT
    d. most frequent in babies born to O mothers

11. Which of the following requirements is NOT important when selecting blood for exchange transfusion?
    a. irradiated blood
    b. CMV-negative blood
    c. leukocyte-reduced blood
    d. blood less than 7 days old

12. A mother is group A, Rh negative with anti-D in her serum. Which of the following units should be selected for an intrauterine transfusion?
    a. group O, D negative
    b. group O, D positive
    c. group A, D negative
    d. group A, D positive

13. The rosette test is:
    a. performed on a cord blood sample
    b. used to screen for FMH
    c. a quantitative test used to calculate the volume of FMH
    d. an acid elution used to estimate the volume of FMH

14. Which of the following tests is NOT necessary when testing a cord blood?
    a. ABO
    b. Rh
    c. DAT
    d. antibody screen

REFERENCES

1. Mollison PL, Engelfriet CP, Contreras M: *Blood transfusion in clinical medicine,* ed 9, London, 1993, Blackwell Scientific.
2. Chavez GF, Mulinare J, Edmonds LD: Epidemiology of Rh hemolytic disease of the newborn in the United States, *JAMA* 265:3270, 1991.
3. Vengelen-Tyler V, editor: *Technical manual,* ed 12, Bethesda, Md, 1996, American Association of Blood Banks.
4. Henry JB: *Clinical diagnosis and management by laboratory methods,* ed 19, Philadelphia, 1996, WB Saunders.

5. Judd WJ, Luban NL, Ness PM, et al: Prenatal and perinatal immunohematology: recommendations for serologic management of the fetus, newborn infant, and obstetric patient, *Transfusion* 30:175, 1990.
6. Ness P, Menitove J, Snyder EL: Guidelines for the use of intravenous RhIG. In *News briefs*, Bethesda, Md, 18:2, 1996, American Association of Blood Banks.
7. Bryant B, editor: Association bulletin No. 98-2. In *News briefs*, Bethesda, Md. 20:16, 1998, American Association of Blood Banks.
8. Menitove JE, editor: *Standards for blood banks and transfusion services*, ed 18, Bethesda, Md, 1997, American Association of Blood Banks.

TRANSFUSION THERAPY IN SELECTED PATIENTS

14

Kathy D. Blaney
Dorilyn Hitchcock

CHAPTER OUTLINE

LEARNING OBJECTIVES

Upon completion of this chapter, the reader should be able to:

1. Discuss the pathophysiology and transfusion needs of patients with sickle cell disease, aplastic anemia, and autoimmune disease.
2. Explain the transfusion requirements of oncology patients.
3. Describe the pathophysiology of acute blood loss and massive transfusion therapy.
4. Discuss the transfusion requirements and causes of bleeding during cardiac surgery.
5. Describe the unique hematologic problems and transfusion therapy issues associated with the neonate.
6. Compare and contrast bone marrow, progenitor, and cord blood transplantation and the required transfusion support for each.
7. List the acquired and congenital disorders of hemostasis and the appropriate transfusion support for each type of disorder.
8. Define *therapeutic hemapheresis* and the conditions and diseases associated with its use.
9. Discuss the transfusion issues unique to chronic renal disease patients and how the use of erythropoietin affects the need for red blood cell transfusions.

One of the benefits of blood component therapy is the ability to provide transfusion support for patients with many unique hematologic problems. For some patients, such as those with sickle cell disease, the need for this support extends throughout their life. For others it may be an urgent requirement resulting from surgery or trauma. By understanding the various patient clinical conditions, laboratory professionals can appreciate the focus of their treatment and be more aware of the value of the blood components they are providing. A description of blood components, their therapeutic value, and the indications for their use is reviewed in Chapter 11. This chapter summarizes the pathophysiology of selected clinical conditions that commonly require transfusion support.

URGENT AND MASSIVE TRANSFUSION

Hemorrhage: bleeding through ruptured or unruptured blood vessel walls.

Rapid blood loss or **hemorrhage** initiates a series of complicated physiologic responses that involve the nervous, hormonal, and circulatory systems. This response, called *hemorrhagic shock,* complicates the treatment of acute blood loss.[1] Characteristic signs and symptoms of shock are listed in Box 14-1. The duration and magnitude of shock are critical factors affecting the mortality in trauma.[2] Severe hemorrhage affects electrolyte metabolism and oxygen transport, which ultimately increases the heart rate and the stress on internal organs. Prolonged shock, hypotension, and extensive tissue damage can result in cardiac and renal failure. Disseminated intravascular coagulation (DIC) is a pathologic activation of the coagulation cascade and may also be caused by hemorrhage, which would further complicate the ability to control bleeding.

BOX 14-1

Symptoms of Hemorrhagic Shock

- Hypotension
- Tachycardia
- Pallor, cyanosis
- Cold or clammy skin
- Oliguria
- Decreased hematocrit
- Decreased central venous pressure
- Central nervous system depression
- Metabolic shock

The most important goal in treating acute blood loss is to correct or prevent hypovolemic shock.[3] Infusing sufficient fluid volume to maintain adequate blood flow and blood pressure for tissue oxygenation is critical. Immediate volume restoration with crystalloid or colloid solutions is usually recommended.[4] Initial blood loss between 1000 and 1200 ml usually does not require red blood cell transfusions. The patient's vital signs, clinical situation, and hematocrit determine the requirement and urgency for red blood cell support. Box 14-2 lists priorities in acute blood loss.[5]

BOX 14-2

Priorities in Massive Transfusion

- Replace and maintain blood volume
- Optimize oxygen-carrying capacity
- Maintain hemostasis: platelets and coagulation factors
- Correct or avoid metabolic disturbances:
  hypocalcemia
  hyperkalemia/hypokalemia
  acid-base disturbances
  hypothermia
- Plasma colloid osmotic pressure

Red blood cell transfusions in trauma situations are usually urgent and of significant quantity. Massive transfusion is defined as the replacement of one or more blood volumes within 24 hours.[6] A blood volume is estimated at 5000 ml, which is about 10 units of whole blood in a 70-kg adult.

Adverse metabolic effects can occur from the transfusion of large quantities of stored blood over a short period of time. One blood volume exchanged within 3 to 4 hours can cause significant acute metabolic disturbances such as citrate toxicity, hypothermia, and coagulation abnormalities. Coagulation abnormalities resulting in microvascular bleeding have been attributed to:

- ◆ Dilution of platelets or coagulation factors occurring with two or three volume exchanges[2]
- ◆ Consumption of platelets and coagulation factors from extensive bleeding
- ◆ Hypotension, which is currently believed to be the principal cause of bleeding[7]

Complications resulting from massive transfusion are summarized in Table 14-1.

Urgent transfusion requirements resulting from trauma or surgery sometimes necessitate the release of uncrossmatched blood if insufficient time to obtain a sample for typing exists. This process of "emergency release" is discussed in Chapter 8. Type O red blood cells should be transfused until the patient's type is

Table 14-1 Complications in Massive Transfusion

PROBLEM	CAUSES	TREATMENTS
Microvascular hemorrhage	◆ Dilution of coagulation factors and platelets ◆ Hypotension ◆ Consumption of factors ◆ Platelet consumption	◆ Platelets ◆ FFP to control defined deficiencies of factors ◆ Control hypotension
Citrate toxicity	◆ Decrease in ionized calcium from effect of anticoagulant in blood products	
Hypothermia	◆ Rapid infusion of blood products	◆ High-flow blood warmers

FFP, Fresh frozen plasma.

Table 14-2 Excessive Blood Loss Following Cardiac Surgery

PROBLEM	CAUSE
Impaired platelet function	Decreased receptors or receptor activity Release of α-granules Presence of fibrin degradation
Increased fibrinolytic activity	Impaired fibrin clot formation Impaired platelet function Lysis of physiologic thrombi
Hypothermia	Platelet sequestration
Heparin effect	Protamine necessary to neutralize heparin is difficult to calculate, since heparin may reappear: heparin rebound
Vascular (anatomic) defects	5% of patients may need to be reexplored for uncontrolled bleeding

known and should be D negative for females with child-bearing potential to avoid sensitization to the D antigen. Transfusion services are required to have guidelines related to releasing uncrossmatched blood components, type-specific red blood cells, and changing blood types during massive transfusion.

CARDIAC SURGERY

During cardiopulmonary bypass surgery the patient's blood circulates through an oxygenating pump outside the patient's body. Hemostasis is altered from the effects of heparin, platelet function, and decreased platelet counts. The platelet count drops to approximately half of the original level.[8] In addition, platelet function is altered from exposure to extracorporeal surfaces, hypothermia, and vasoconstriction. Platelet transfusions should be withheld until the conclusion of bypass.[9] Risk factors for bleeding during cardiac surgery vary substantially among patients and are listed in Box 14-3.

During and following surgery, heparin causes the activated partial thromboplastin time to be prolonged. The thrombin time, or TT, confirms heparin excess. Treatment with protamine rather than fresh frozen plasma (FFP) corrects heparin excess. FFP is usually indicated only for factor deficiency or massive transfusion from severe bleeding during cardiac surgery. The effects of preoperative warfarin therapy contribute to postoperative blood loss and transfusion requirements.[9] A summary of the complications following cardiac surgery appears in Table 14-2.

BOX 14-3

Risk Factors for Bleeding During Cardiac Surgery

FACTORS CAUSING INCREASED BLEEDING

Time on the pump
Previous cardiac surgery
Valve replacement
Preoperative medications: aspirin and warfarin

VARIABLES IN BLEEDING

Effective anticoagulation: reversal of heparin effect
Decreased platelet function: hypothermia
Use of aprotinin and desmopressin
Surgeon

NEONATAL AND PEDIATRIC TRANSFUSION ISSUES

Neonatal and pediatric transfusion issues are significantly different from those for adults because of the small size, hemoglobin changes, and erythropoietin response in early infancy. Ill neonates are more likely than hospitalized patients of any other age group to receive red blood cell transfusions.[10]

Fetal cells contain hemoglobin F, which has a higher affinity or ability to bind oxygen. This affinity is important during the intrauterine period, since it enhances oxygen transfer from maternal red blood cells to fetal red blood cells. The time of conception determines the shift from fetal to adult hemoglobin.[3] For this reason, preterm infants have a higher level of fetal hemoglobin than those born at term. The change from fetal to adult hemoglobin occurs during the first few weeks of life, and the process causes a condition called *physiologic anemia of infancy*. In a full-term infant of normal birth weight, this change is well tolerated; however, in an infant born prematurely with low birth weight, treatment is often necessary.

Iatrogenic blood loss: blood loss caused by treatment (e.g., collection of samples for testing).

In addition to the shift in hemoglobin, the need for frequent laboratory tests contributes to the need for transfusions. **Iatrogenic blood loss** is the most common indication of transfusion in the preterm infant with low birth weight.[11] Newborns do not compensate for hypovolemia as well as adults do.

Erythropoietin in adults is released from the kidneys in response to diminished oxygen delivery. This growth factor triggers the bone marrow to increase red blood cell production and release more erythrocytes into the circulation. Erythropoietin production in an infant is believed to occur in the liver, which is less responsive to low levels of oxygen. The lower level of response to hypoxia protects the infant from becoming polycythemic during fetal life but does not allow an effective response to anemia in the immature infant.

A newborn's response to hypothermia is also different from an adult's response. The metabolic rate, hypoglycemia, and acidosis can cause apnea and lead to hypoxia, hypotension, and cardiac arrest. For this reason, a monitored blood warmer is often used to administer red blood cells, especially for exchange transfusions.

The ability to metabolize citrate and potassium is more difficult for newborns because of their immature liver and kidneys. For this reason washed or fresh blood is often indicated for newborns. Since potassium increases when blood is irradiated, washing irradiated red blood cells is also recommended. The transfusion of fresh blood to maximize the level of 2,3-diphosphoglycerate (2,3-DPG), which decreases during storage, is also important in newborns because of their limited ability to compensate for hypoxia.

In newborns, hemoglobin less than 13 g/dl indicates severe anemia during the first 24 hours of life. Red blood cell transfusions are usually given in small volumes prepared from multiple pack systems that allow preparation of several aliquots from a single donor unit. Since infants do not form red blood cell antibodies during the first 4 months, crossmatching is not necessary. If an antibody exists in the baby's or mother's serum, antigen-negative blood must be provided. ABO-identical or ABO-compatible blood that is Rh negative or the same as the infant's can be released during the first 4 months.

Transfusion-transmitted cytomegalovirus (CMV) is a risk to preterm infants weighing less than 1200 g who are born to seronegative mothers or to mothers whose CMV status is unknown.[12] This risk is avoided by providing CMV antibody–negative blood to neonates. In addition, leukoreduction, using highly efficient leukocyte removal filters, is recommended, since the CMV virus resides within the white blood cell.[13]

The transfusion issues unique to infants are summarized on Box 14-4. Familiarity with these problems provides an understanding of the transfusion requirements for preterm babies and infants.

BOX 14-4

Transfusion Issues Unique to Neonates

Fetal to adult hemoglobin change causing physiologic anemia of infancy
Iatrogenic blood loss
Decreased response of erythropoietin
Less tolerance of hypothermia
Greater CMV risk
Less ability to metabolize citrate and potassium
Decreased ability to restore 2,3-DPG in older units

CMV, Cytomegalovirus; *2,3-DPG*, 2,3-diphosphoglycerate.

TRANSPLANTATION

The transfusion service and blood bank provide support for transplantation of organs and bone marrow. This section describes the issues surrounding transplantation and transfusion requirements.

Organ Transplants

Massive blood loss and hemostatic problems are major complications of liver transplant because of the important role the liver plays in hemostasis. The preexisting liver disease also contributes to the hypocoagulability of the procedure. Surgery can last for 6 to 8 hours.[3] Blood product requirements in adult liver transplantation average 20 units of red blood cells, 25 units of FFP, 17 units of platelets, and 5 units of cryoprecipitated antihemophilic factor (CRYO).[14]

Graft survival is enhanced with human leukocyte antigen (HLA)–matched donor-recipient combinations. ABO compatibility is important in vascularized grafts, such as livers, kidneys, and hearts, but not important in tissue grafts, such as bone, heart valves, skin, and cornea. Minor ABO incompatibility (an O donor to an A recipient) is not critical, but it can be associated with hemolytic anemia associated with antibody production by passenger graft lymphocytes.[6]

BOX 14-5

Conditions Treated with Progenitor Cell Transplants

CONGENITAL IMMUNE DEFICIENCIES
Severe combined immunodeficiency disease
Wiskott-Aldrich syndrome

ANEMIAS
Acquired severe aplastic anemia
Fanconi's anemia
Thalassemia
Sickle cell disease

MALIGNANCY
Acute leukemia
Chronic myelogenous leukemia
Lymphoma
Myelodysplastic/myeloproliferative disorders
Multiple myeloma

SOLID TUMORS
Neuroblastoma
Breast cancer
Ovarian cancer
Testicular cancer

Progenitor Cell Transplantation

Progenitor cell transplants can be allogeneic or autologous. They can be derived from the following:

- Bone marrow (iliac crest)
- Peripheral blood (mononuclear cell fraction separated by apheresis equipment)
- Umbilical cord blood

Before transplantation transfusion support should include leukocyte-reduced blood products to avoid alloimmunization to histocompatibility antigens and subsequent graft rejection.[6]

Following transplantation patients usually require extensive platelet and red blood cell support for about 2 weeks. If the patient's and donor's ABO types are not matched, careful monitoring by the transfusion service is necessary, and additional red blood cell support may be necessary if hemolysis occurs.

Because of the immunosuppression of the patients undergoing transplants, the risk of graft versus host disease is serious. Blood products received after transplant should be irradiated. The progenitor cell product must never be irradiated, however, since this would prevent engraftment.[6] CMV infection is another potential problem because of immunosuppression, which can be avoided with leukopoor or seronegative blood products. Box 14-5 lists diseases treated with progenitor cell transplants.[3]

THERAPEUTIC HEMAPHERESIS

Therapeutic hemapheresis involves the removal of abnormal cells, plasma, or plasma constituents from a patient's blood to achieve a clinical benefit. The

Table 14-3 Indications for Therapeutic Hemapheresis

CONDITION	GOALS OF HEMAPHERESIS
Multiple myeloma; Waldenström's macroglobulinemia	Reduces abnormal proteins to improve circulation
Hyperleukocytosis	Reduces cell burden before chemotherapy
Thrombocythemia	Reduces the risk of thrombosis or stroke
TTP/HUS	Lessens the development of microthrombi
Sickle cell disease	Reduces severe symptoms, such as stroke, priapism, and acute chest syndromes
Myasthenia gravis	Reduces autoantibody concentration that attacks acetylcholine receptors
Acute Guillain-Barré syndrome	Reduces autoantibodies associated with nerve cells

TTP, Thrombotic thrombocytopenic purpura; *HUS*, hemolytic uremic syndrome.

replacement fluid varies with the condition and the portion that is removed. The goal may be to:

- Supply an essential substance that is absent
- Reduce the quantity of a particular antibody
- Modify mediators of inflammation
- Clear immune complexes
- Replace cellular elements

A list of conditions commonly treated with hemapheresis is found in Table 14-3.

Replacement fluids include crystalloids, albumin, plasma protein fraction, or FFP in the case of a plasma exchange. When exchanges necessitate FFP or red blood cell support, large quantities are used and necessitate adequate planning and communication with the transfusion service. A more comprehensive description of therapeutic hemapheresis is found in the American Association of Blood Banks' *Technical Manual.*

ONCOLOGY

The patient undergoing chemotherapy or radiation treatment for cancer relies on the transfusion service for a number of blood products. Cancers involve the unregulated, uncontrolled growth and division of a clone of cells from an organ or tissue. These clones of cells may divert the blood supply or crowd out the organ or neighboring organ(s), thus causing undesirable effects to the patient. Depending on where the abnormal cell originated, the cells, if left untreated, migrate and take hold in other organ systems in a process known as metastasis. The oncology patient is brought to the hospital for a combined treatment regimen of physical (radiation) and chemical therapies mostly targeting rapid cellular division. These patients usually have high uric acid levels, lactate dehydrogenase, and varying blood count levels.

The majority of chemotherapeutic agents (Table 14-4) act by:

- Interfering with DNA synthesis
- Slowing down or inhibiting DNA replication
- Interfering with translation (RNA synthesis)

Chemotherapeutic agents have a problem in that they are not specific for the target cancer or clone of cells. In essence they affect every cell actively involved in replication. Blood-forming cells of the bone marrow, epithelial cells of the gas-

Table 14-4 Chemotherapeutic Agents

DRUG	CLASS	ACTION
Cytosine arabinoside	Pyrimidine antimetabolite	Inhibits DNA synthesis
Daimpribocin	Anthracycline antibiotic	Inhibits DNA and RNA synthesis
Doxorubicin	Anthracycline antibiotic	Inhibits DNA and RNA synthesis
5-Azacytidine	Pyrimidine antimetabolite	Inhibits DNA and RNA synthesis
6-Thioguanine	Purine antimetabolite	Inhibits purine synthesis
Methylglyoxal bis (guanylhydrazone)	Unknown	Unknown
4′-(9-Acridinylamino) methanasulfon-m-anisidide	Unknown	Binds to DNA
Prednisone	Synthetic glucocorticoid	Lyses lymphoblasts
Vincristine	Plant alkaloid	Inhibits RNA synthesis and assembly of mitotic spindles
Asparaginase	*Escherichia coli* enzyme	Depletes endogenous asparagine
Daunorubicin	Anthracycline antibiotic	Inhibits DNA and RNA synthesis
Doxorubicin	Anthracycline antibiotic	Inhibits DNA and RNA synthesis
Methotrexate	Folic acid antimetabolite	Inhibits pyrimidine synthesis
6-Mercaptopurine	Purine antimetabolite	Inhibits pyrimidine synthesis
Cyclophosphamide	Synthetic alkylating agent	Cross-links DNA strands
Cytosine arabinoside	Pyrimidine antimetabolite	Inhibits DNA synthesis

DNA, Deoxyribonucleic acid; *RNA*, ribonucleic acid.
From McKenzie SB: *Textbook of hematology*, ed 2, Baltimore, 1996, Williams & Wilkins.

Table 14-5 Alternatives to Transfusion: Hematopoietic Growth Factors

FACTOR	NAMES	USES
Erythropoietin	EPO rHuEPO (prepared by recombinant technology)	Chronic renal failure AZT treatment in HIV Cancer patients on chemotherapy
Colony-stimulating factors (CSF)	Granulocyte-CSF Granulocyte-macrophage-CSF	Decreased infection in patients undergoing chemotherapy Congenital agranulocytosis Acute leukemia Myelodysplastic syndrome Aplastic anemia in children Autologous and allogeneic bone marrow transplant

EPO, Erythropoietin; *rHuEPO*, human recombinant erythropoietin; *AZT*, azidothymidine; *HIV*, human immunodeficiency virus.

trointestinal tract, and germinal epithelium of the hair follicles are particularly affected. In the bone marrow, megakaryocytes (from which platelets are derived) are some of the first affected. They are few in number compared to myeloid and erythroid precursors, thus the quick disappearance of platelets from peripheral blood. As treatment progresses, leukocyte, hemoglobin, and hematocrit levels fall. The most common complications are bleeding and infection. Careful monitoring of laboratory results and clinical conditions associated with bleeding and anemia is necessary to determine component therapy. Colony-stimulating factors are becoming more widely used in preventing infection and bleeding risks associated with chemotherapy (Table 14-5).

CHRONIC RENAL DISEASE

Table 14-6 Chronic Renal Disease

Cause	Effect
Elevated uremia	Altering of red blood cell shape, thus causing their premature removal
Dialysis procedure	Shearing of red blood cells
Low erythropoietin level	Low red blood cell production

The dialysis patient has many hematologic complications that necessitate transfusion therapy, usually in the form of red blood cell support. The high uremic content of the blood leads to altered red blood cell shapes; this prevents the red blood cells from traversing the spleen without being removed prematurely by macrophages, which results in hemolytic anemia. The act of dialysis itself causes a shearing of the red blood cells, which can contribute to hemolysis. These patients, because of the nonfunctioning kidney, fail to produce sufficient levels of erythropoietin; therefore an erythrocyte production problem also adds to the anemic condition. Factors contributing to transfusion needs in the dialysis patient are summarized on Table 14-6. Careful monitoring of hemoglobin and hematocrit levels that contribute to clinical symptoms determines transfusion therapy. The use of recombinant erythropoietin has significantly reduced the need for transfusion; however, in acute anemia, red blood cell transfusions are required. Transfusions are usually given while the patient is on dialysis equipment to reduce the need for an additional venipuncture.

HEMOLYTIC UREMIC SYNDROME AND THROMBOTIC THROMBOCYTOPENIC PURPURA

Hemolytic uremic syndrome (HUS) and thrombotic thrombocytopenic purpura (TTP) are classified together because of the numerous overlaps in clinical symptoms. The latter usually has a fever accompanying the other symptoms. Clinical symptoms include:

- Thrombocytopenia
- Microangiopathic hemolytic anemia
- Renal dysfunction
- Central nervous system involvement

In both of these disorders damage to the vessel endothelium has activated and consumed platelets and coagulation proteins, thus causing microthrombi to become lodged in the kidney. These patients have a hemolytic anemia and decreased platelet counts. Vessel damage is believed to be somehow immune related. HUS usually affects young children, often before their first year. It usually follows a severe viral infection or bacterial gastroenteritis. With supportive therapy mortality has dropped to 10% to 15%. TTP usually affects young adults after they have experienced a severe infection. TTP has a much higher mortality rate of as high as 90% without supportive therapy because of multiple organ failure. Blood transfusions and FFP are standard treatment and can even reverse some of the symptoms. Therapeutic apheresis is a common treatment in severe acute disease states.

ANEMIAS REQUIRING TRANSFUSION SUPPORT

Sickle Cell Anemia

Sickle cell disease (hemoglobin S) is one of the most prevalent hemoglobinopathies occurring in Africa, the Middle East, the Mediterranean Basin, India, and South America. A correlation seems to exist between the geographic location of malaria and the presence of sickle cell disease. The anomaly is a structural variant in the β-chain of the hemoglobin molecule. An amino acid substitution in the sixth position of the polypeptide chain (valine for glutamic acid) on the surface of the molecule alters the solubility of the hemoglobin molecule. The hemoglobin polymerizes in the deoxy state, thus causing the characteristic sickling of the cell. The resulting hemolytic anemia occurs because of extravascular hemolysis of the sickled cells, which causes the decreased life span of the erythrocytes. Blockage of the microvasculature by these sickled cells causes "sickle cell crisis," with the resulting onset of pain. Laboratory findings are a normochromic, normocytic anemia with a reticulocytosis, sometimes appearing macrocytic and with the presence of sickled cells.

Hemoglobin and hematocrit values can be low in sickle cell patients before transfusions are provided. Clinical symptoms associated with cardiac insufficiency indicate when red blood cell transfusions are necessary. In situations of severe pain and crisis, red blood cell exchange is often therapeutic.

Since patients with sickle cell disease require red blood cell support throughout most of their life, the potential for alloantibody production is high. One reason for the high rate of alloantibodies is that the red blood cell antigens from the predominantly White donor populations are different from the antigens inherited in the Black population. To avoid this problem, many hematologists consider phenotypically matched red blood cells early in the treatment of sickle cell disease. This reduces the chance of potentially life-threatening hemolytic reactions. Encouraging support from Black donors in areas where sickle cell disease is common is extremely beneficial for meeting the need for phenotypically matched red blood cells.

Thalassemia

Thalassemia, though not a hemoglobinopathy, has a similar geographic occurrence and potential evolutionary benefit of fighting off malaria as does sickle cell disease. Thalassemias are classified differently from the hemoglobinopathies, since the anomaly is not a structural defect in one or more of the hemoglobin chains but a decrease in the *rate* of synthesis of either the α-chain or β-chain of the hemoglobin molecule. The rate decrease causes an imbalance of chain formation, with the excess of the nonaffected chain building up in the cytoplasm of the erythrocyte. The resulting hemolytic anemia is due to precipitation of the excess chains, which causes membrane damage or decreased erythrocyte deformability. These red blood cells with abnormal hemoglobin chains are destroyed prematurely in the spleen or by bone marrow macrophages before the cells are even released from the bone marrow. Hemoglobin and hematocrit values are monitored to determine whether transfusion therapy is needed.

With both sickle cell disease and thalassemias, iron chelation therapy must accompany blood transfusions to prevent the iron overload these patients experience because of the multiple transfusions. The iron from normal red blood cell kinetics is neutralized, but the constant addition of cells of varying ages creates the iron excess that becomes stored and detrimental to many tissues.

Aplastic Anemia

Aplastic anemia is characterized by a hypocellular bone marrow (less than 25% cellularity), peripheral blood granulocytes less than $0.5 \times 10^9/L$, and platelets less than $20 \times 10^9/L$ with a corrected reticulocyte count less than 1%.[8] The bone marrow is essentially incapable of supporting the production of blood cells. Pathophysiology can be classified as:

- Stem cell deficiency or dysfunction

BOX 14-6

Aplastic Anemia

CHARACTERISTICS

Bone marrow: less than 25% cellularity
Peripheral granulocytes: less than $0.5 \times 10^9/L$
Platelets: less than $20 \times 10^9/L$

PATHOPHYSIOLOGY

Stem cell deficiency or dysfunction
Damaged or altered bone marrow
Immune suppression

- Bone marrow microenvironment dysfunction
- Immune suppression

Two types of aplastic anemia exist: congenital and acquired. The number of individuals with aplastic anemia has steadily increased since the beginning of the twentieth century, which suggests an environmental influence. Prognosis even with supportive transfusion therapy is usually less than 5 years. Bone marrow transplants are the therapy of choice (e.g., replacing needed stem cells). In the future peripheral stem cells have a potential for being harvested and used for therapy. Box 14-6 summarizes the characteristics and pathophysiology of aplastic anemia.

Immune Hemolytic Anemias

The immune hemolytic anemias belong to a group of disorders characterized by decreased survival of the erythrocyte because of antibody coating of the red blood cell membrane. This coating causes the cell to be less pliable and fit through the small sequestrations of the spleen, hence removed from the circulation much sooner than the average 120 days. These disorders are classified into three groups:

- *Autoimmune hemolytic anemia*: The antibody is reacting to a self-antigen on the red blood cell, which results in removal by the spleen and causes anemia. Based on serologic tests this category is further divided into cold or warm autoantibodies.
- *Drug-induced hemolytic anemia*: Either the drug is adsorbed directly onto the membrane, or the drug-antibody combination becomes adsorbed onto the red blood cell. Some medications can also induce the production of an autoantibody.
- *Alloimmune hemolytic anemia*: This occurs when red blood cell clearance from alloantibodies is produced against transfused red blood cells or against fetal cells in hemolytic disease of the newborn.

Transfusion therapy in hemolytic anemia includes transfusions of red blood cells dependent on the extent of the anemia. In all cases identification of the causative agent should be the first step in treatment. The severity of the anemia depends on the response by the bone marrow to keep up with increased destruction. In compensated anemia, the hemoglobin may be low; however, without clinical symptoms, transfusions should be avoided.

Pretransfusion testing in patients with autoimmune hemolytic anemias caused by medications or disease can be challenging and time consuming. The risk of an underlying alloantibody makes the serologic tests confusing and necessitates adsorption procedures to rule out the possibility of underlying alloantibodies. Tests associated with warm and cold autoantibody problems are outlined in Chapter 7.

HEMOSTATIC DISORDERS

This group of disorders is characterized in two ways:

- A decrease in or lack of production of one or more of the coagulation proteins
- Normal production but an abnormal structure resulting in a nonfunctioning protein

The most common deficiencies are Factors VIII and IX, which are needed for the intrinsic pathway of fibrin formation. The clinical characteristics of coagulation deficiencies are prolonged bleeding, bleeding into joints, and subcutaneous bleeds. The administration of exogenous factors has the potential to cause the development of antibodies or "inhibitors" to one or more of the factors, which can lead to further bleeding episodes.

DIC is an acquired hemostasis disorder in which the patient develops microthrombi, which consume platelets and fibrinogen when the coagulation mechanism is turned on inappropriately, such as during surgery, massive blood loss, or after a snake or insect bite. Strands of fibrin actually trap platelets. DIC patients can spontaneously bleed or form a thrombus. The therapy, as with all other secondary manifestations, is to determine and treat the cause while stabilizing the patient.

ALTERNATIVES TO TRANSFUSION

Blood is a limited resource and contains risks associated with transfusion-transmitted diseases and adverse reactions. For this reason ongoing research exists to substitute blood products with safer, more effective, and more readily available products. Tables 14-5, 14-7, and 14-8 summarize three categories of these substitutes for blood, which include hematopoietic growth factors, blood derivatives, and volume expanders.

Essential components or factors involved in the coagulation cascade, including Factor VIII, Factor IX, and antithrombin concentrate, are blood derivatives formulated to replace factor deficiencies and overcome the effects of inhibitors. The risk of transmitting viruses has been reduced with the use of heat and detergent treatment. Recombinant technology has eliminated the risk; however, these products are substantially more costly. The factor concentrates are sterile, stable, and lyophilized, which makes administration more convenient than that of blood components. Each product differs in terms of purity and the method of treatment to inactivate potential viruses. The clotting factor per milligram of protein or specific activity differs and is indicated on the vial.[6]

Table 14-7 Alternatives to Transfusion: Blood Derivatives

DERIVATIVE	GENERAL INFORMATION	INDICATIONS
Factor VIII	Pasteurized Solvent detergent Monoclonal antibody purified, recombinant	Hemophilia A von Willebrand disease
Factor IX	Factor IX complex (prothrombin complex) contains II, VII, and X Coagulation Factor IX: only Factor IX	Factor II, IX, and X deficiency Hemophilia B (Christmas disease)
Antithrombin concentrate	Inhibitor of coagulation Prepared from pooled plasma	Surgical or obstetric procedures Antithrombin deficiency
Protein C concentrate	Inhibitor of coagulation	Protein C deficiency
C1-esterase inhibitor	Regulates complement cascade	Hereditary angioedema
API	α_1-Antitrypsin Inhibitor of fibrinolysis	API deficiency

AT, Antithrombin; *API,* alpha$_1$-proteinase inhibitor.

Table 14-8 Alternatives to Transfusion: Volume Expanders

TYPE	NAME	CONTENT	USE
Crystalloids	Normal saline Ringer's lactate	Na and Cl ions in water K^+, Ca^{++} ions, and lactate	Shock from hemorrhage and burns
Colloids	Dextran	Polymerized glucose in dextrose or saline	Prolonged intravascular volume expansion
	Hydroxyethyl starch	Synthetic polymer: amylopectin in saline	
Albumin	Albumin	96% albumin, 4% globulin	
Plasma protein fraction (PPF)	PPF	83% albumin, 17% globulin	

Na, Sodium; *Cl*, chloride; *K*, potassium; *Ca*, calcium.

Volume expanders include crystalloids, colloids, albumin, and plasma protein fraction. They are usually dispensed by the pharmacy rather than the transfusion service and are used with or in place of blood for hypovolemia.

Hematopoietic growth factors stimulate the bone marrow to produce erythrocytes, platelets, and leukocytes for patients with chronic anemia and various conditions, thus causing low cell counts. Their uses for chronically transfused renal dialysis and in patients undergoing chemotherapy have been well documented.

CHAPTER SUMMARY

Transfusion therapy provides patients with the correct component of critical value for many types of diseases and conditions. The major focus of transfusion support for the selected patient discussed in this chapter is summarized below.

SUMMARY OF TRANSFUSION SUPPORT

Disease or Condition	Problem	Transfusion Therapy
Massive transfusion	Hypovolemic shock	RBCs
Cardiac surgery	Heparin; hypothermia; platelet destruction	RBCs; platelets
Premature infant	Iatrogenic blood loss; hemoglobin F; low erythropoietin response	Washed or fresh RBCs
Liver transplant	Low levels of vitamin K–dependent factors; bleeding	RBCs; FFP platelets; CRYO
Progenitor cell transplant	Immunosuppression; irradiation of bone marrow	Irradiated platelets and RBCs
Oncology	Chemotherapy and irradiation treatment reduce red blood cell and platelet production	Platelet and RBCs; colony stimulating factors
Chronic renal disease	Unable to produce erythropoietin; red blood cell damage from dialysis and increases in uremia	Erythropoietin; RBCs
TTP and HUS	Platelet and coagulation factors are consumed	Therapeutic apheresis, FFP, and RBCs
Sickle cell anemia	Chronic red blood cell destruction from sickling of cells	RBCs, often phenotypically matched to prevent alloantibody production

SUMMARY OF TRANSFUSION SUPPORT—CONT'D

Aplastic anemia	Stem cell deficiency	Bone marrow transplant or peripheral stem cells
Hemostatic disorders	Factor deficiencies: hemophilia, Christmas disease	Factor derivatives specific for factor that is lacking

RBCs, Red blood cells; *FFP*, fresh frozen plasma; *CRYO*, cryoprecipitated antihemophilic factor; *TTP*, thrombotic thrombocytopenic purpura; *HUS*, hemolytic uremic syndrome.

CRITICAL THINKING EXERCISES

◆ ***EXERCISE 14-1***

A trauma patient in the emergency room has received 6 units of O-negative red blood cells by emergency release. The physician has requested 10 more units of type-specific red blood cells, since a sample has been obtained and sent to the blood bank. What may be some potential problems in determining an ABO/Rh type? At what point will the sample from this patient not reflect his own red blood cells?

◆ ***EXERCISE 14-2***

A 68-year-old man is undergoing a second cardiac surgery, this time to replace a valve. He has been in surgery 4 hours, and there has been a recent request for platelets, red blood cells, and FFP. What are the potential problems that this patient may be undergoing, and what factors make this type of surgery a challenge?

◆ ***EXERCISE 14-3***

A 4-day-old premature infant has been using small aliquots of red blood cells. The parents of the infant would like to donate blood for their child. Can they be potential donors? What special requirements are necessary for red blood cells during the neonatal period? Are crossmatches required? What needs to be done to make blood products from family members safer?

◆ ***EXERCISE 14-4***

A kidney dialysis center requested 2 red blood cell units stat for a patient with a 7-gram hemoglobin. The center is an outpatient clinic, and three other stats for preoperative procedures need to be completed before the shift ends. The technician fills the order but would like to know why the request did not come earlier. What are the unique transfusion needs of kidney dialysis patients, and why was this ordered as a stat? Does erythropoietin eliminate the need for all red blood cell transfusions for renal patients? What contributes to their anemia?

◆ ***EXERCISE 14-5***

The oncology unit has requested that platelets be available for a patient scheduled to undergo chemotherapy for breast cancer. The request for leukopoor platelets, pheresis is common and often extends for a week or more every 2 to 3 days. Why is this product necessary, and what are potential problems associated with platelet transfusions with regard to antibodies?

◆ ***EXERCISE 14-6***

A sample from a 4-year-old sickle cell patient was sent to the blood bank with a request for 1 unit of phenotypically matched red blood cells. The patient needs to be typed, and a unit needs to be located. Why are closely matched red blood cells important for this child? Will it be difficult to find red blood cells for this patient population?

STUDY QUESTIONS

1. Plasmapheresis has been reasonably effective in treating:
   a. TTP
   b. hemolytic disease of the newborn
   c. sickle cell disease
   d. renal patients

2. Finding compatible blood for patients with autoimmune disease is difficult because of the:
   a. potential of underlying alloantibodies
   b. positive DAT
   c. reactive eluate
   d. hemolysis in the serum

3. Infants do not require crossmatching during:
   a. the first 4 months
   b. the first 6 months
   c. the first year
   d. an indefinite period if the parents' blood is used

4. An example of a crystalloid solution used to treat hypovolemia is:
   a. PPF
   b. albumin
   c. Ringer's lactate
   d. dextrose solution

5. Hemophilia A patients are treated for bleeding with:
   a. CRYO
   b. FFP
   c. red blood cells
   d. Factor VIII

6. Common complications of chemotherapy include:
   a. bleeding
   b. infection
   c. anemia
   d. all of the above

7. In the adult, erythropoietin to stimulate red blood cell production is produced in the:
   a. bone marrow
   b. liver
   c. kidneys
   d. spleen

8. Transfusion of red blood cells in the neonate is usually needed to compensate for:
   a. iatrogenic blood loss
   b. hemoglobin F
   c. insufficient erythropoiesis
   d. physiologic anemia of infancy

9. HLA-matched organ transplants are *not* critical in which of the following transplants?
   a. kidneys
   b. liver
   c. heart
   d. bone

10. Colony-stimulating factors are an important therapy for cancer patients, because they stimulate which of the following cells?
    a. erythrocytes
    b. megakaryocytes
    c. granulocytes
    d. lymphocytes

REFERENCES

1. Shoemaker WC, Walker WF: *Hemorrhagic shock: clinical evaluation, monitoring and therapy*, Costa Mesa, Calif, 1977, Hyland, Division Travenol Laboratories.
2. Jeter EK, Spivey MA: *Introduction to transfusion medicine: a case study approach*, Bethesda, Md, 1996, American Association of Blood Banks.
3. Vengelen-Tyler V, editor: *Technical manual*, Bethesda, Md, 1996, American Association of Blood Banks.
4. Collins JA: Massive blood transfusion, *Clin Haematol* 5:201, 1976.
5. Hewitt PE, Machin SJ: Massive blood transfusion. In Contreras M: *ABCs of transfusion*, Great Britain, 1990, British Medical Journal.
6. Lane TA, editor: *Blood transfusion therapy, a physician's handbook*, ed 5, Bethesda, Md, 1996, American Association of Blood Banks.
7. Ross S, Jeter E: Emergency surgery-trauma and massive transfusion. In Petz LD, Swisher SN, Kleinman S, et al, editors: *Clinical practice of transfusion medicine*, ed 3, New York, 1996, Churchill Livingstone.
8. McKenzie SB: *Textbook of hematology*, ed 2, Baltimore, Md, 1996, Williams & Wilkins.
9. Sobel M, NcNeill PM: Diagnosis and management of intraoperative and postoperative hemostatic defects. In Rossi EC, Simon TL, Moss GS: *Principles of transfusion medicine*, Baltimore, Md, 1991, Williams & Wilkins.
10. Strauss RG: Transfusion therapy in neonates, *Am J Dis Child* 145:904, 1991.
11. Obladen M, Sachsenweger M, Stahnke M: Blood sampling in very low birth weight infants receiving different levels of intensive care, *Eur J Pediatr* 147:399, 1988.
12. Strauss RG: Neonatal transfusion. In Anderson KC, Ness PM, editors: *Scientific basis of transfusion medicine: implications for clinical practice*, Philadelphia, 1994, WB Saunders.
13. Goldman M, Delage G: The role of leukodepletion in the control of transfusion-transmitted disease, *Transfus Med Rev* 9:9, 1995.
14. Ramsey G, Sherman LA: Transfusion therapy in solid organ transplantation, *Hematol Oncol Clin North Am* 8:1117, 1994.

VI

QUALITY AND SAFETY ISSUES

QUALITY ASSURANCE AND REGULATION OF THE BLOOD INDUSTRY

15

Awilda Orta

CHAPTER OUTLINE

Good Manufacturing Practices
Records
Record Keeping
Document Control
Process Control
Standard Operating Procedures
Change Control
Personnel Qualifications
Selection Criteria and Job Descriptions
Training
Competency Assessment
Supplier Qualification
Error Management
Root-Cause Analysis and Problem Solving
Recalls
Validation
Facilities and Equipment
Design
Calibration
Quality Control
Preventive Maintenance
Proficiency Testing
Housekeeping
Lot Release and Label Control
Quality Assurance Department
Responsibilities
Internal Quality Auditing
Regulatory and Accrediting Agencies
American Association of Blood Banks
Food and Drug Administration
International Standards Organization 9000
Background
Objective
Registration

LEARNING OBJECTIVES

Upon completion of this chapter, the reader should be able to:

1. Define and list the elements in good manufacturing practices.
2. Compare and contrast proficiency and competency testing.
3. Differentiate quality assurance from quality control.
4. Discuss the importance of job descriptions and personnel qualifications.
5. List the elements of, and explain the importance of, a well-written standard operating procedure.
6. Define the benefits of adopting good manufacturing practices and other quality assurance philosophies.
7. Compare good record keeping with bad record keeping.
8. Explain what external auditors or inspectors look for with regard to documents and standard operating procedures.
9. Describe the elements of a good training program.
10. Give examples of methods used to evaluate competency.
11. Explain the importance of prospective validation and the consequence of not validating a system.
12. Define *calibration, preventive maintenance,* and *quality control requirements;* discuss the importance to each in reporting accurate results.
13. Define and describe the purpose behind root-cause analysis in error management.
14. Explain the recall classifications as stipulated by the Food and Drug Administration.
15. Compare the American Association of Blood Banks' quality essentials versus International Standards Organization 9000.
16. Identify the responsibilities of the quality assurance department.

In the years before the human immunodeficiency virus (HIV) epidemic and the changes created by managed care issues, blood banks were perceived as organizations providing a community service to patients, hospitals, and donors. Donor testing included only hepatitis B and syphilis, and the public did not perceive the blood supply as being "unsafe." The increasing occurrence of HIV, however, created an atmosphere of increased public scrutiny and stricter Food and Drug Administration (FDA) regulations. As a result blood banks are now viewed as drug manufacturing firms that produce and distribute a variety of injectable products. Consequently, health care cost issues, public scrutiny, and FDA regulatory oversight have resulted in an increased effort to provide a safe, high-quality product at the lowest possible cost.

The FDA describes industry standards through good manufacturing practices (GMPs) that guarantee the quality, purity, and safety of blood products. For many blood banks compliance with these rules and the adoption of other quality philosophies have been challenging. The high price of new and ever-changing technology, increased donor testing, corporate downsizing, fierce competition, and increasing regulatory oversight sometimes places quality assurance (QA) as a low priority.

Continuous quality improvement/total quality management: plans that provide the framework for establishing quality assurance in an organization.

The benefits of a serious commitment to GMPs and QA programs, such as **continuous quality improvement** and **total quality management,** are worthwhile and profitable. Allocating time and effort to the identification and elimination of unnecessary and costly steps that do not add value to the end product ultimately increases efficiency and decreases cost. In addition, value exists in reviewing manufacturing errors and accidents. Taking appropriate corrective and preventive measures reduces the cost of rework. In summary, quality efforts and activities enhance efficiency and customer relations, satisfy regulatory requirements, and ultimately provide a safe product. This chapter discusses the elements of a QA program as it applies to blood banks and the current GMPs that guide these efforts.

BOX 15-1

Good Manufacturing Practices

- Write standard operating procedures
- Follow standard operating procedures
- Record and document all work performed
- Qualify personnel by training and education
- Design and build proper facilities and equipment
- Clean by following a housekeeping schedule
- Validate equipment, personnel, processes, etc.
- Perform preventive maintenance on facilities and equipment
- Control for quality
- Audit for compliance with all of the above

GOOD MANUFACTURING PRACTICES

Good manufacturing practices are legal requirements established by the FDA. These regulations itemize "what" needs to be done without necessarily specifying "how." In other words each organization must determine the best way to implement all of these practices. Box 15-1 lists the elements of GMPs. The GMPs applicable to the blood industry are found in the *Code of Federal Regulations* (CFR), specifically Title 21, parts 600. Parts 200, intended for the pharmaceutical industry, are also applicable. GMPs are only a part of the overall QA program in any given facility. In fact QA comprises the combined activities performed by an organization to ensure the quality of products and services they offer, which must include GMPs. The basic components of a blood center's QA program are listed in Box 15-2. These activities must be planned and documented by written policies and procedures. They also must be fully supported by all levels of management. *Without management commitment and support, a QA program will not be effective.*

BOX 15-2

Components of a Quality Assurance Program in a Blood Center

- Record keeping and standard operating procedures
- Personnel selection and training
- Validation, calibration, preventive maintenance, proficiency testing
- Supplier qualification
- Error management
- Process improvement
- Process control
- Label control
- Internal auditing

RECORDS

Record Keeping

If it is not recorded, it never happened. The concept seems simple; however, bad record keeping is the most common violation identified by regulatory and accrediting agencies. Good record keeping, whether manual or automated, allows tracing of all products collected or transfused by an organization. A thorough record-keeping system recreates every step related to the production and distribution of a unit of blood and all its components (Box 15-3). This concept is known as an **audit trail** and is important when investigating errors and accidents, as discussed later in this chapter.

Good record-keeping habits are outlined in Table 15-1. Some common record-keeping errors often encountered in laboratories are also listed. Error correction, for example, is a critical issue. The original data must not be obliterated or deleted when making a correction (Fig. 15-1). The identity of the person making the change also needs to be recorded. A standard practice is to circle or cross off with a single line the item that is incorrect and write the correct data or information next to it, followed by the date and initials of the person making the correction. A mechanism to trace back the original entry and the person making the correction is also necessary in computer systems.[1]

BOX 15-3

Steps in Blood Product Manufacturing

- Donor recruitment
- Donor suitability
- Donor collection
- Component processing
- Donor testing
- Lot release and labeling
- Component storage and distribution
- Compatibility testing
- Blood administration

Audit trail: record-keeping system that recreates every step in the manufacturing process.

NOT ACCEPTABLE

Anti-A	Anti-B	Anti-D	A1 Cells	B Cells	Interpretation
0	0	3+	4+	4+	AB positive (obliterated) O positive

ACCEPTABLE

Anti-A	Anti-B	Anti-D	A1 Cells	B Cells	Interpretation
0	0	3+	4+	4+	~~AB~~ O positive Rm 9/1/99

Fig. 15-1 Correcting a manual record.

Table 15-1 Good Record Keeping versus Bad Record Keeping

GOOD RECORD KEEPING	BAD RECORD KEEPING
◆ Use of indelible (permanent) ink	◆ Use of correction fluid or white tape when making a correction ◆ Use of pencil or nonindelible (nonpermanent) ink
◆ Recording data on appropriate form or log	◆ Recording data on a piece of scratch paper
◆ Recording date and the initials of the person making the correction.	◆ NOT recording the date or the initials of the person making the correction ◆ Recording data for someone else
◆ Recording data immediately	◆ Recording data later or not immediately following performance
◆ Not obliterating or deleting the original entry when making a correction	◆ Obliterating or deleting original entry when making a correction
◆ Indicating "broken," "closed," or "not in use" when appropriate	◆ NOT recording "broken," "closed," or "not in use" when appropriate
◆ Not using dittos	◆ Use of dittos

Document Control

Regulatory and accrediting agencies expect documentation to be thorough, well organized, appropriately stored, retrievable in a reasonable amount of time, and protected from unauthorized access, modification, and destruction.[1] **Document control** programs should specify and describe acceptable media to be used, types of documents to be kept, and record retention intervals (Boxes 15-4 and 15-5).[1] Alternate methods should be in place to handle situations when the automated systems become unavailable. Finally, all record systems, including their control, handling, and disposal, must be described thoroughly in the facility's **standard operating procedures** (SOPs).

Document control: plan for the management of all documents in an organization that addresses the design, responsibility, storage, removal, and revision of all records, forms, and procedures.
Standard operating procedures: written procedures to help ensure the complete understanding of a process and achieve consistency in performance from one individual to another.

PROCESS CONTROL

Standard Operating Procedures

SOPs describe how a particular task is to be accomplished. Established methods for performing and administering processes ensure the consistent quality of the final product or result. Internal and external auditors carefully assess noncompliance with written SOPs, one of the most serious violations that can be identified during an inspection. Facilities need to say what they do (write SOPs) and do what they say (follow SOPs).

BOX 15-4
Types of Record Media and Examples

PAPER
Manual logs
Worksheets
Computer printouts
Temperature charts

ELECTRONIC
CD-ROM
Floppy disks
Computer tapes

FILM
Microfilm
Microfiche
Photography
Videotape

BOX 15-5 ***Blood Bank Records and Retention Intervals***

INDEFINITE
- Donor's identifying information, medical history, physical examination, consent, and interpretations of tests for disease markers
- Blood and components from outside sources, including numeric or alphanumeric identification of the blood unit, and identification of the collecting facility; however, the information from an intermediate facility may be used if the intermediate facility retains the unit number and identification of the collecting facility
- Information to identify facilities that carry out any part of the preparation of blood components and the functions they perform
- Final disposition of each unit of blood or blood component
- Notification to donors of permanent deferral
- Records of prospective donors who have been placed on surveillance or indefinitely deferred for the protection of the potential recipient
- Notification to transfusing facilities of previous receipt of units from donors subsequently found to be confirmed positive for HIV or HTLV
- Difficulty in blood typing, clinically significant antibodies, and adverse reactions to transfusion
- Notification to recipients of potential exposure to disease transmissible by blood
- Names, signatures, initials or identification codes, and inclusive dates of employment of those authorized to sign or review reports and records

MINIMUM OF 5 YEARS OF RETENTION
- Donor's ABO and Rh type, difficulty in blood typing, severe adverse reactions to donation, and apheresis procedure clinical record
- Records of blood component inspection before issue

BOX 15-5 Blood Bank Records and Retention Intervals—cont'd

- Patient's ABO and Rh type, interpretation of compatibility testing, therapeutic procedures including phlebotomy, apheresis, and outpatient transfusion
- All superseded procedures, manuals, and publications
- Temperatures of storage and results of inspection before issue of blood and blood components
- Control testing of components, reagents, and equipment
- Proficiency testing surveys, including dates, performed tests, observed results, interpretations, identification of personnel carrying out the tests, and any appropriate corrective action taken
- Documentation of staff qualifications, training, and competency
- Quality systems audits and internal assessment records

HIV, Human immunodeficiency virus; *HTLV*, human T-cell lymphotropic virus.
From Vengelen-Tyler V, editor: *Technical manual*, ed 12, Bethesda, Md, 1996, American Association of Blood Banks.

SOPs are important training tools for new employees. These documents should be written using a standard format, such as that in Box 15-6. They need to be written following reagent and equipment manufacturers' recommendations and in compliance with other GMPs and industry standards as appropriate. Effective procedures do not need to be wordy. In fact the more user-friendly they are, the more likely they are to be used by staff. In summary, well-written procedures include all those steps that ensure process control and contribute to the safety, purity, and potency of the blood product.

BOX 15-6 Suggested Elements of a Procedure

- Principle or purpose
- Specimen requirements
- Supplies, reagents, and equipment requirements
- Quality control requirements
- Calibration requirements
- Procedure instructions
- Interpretation and reporting
- Acceptable values or results
- Procedure notes
- References

Change Control

The blood industry is in a constant state of change. Blood banks and transfusion services are being challenged routinely by new and ever-changing technology and new regulatory and accrediting requirements. Box 15-7 lists areas that are continually requiring modification because of industry changes. In addition, facilities also have to keep up with internal trends and business issues, such as mergers, acquisitions, employee turnover, expansion, and downsizing. These changes need to be controlled to prevent oversights that may affect multiple aspects of the organization. Manufacturing changes, especially, need to be well thought out and planned *before* implementation to guarantee their success and effectiveness. **Change control,** just like validation (discussed later in this chapter), needs the allocation of time, money, and manpower. However, the many benefits outweigh the cost.

Change control programs are used by manufacturing firms to ensure nothing "falls through the cracks." For example, the addition of a new blood storage refrigerator would seem straightforward; however, the installation goes beyond the purchase and plug-in steps. Box 15-8 illustrates a change protocol for a new refrigerator that addresses critical steps in equipment installation to prevent potential problems. Thus the key in change control is the anticipation and prevention of problems.

BOX 15-7 Areas of Constant Change in the Blood Bank

- Labeling
- Donor screening or criteria
- Component preparation methods
- Donor and patient test methodology
- Equipment
- Computer software and hardware

Change control: system to plan and implement changes in procedures, equipment, policies, and methodologies to increase effectiveness and prevent problems.

BOX 15-8 *Change Control Plan for New Refrigerator*

- Installation qualification protocols: What are the refrigerator specifications regarding temperature, size, alarms, power supply, storage capacity, etc.?
  (Decided before purchase or installation)
- Validation test plan: Plan for the evaluation of equipment. Parameters: alarm test and temperature monitoring.
  (Written, executed, and reviewed before being put into use)
- Initial calibration and quality control: Results of testing and alarm quality control
  (Usually performed concurrently or as part of the test plan)
- SOPs addressing operation, calibration, QC, and preventive maintenance for equipment
- Training of staff on operating the new piece of equipment
- How to operate and maintain the new piece of equipment

SOPs, Standard operating procedures; *QC*, quality control.

PERSONNEL QUALIFICATIONS

Selection Criteria and Job Descriptions

Good employees are essential to the success of any given organization. Hiring unqualified individuals can add significant expense to the organization and create a demoralizing environment to coworkers who have to accommodate poor performance. The selection process must be thorough, and minimal preestablished criteria should be identified. These criteria must be identified for each type of position in the organization, which addresses the experience, background, skills, and credentials (e.g., degrees, licensure, certification) deemed necessary to perform the job. The selection criteria are not stagnant. They should be revised as changes in job duties or tasks occur.

Job description documents should be developed for each type of position in the organization. These documents describe the tasks for which the employee is responsible and outline the areas of knowledge and skill that need to be acquired during training to perform the job. These documents also necessitate updating as appropriate to reflect all employee duties.

Training

Training is a critical aspect of compliance with GMPs that necessitates a significant organization-wide commitment for success. Facilities that allocate time and resources for training and education benefit by reducing rework and inconsistency. When developing a training program the designation of trainers is important. Individuals selected as trainers should be able to convey information clearly, be respected by their peers, enjoy sharing expertise, and have a positive attitude toward building teams.

Training is provided during new employee orientation and is also necessary whenever there are procedure changes or evidence of poor performance. Training activities usually include, but are not limited to, the following activities:

- Employee's review of SOP documents and associated materials
- Trainer's demonstration of task or procedure
- Employee's performance of task or procedure with the trainer's assistance

- Employee's demonstration of knowledge and application of the learned skill without the trainer's assistance

Good training programs allow the trainer to explain all functions and demonstrate the task before employee performance. Repetition of tasks in a "test" environment or with supervision is necessary before the trainee is allowed to perform the procedure independently. Throughout the training process the employee must have ample opportunities to ask questions and receive explanations. Finally, training is not complete until it is documented, which typically takes place in the form of a checklist signed by the trainee, trainer, or supervisor.

Competency Assessment

Training is concluded only when documented evidence exists that the employee is able to demonstrate his or her knowledge and application of the new skill (Box 15-9). This is the purpose of **competency assessment.**

Initial competency assessment refers to the evaluation of the level of knowledge and skill an employee has gained during training to determine whether he or she is ready to perform a procedure. In addition, *periodic* competency is used to determine whether the employee has maintained the level of knowledge and skill necessary to perform the job or task as described in the facility's SOP. The Health Care Financing Administration (HCFA) and the American Association of Blood Banks (AABB), through the Clinical Laboratory Improvement Amendments of 1988, have established requirement of proof of competency for testing personnel twice during the first year of employment and annually thereafter.[2] Most regulatory and accrediting agencies require retraining for those employees who fail to prove competency. The employee must not be allowed to perform the procedure(s) until retraining is provided and subsequent competency assessment proves to be satisfactory.

In the case of unacceptable performance, corrective actions should be taken. Again, actions include retraining and redocumenting performance and competency assessment. The employee cannot perform the tasks in which unacceptable performance was demonstrated.

BOX 15-9

Competency Assessment Tools

- Direct observation of performance
- Written tests
- Review of results, records, and worksheets
- Blind samples (e.g., proficiency testing)

Competency assessment: evaluation of the employee's ability and knowledge to perform a procedure or skill.

Supplier Qualification

The quality of any given product is as good as the quality of the raw materials that go into its production. Supplier qualification has become a standard practice among many blood banks and transfusion services. These facilities have established procedures to evaluate whether the quality of critical products and services received from suppliers is meeting preestablished criteria (Box 15-10). Written agreements between blood banks and their suppliers are common practice. These documents, among many things, usually specify terms, including expectations between the involved parties. In some instances facilities choose to audit their suppliers on an ongoing basis to determine the level of compliance with product specifications (Box 15-11). This practice also should be included in written agreements. In addition, facilities should have procedures for inspecting and testing incoming materials (when applicable). These procedures should specify acceptable criteria and the course of action to be taken when they are not met.

BOX 15-10

Examples of Critical Products or Services Received from Suppliers

- Blood products
- Test reagents (antisera, red blood cells, viral marker testing reagents, etc.)
- Blood bags
- Reference laboratory donor testing
- Labels

BOX 15-11

Examples of Product Specifications

- Size
- Color
- Container type
- Temperature
- Purity
- Potency

ERROR MANAGEMENT

Root-Cause Analysis and Problem Solving

As part of a QA plan, facilities must have in place mechanisms for the detection and management of errors and their consequences. Errors, incidents, variances, and nonconformances should be thoroughly documented and investigated. Employees must be actively involved in the problem-solving stages for the process to be successful. Once a problem is identified, an immediate response follows to correct the problem. The facility should then initiate a **root-cause analysis** to identify what factor(s) contributed to its occurrence. Once the cause is identified, a proposed plan for prevention should be drafted. After changes are made and the process is fine-tuned or adjusted, a subsequent review should be made to evaluate the effectiveness of the preventive corrective action. If the error recurs, another root-cause analysis is indicated. The adoption of this strategy ensures continuous quality improvement of all processes. Errors should be viewed as opportunities for improvement, and employees should be encouraged to report errors without concern for reprisal.

Root-cause analysis: investigation and subsequent identification of the factors that contributed to an error.

Errors can be identified internally by employees or externally by customers. Box 15-12 lists the classification of some types of errors. Errors must be logged and their frequencies tracked and monitored. Graphing incidences of occurrence and subsequent recurrences can provide QA departments with a comprehensive understanding of the reliability of a given process or individual and the effectiveness of a corrective action taken. Tracking can also help identify where quality efforts should be focused and which areas need to be addressed and corrected first.

BOX 15-12

Error Classifications

- Incidents
- Variances
- Nonconformances
- Deviations
- Complaints

Recalls

The FDA requires that licensed and registered facilities report any instances of an error or accident that compromises the safety of the donor or patient (Box 15-13). Notification to the FDA is required (under 21 CFR 600.14) if the investigation reveals that the release of the implicated unit(s) was the result of an error in manufacturing.[3] **Recalls** are usually issued by manufacturers in an attempt to remove products from the market that might compromise the safety of the recipient. They can be initiated voluntarily by the organization or at the request of the FDA. In some instances recalls are issued months and even years after the product has

Recalls: manufacturers' removal of products from the market that may compromise the safety of the recipient.

BOX 15-13 ***Food and Drug Administration Reportable Errors and Accidents***

The following errors and accidents should be reported regarding the release of blood units:

- Repeatedly reactive to viral marker testing
- From donors for whom test results were improperly interpreted because of testing errors related to improper use of equipment or failure to strictly follow the reagent manufacturer's direction for use
- From donors who are, or should have been, either temporarily deferred because of medical history or history of repeatedly reactive results to viral marker tests
- Released before completion of all tests
- Incorrectly labeled
- Microbially contaminated

been transfused or has expired. In this case the objective of the recall notification is to alert the client of possible hazards or adverse consequences the recipient might have incurred by receiving the product. Recalls are classified based on the degree of danger or hazard they impose (Box 15-14).

VALIDATION

Validation is a process that establishes documented evidence providing a high degree of assurance that a specific process consistently produces a product that meets its preestablished quality and performance specifications.[4] Even if regulatory and accrediting agencies did not make it necessary, validation is a good business practice. Procedures, equipment, personnel, new methodology, and computer information systems must be proven reliable before being put into use. The best way to prove reliability is by stressing and challenging the process or system *before* it is implemented.

Validation: establishing that a specific process consistently produces a product that meets predetermined specifications.

Validation necessitates the commitment of time, resources, and manpower, and it must be planned and thoroughly documented. It is usually accomplished by executing detailed test plans prospectively. In other words, validation efforts are intended to discover any flaws before they occur in the manufacturing and testing process. Going live with a system or a process that has not been validated can turn into an embarrassing and costly problem for the organization.

FACILITIES AND EQUIPMENT

Design

Facilities and equipment should be designed in compliance and in support of GMPs and constructed to prevent errors and accidents, mix-ups, and contamination. Work areas in blood manufacturing should be free from clutter, should be organized in a logical manner, and should have enough space to reduce interruptions in the workflow.

Calibration

In the laboratory setting, **accuracy** refers to the degree to which a measurement represents the true value. Accuracy is determined by comparing results of the test

Accuracy: degree to which a measurement represents the true value of the attribute being measured.

BOX 15-14 ***Food and Drug Administration's Product Recall Classifications***

CLASS I
A reasonable probability exists that the use of the product will cause serious adverse health consequences or death

CLASS II
The use of the product may cause temporary or medically reversible adverse health consequences, or the probability of serious adverse health consequences is remote

CLASS III
The use of the product is not likely to cause adverse health consequences

Calibration: process of standardizing an instrument against a known value.

in question with results from an established reference method. The closer the two values, the more accurate the test result. To obtain accurate results, instruments and equipment require calibration. **Calibration** is the process of standardizing an instrument. In the process of calibration, the instrument value is first compared with a known measurement standard. Variation is then eliminated by adjusting the instrument or procedure to obtain the true value.[4] Equipment used in the collection, processing, compatibility testing, storage, and distribution of blood components must be standardized and calibrated on a regularly scheduled basis.[5] Calibration helps eliminate errors that could harm a donor or a patient. For example, as discussed in Chapter 11, optimal centrifugation time and speed are critical when using tube methodology. Too hard or too light a spin could cause false test results. For this reason centrifuges, like many other pieces of equipment in the laboratory, require calibration.

Quality Control

Quality control: testing to determine the accuracy and precision of the equipment, reagents, and procedures.

For many years the terms *quality assurance* and **quality control** (QC) were used interchangeably. The current philosophy includes QC as one of the many components of a QA program. QC helps to manage the test process by confirming accuracy and reproducibility. QC also monitors equipment functionality and reagent specificity and sensitivity.[6]

Preventive Maintenance

Preventive maintenance: maintenance that maximizes the duration of the equipment or facility, decreases "downtime," and avoids unnecessary costly repairs.

Preventive maintenance maximizes the duration of the equipment or facility, decreases "downtime," and avoids unnecessary costly repairs. In the laboratory, scheduled or periodic preventive maintenance tasks performed on equipment also guarantee the reliability of test results reported by ensuring the proper performance of the equipment.

Proficiency Testing

Proficiency testing: surveys performed to ensure that a laboratory's test methods and equipment are working as expected.

Proficiency testing is a required component of the QA program for testing laboratories. It is used to ensure that test methods and equipment are working as expected and that staff members are following procedures.[1] Proficiency surveys are prepared by accredited agencies that distribute samples for testing to requesting laboratories. A common proficiency test is the "CAP Survey," issued by the College of American Pathologists. Tests are run by routine testing personnel, using routine test equipment, during regular test runs, and in conformance with the facility's SOP. The results are recorded on standard forms and submitted to the agency within a given period. The test results are evaluated and scored, and a report is returned to the institution for review. Corrective action is implemented and monitored for improvement when results are not acceptable. Proficiency tests can be used to prove competency; however, competency tests cannot replace proficiency testing.

Housekeeping

GMPs address the necessity to clean, following a regular housekeeping schedule. An untidy and unclean work environment adversely affects employees, customers, donors, inspectors, and test results. Facilities that fail to maintain clean work areas also risk contamination and equipment problems.

LOT RELEASE AND LABEL CONTROL

Many of the blood product recalls are due to mislabeling. If the incorrect label is placed on a unit of blood, the product is called *misbranded*. Like other recalls, mislabeling errors are not only time consuming but also embarrassing. For this reason blood banks, just like pharmaceutical firms, have instituted label control programs. In many facilities it is the QA department's responsibility to inspect and approve all labels upon receipt and before they are put into use, ensuring all labels are in compliance with requirements. Labeling is a critical step in manufacturing and should be done in areas designed only for that purpose.

In the blood industry a **lot** is defined as a unit of blood and all its parts. Before a lot of blood is released, records are reviewed for accuracy, completeness, and compliance with established standards.[7] Ideally a second review of each significant manufacturing step should be done before the lot release and labeling. Any discrepancy must be documented and investigated.

Lot: unit of blood from one donor and all of its parts or components.

QUALITY ASSURANCE DEPARTMENT

Responsibilities

Blood banks are required to establish QA departments separate from manufacturing and should report to upper management. QA responsibilities include:

- Compliance with GMPs
- Review and approval of all SOPs
- Specifications and validation protocols
- Development, review, and approval of training programs
- Investigation of product recalls, errors, and complaints
- Coordination of internal auditing programs

Internal Quality Auditing

The QA department performs internal quality **audits** to evaluate the effectiveness of the quality system in the organization. Audits should be performed periodically and are intended to be systematic investigations to confirm the level of compliance with established SOPs. They are useful in the early identification of problems and ensure continuous quality improvement.

Audits: systematic investigations to determine whether policies and procedures are being performed and supported properly.

REGULATORY AND ACCREDITING AGENCIES

The blood industry is monitored by many regulatory and accrediting agencies. Compliance with industry, federal, state, and local requirements is reviewed by these agencies. Although the rules are presented in different formats, they focus on ensuring product quality and donor and patient safety. Regulatory and accrediting agencies listed in Box 15-15 address similar issues regarding QA and quality improvement. The agencies differ in the degree of authority they have to enforce the standards. Compliance with standards set by governmental agencies, such as FDA, HCFA, and state agencies, are enforceable by law. Accrediting agencies such as AABB are considered industry associations, and compliance with their requirements is voluntary and evaluated by peer review.

BOX 15-15

Agencies with Quality Assurance and Quality Improvement Requirements

REGULATION

Food and Drug Administration
Health Care Financing Administration

ACCREDITATION

American Association of Blood Banks
American Association of Tissue Banks
College of American Pathologists
Joint Commission on Accreditation of Healthcare Organizations

American Association of Blood Banks

AABB is a voluntary accrediting agency. Its publications serve as guidelines for members seeking accreditation. These include the *Standards for Blood Banks and Transfusion Services*, the *Technical Manual*, and the *Accreditation Requirements Manual*. In recent years AABB has increased the emphasis on quality principles. AABB has supported its members by designing documents that facilitate the implementation of QA programs, such as the *Quality Essentials*. Compliance with the AABB *Quality Essentials* became mandatory as of January 1, 1998, for those organizations seeking accreditation. The *Quality Essentials* itemizes all the elements of QA appropriate for blood banks or transfusion services.

Food and Drug Administration

The FDA is a federal agency within the Department of Health and Human Services. Many industries fall within the FDA's jurisdiction, including drugs, cosmetics, food, and blood. The agency is involved in three areas:

- Surveillance of facilities (inspections)
- Policy enforcement
- Establishment and issue of regulations

FDA uses several tools to enforce its policy: regular unannounced inspections, warning letters, license suspension, license revocation, and injunction (consent decree). The last four are used only when the violations identified during an establishment inspection are considered serious enough to compromise public safety or when a persistent history of noncompliance with the organization exists.

INTERNATIONAL STANDARDS ORGANIZATION 9000

Background

ISO 9000: quality philosophy that establishes standards for manufacturing, trade, and communication.

International Standards Organization (ISO) 9000 is the most recent quality philosophy with increasing recognition among blood bank organizations. (ISO can also stand for the International Standard for Organization, the International Organization for Standardization, or the Greek term meaning equal.[8]) ISO was founded in 1946 in Geneva, Switzerland with the purpose of developing standards for manufacturing, trade, and communication. The international agency consists of almost 100 member countries, with an equal vote given to each of them. The United States' representative to ISO is the American National Standards Institute.

Objective

The core of the ISO 9000 Quality Systems Standard is a series of five international standards (Table 15-2) that provide guidance in the development and implementation of an effective quality management system. ISO is not specific to any particular product or industry; these standards are applicable to all manufacturing and services industries. Blood banks that request ISO registration must comply with two documents: ISO 9000-1 (the umbrella document) and ISO 9002. Compliance with ISO 9000 standards does not indicate that every product or service meets the customer's requirements, but only that the quality system in use is capable of meeting them.

Table 15-2 International Standards Organization (ISO) 9000 Series

ISO 9000-1	This standard provides guidelines and basic definitions that describe what the series is about and helps in the selection and use of the appropriate ISO standard (ISO 9001, 9002, or 9003) for any organization.
ISO 9001	This standard is a model for use by manufacturing and service organizations to certify their quality system from initial design and development of a desired product or service through production, installation, and servicing.
ISO 9002*	This standard is identical to ISO 9001, except it omits the requirement of documenting the design and development process.
ISO 9003	This standard is used by organizations that need only to show, through inspection and testing, that they are delivering the desired product or service.
ISO 9004-1	This standard is a basic set of guidelines that organizations can use to help them develop and implement their quality management system.

*ISO 9002 is the conformance model for blood manufacturing firms.

Registration

Conformance of a blood bank's quality management system to ISO 9000 is becoming a customer service issue, similar to other industry standards. To become "registered," an independent "third party" called the "registrar" performs an onsite audit to verify that such a system exists. When the "registrar" finds proof that the organization fulfills ISO 9000 requirements, the blood bank organization becomes "registered." Independent registrars reevaluate ISO compliance every 6 months thereafter.

CHAPTER SUMMARY

GMPs are the minimum federal requirements that guarantee the safety, potency, purity, and quality of blood products. GMPs are only a part of the QA program for a manufacturing firm. QA encompasses all other planned activities that, when executed, ensure the quality of the products or services offered. These include: record keeping and SOPs, personnel selection and training, validation, supplier qualification, calibration, preventive maintenance, proficiency testing, error management, process improvement, process control, label control, and internal auditing.

The blood industry is regulated by multiple regulatory and accrediting agencies. All of these entities require compliance with QA and quality improvement concepts. However, only regulatory agencies have the lawful authority to enforce their requirements.

CRITICAL THINKING EXERCISES

◆ ***EXERCISE 15-1***

PEC is a relatively successful and modern blood center located in the northeastern region of the United States. Its management style has always stood out among other blood centers in the country because of its modern and progressive views. It has been well known for embracing changes in manufacturing with a positive approach by appropriately planning and allocating resources to ensure things are done the right way. However, in the last few years, both employees and customers have noticed a steady decline in control and quality. The number of manufacturing errors and product and service complaints reported by customers has drastically increased. PEC has tripled in size in the last 3 years, following the acquisition of several small blood banks in the state. Changes have occurred quickly to accommodate this growth, and thorough planning before their implementation has not always been possible. Among many of its growing pains, PEC employees finally realized that their blood bank computer system was outdated and unable to handle the workload volume increase in the last few years. Even FDA investigators pointed out the problem during their most recent inspection in October 1997. Something had to be done. By the end of December 1997, PEC's management had chosen EJO, Inc., as the new software vendor. Even though EJO's experience, reputation, expertise, and client support were well known, its new blood banking software was not. However, the cost of implementing this new software fit well within the approved 1998 budget. With full management support, validation and training efforts began early in 1998 with a proposed "live" date for September of that year. This new project placed even more stress on managers, supervisors, and employees, who were already overwhelmed by the increase in work and the recent cuts in personnel. By June multiple "bugs" had been identified during system testing. EJO's technical support was excellent, but with so many problems to be addressed and corrected, management was getting anxious. They wanted the new system to go "live" before their next FDA inspection. September came and went and the system was not ready for implementation. Finally, in March 1999, parallel testing was completed. Because of time constraints, not all functions were tested, especially those pertaining to the issue of products. Management was aware of this but decided to go ahead with the system's implementation. On April 1, 1999, PEC's new system was implemented with no major problems. Everything was okay until 3 months later, when the distribution supervisor noticed that the system had allowed the release of several HTLV-I/II, repeatedly reactive units. PEC's QA department was immediately notified, and recall procedures were initiated. By then 35 units and all their parts had been released.

1. What did PEC fail to do? What were the consequences?
2. What are some of the factors that contributed to the release of unacceptable units?
3. What can be done to prevent this from happening again?

◆ ***EXERCISE 15-2***

AKC Blood Bank collects over 600 platelets, pheresis products each month. Platelet counts for donors and these products are determined using KB1, a state-of-the-art automated hematology counter. This piece of equipment, like many others, requires extensive quality control and preventive maintenance by the manufacturer. During the last 4 days, Fred, the medical technologist assigned to run the instrument, has failed to notice that the low-level control has consistently fallen below the mean. Fred has been too busy trying to train new personnel in the department and has had no time to plot his results on the quality control chart, which is a departmental procedure requirement. Had he done that, he would have noticed the obvious shift.

Today the new trainee, Francie, is running platelet counts with Fred's assistance. Once again the low-level control falls below the mean, but this time it is outside the manufacturer's range altogether. Francie notices the value is being flagged by KB1 and notifies Fred of the problem. Fred is too busy on the phone and tells Francie to "keep running it until it falls in. You know, sometimes it takes a while for controls to come in."

1. If you were Fred's supervisor, what would you do?
2. What is the root cause of the problem?
3. What can be done to prevent this from happening again?
4. What can be said about Fred's results since he started using the instrument?

◆ *EXERCISE 15-3*

The transfusion services department at PSB Medical Center has always been happy with the level of service offered by YR Blood Center. However, during the last 3 months, they have noticed quite a few platelet units with visible agglutinants. If you worked for the QA unit at YR Blood Center and were told to investigate this problem, what areas would you investigate to identify the root cause of the problem?

◆ *EXERCISE 15-4*

Prepare a list of all the things that need to be done before the implementation of a new component centrifuge.

◆ *EXERCISE 15-5*

Identify the consequences of the following GMP violations:

1. NOT taking daily temperature reading for a blood refrigerator
2. Extending test incubation times beyond what the SOP states
3. Overloading a refrigerator beyond its capacity
4. Cutting an employee's training short
5. Running proficiency samples over and over until the sample is used up
6. Using expired reagents
7. Reporting test results when controls are out of range
8. Not performing preventive maintenance on an instrument as required by the manufacturer

STUDY QUESTIONS

1. Which of the following is not a basic component of a QA program?
   a. calibration
   b. preventive maintenance
   c. viral marker testing
   d. record keeping

2. Manual records can be corrected as long as:
   a. the original entry is neither obliterated nor deleted
   b. the person making the correction dates and initials the change
   c. the item to be corrected is crossed off with a single line
   d. all of the above

3. All of the following statements are true about SOPs EXCEPT that they are:
   a. step-by-step instructions
   b. used to monitor accuracy and precision
   c. written in compliance with GMPs
   d. written in compliance with manufacturer's recommendations

4. What is the purpose of competency assessment?
   a. identify employees in need of retraining
   b. evaluate an individual's level of knowledge during a job interview
   c. identify those employees who need to be fired
   d. all of the above

5. All of the following statements are true regarding internal audits EXCEPT that they:
   a. help identify problems early
   b. ensure continuous quality improvement efforts
   c. are used solely for the purpose of identifying "troublemakers"
   d. are one of the many responsibilities of the QA unit

6. Employees are the core of an organization, and they therefore:
   a. must be trained
   b. must report errors without fear of reprisal
   c. can deviate from SOPs only after obtaining supervisor's approval
   d. are a key part of problem-solving
   e. all of the above

7. GMPs applicable to the blood industry can be found in the:
   a. AABB *Standards*
   b. Standard operating procedure manual
   c. FDA's *Code of Federal Regulations*
   d. QA manual

8. Early identification of problems by evaluating the compliance with established SOP is the purpose of:
   a. internal audits
   b. accident reports
   c. root-cause analysis
   d. FDA inspections

Match the following descriptions with the appropriate organization:

Description	Organization
9. internal quality philosophy	a. FDA
10. voluntary peer review organization	b. AABB
11. government agency that regulates blood banks	c. ISO

REFERENCES

1. Vengelen-Tyler V, editor: *Technical manual,* ed 12, Bethesda, Md, 1996, American Association of Blood Banks.
2. Sazana K, editor: *Accreditation requirements manual,* ed 6, Bethesda, Md, 1995, American Association of Blood Banks.
3. Food and Drug Administration: *Memorandum: responsibilities of blood establishments related to errors and accidents in the manufacture of blood and blood components,* Rockville, Md, March 20, 1991, Congressional and Consumer Affairs.
4. Quinley ED, Caglioti TA: *GMP fundamentals,* Raritan, NJ, 1994, Ortho Diagnostic Systems.
5. Food and Drug Administration: *Code of federal regulations,* 21 CFR 600-799, Washington, DC, 1997, US Government Printing Office.
6. Hammering D, editor: *Modern blood banking and transfusion practices,* ed 4, Philadelphia, 1999, FA Davis.
7. Food and Drug Administration: *Guideline for quality assurance in blood establishments,* Rockville, Md, July 11, 1995, Congressional and Consumer Affairs.
8. Oddo F, editor: *The memory jogger,* Methuen, Mass, 1996, GOAL/QPC.

SAFETY ISSUES IN THE BLOOD BANK 16

Jo Ann Wilson

CHAPTER OUTLINE

LEARNING OBJECTIVES

Upon completion of this chapter, the reader should be able to:

1. Describe regulatory agencies that govern activities in the blood bank.
2. Interpret federal regulatory safety standards.
3. Apply federal regulatory safety standards to the workplace.
4. Describe voluntary agencies.
5. Interpret voluntary agency compliance guidelines.
6. Apply voluntary agency compliance guidelines to the workplace.
7. Define *universal precautions*.
8. Properly dispose of laboratory waste material.
9. Use a material safety data sheet.
10. Assist in the preparation of a laboratory safety program.
11. List safety equipment and protective devices.
12. Recognize chemical hazards.
13. Recognize the need for accident reporting.
14. Encourage employee education in safety.

SAFETY FACT
Safety is not only a matter of regulations and standards; it is common sense.

Safety concerns everyone. Employer and employee must understand their respective roles in the issues of compliance in blood banking safety. This understanding centers on the need to decrease infection risk and physical and chemical hazards in the workplace. The blood bank is governed by many regulatory bodies, including federal, state, and local authorities, and may choose to voluntarily comply with the standards of conduct of accrediting agencies or the acceptable practices recommended by professional organizations. The responsibility by law for employee safety ultimately resides with the employer or director of the laboratory. The employer has an obligation to provide a safe work environment by following the imposed standards of care. However, the individual employee must assume responsibility for his or her health and safety and the safety of coworkers by following laboratory safety policies and procedures. When safety is endorsed and practiced by everyone in the blood bank, fewer errors and accidents occur.

FEDERAL, STATE, AND LOCAL SAFETY REGULATIONS IN THE BLOOD BANK

Many government agencies impose standards in clinical laboratories through federal, state, and local laws. State and local laws must be as stringent as federal standards. In addition, state and local governments may impose additional safety requirements.

Food and Drug Administration

The Food and Drug Administration (FDA) enforces regulations to ensure the safety and efficacy of biologics, drugs, and devices, including blood and blood components and diagnostic reagents used or manufactured by blood establishments. The regulation of biologics products in the United States began when Congress passed the Biologics Control Act of 1902.[1] Provisions of the act include requirements for the licensing of manufacturers and products, labeling, facility inspections, suspension or revocation of licenses, and penalties for violation. Current implementation of the law is placed under the Public Health Service (PHS) Act 42 USC §262.[2]

The FDA is the agency for the enforcement of the regulations of the PHS Act and the federal Food, Drug and Cosmetic Service Act.[3] Each inspection is designed to follow a unit of blood or a blood product from donor to patient. The inspection includes many elements of safety: errors, accidents and fatalities, facilities, equipment, personnel, and disposal of infectious waste.

Occupational Safety and Health Act

The Occupational Safety and Health Act was passed by Congress in 1970 "to assure safe and healthful working conditions for working men and women; by authorizing enforcement of the standards developed under the act; by assisting and encouraging the states in their efforts to assure safe and healthful working conditions; by providing for research, information, education, and training in the field of occupational safety and health; and for other purposes."[4] The act is enforced by the **Occupational Safety and Health Administration (OSHA).**

Occupational Safety and Health Administration: agency responsible for ensuring safe and healthful working conditions.

Each year updated regulations are published in the Code of Federal Regulations (CFR), and standards are enforced under OSHA by workplace inspections.

Most clinical facilities are inspected following employee or consumer complaints. However, OSHA may choose under authority of the Occupational Safety and Health Act to inspect any facility at any time. Employers are responsible for informing employees of the OSHA standards and must post OSHA literature that informs employees of their rights and responsibilities.

Twenty-three states and territories operate their own job safety and health plans under OSHA. These standards are identical to, or as stringent as, the federal OSHA standards and must cover state and local government employees.[5] In addition, state and local governments may impose additional requirements for safety.

Centers for Disease Control and Prevention

The concept of **universal precautions** was first introduced in 1987 by the Centers for Disease Control and Prevention (CDC) to decrease the occupational risks of bloodborne diseases, such as acquired immunodeficiency syndrome and hepatitis B virus (HBV), to healthcare workers.[6] In 1991 OSHA issued its final standard on occupational exposure to bloodborne pathogens, which mandated the use of universal precautions. Current universal precautions focus on treating all body substances as potentially harmful and applying appropriate safety measures to decrease possible exposure and infection. The use of protective measures is now based on the healthcare worker's contact with body fluids rather than on a patient's diagnosis. This concept, originally known as body substance isolation, has been adapted and incorporated into CDC's two-tiered isolation guidelines as standard precautions (Box 16-1).[7]

The standards set forth by the CDC are incorporated within the regulations of the Health Care Finance Administration (HCFA) of the Clinical Laboratory Improvement Amendments of 1988.[9] Laboratory compliance inspections are conducted by HCFA in each state or by an accrediting agency with HCFA-deemed status (recognized as equivalent in standards to HCFA).[10]

Universal precautions: policies of treating all body substances as potentially infectious and applying safety measures to reduce possible exposure.

SAFETY FACT

OSHA estimates that the 1991 final standard on occupational exposure to bloodborne pathogens protects more that 5.6 million workers and prevents more than 200 deaths and 9200 bloodborne infections each year.[8]

SAFETY FACT

The EPA estimates that 3.2 million tons of medical waste is generated each year, of which 10% to 15% is potentially infectious.[12]

Environmental Protection Agency

The Environmental Protection Agency (EPA) is involved in the assessment of medical waste as specified in the Medical Waste Tracking Act of 1988.[11] The act requires the EPA to determine types, numbers, and sizes of generators of medical waste in the United States. The EPA examines the present or potential threat of medical waste to human health and the environment. Most medical waste regulations emanate from the individual states or local authorities and are variable, since no national policy exists for the handling of medical waste.

Department of Transportation and the United States Postal Service

The Department of Transportation (DOT) regulates diagnostic materials or etiologic agents shipped between states and to foreign countries. The DOT governs all transportation except shipping by mail, which is covered by the U.S. Postal Service (USPS). The USPS requirements for the mailing of tissue, blood, serum, and cultures are listed in the *Postal Service Manual*. The CDC has set standards for the shipment of etiologic agents, diagnostic specimens, and biologic products.[13] All blood and blood products emanating from the blood bank are considered diagnostic specimens.

BOX 16-1

Centers for Disease Control and Prevention Standard Precautions Isolation Guidelines

TIER I

Blood, all body fluids, secretions, and excretions regardless of the patient diagnosis or evidence of visible blood

TIER II

Airborne, droplet, and contact from patients of documented or suspected infection of highly transmissible or epidemiologic pathogens for which additional precautions are necessary

VOLUNTARY COMPLIANCE

Healthcare facilities and laboratories may choose to be accredited by a private organization. Many laboratories choose accreditation by the College of American Pathologists (CAP) and American Association of Blood Banks (AABB) as recognition of their adherence to the professional standards of practice.

Joint Commission on Accreditation of Healthcare Organizations

The Joint Commission on Accreditation of Healthcare Organizations (JCAHO) is an accrediting agency by which organizations elect to be inspected and accredited. Laboratories are a part of the overall review of medical facilities, and the guidelines are provided in the *Accreditation Manual for Pathology and Clinical Laboratory Services.*[14] Blood banks are included in this inspection and accreditation process. Safety requirements incorporate general safety, hazardous chemicals, security, life safety, emergency preparedness, equipment safety, and utilities, which are outlined in the *Comprehensive Accreditation Manual for Hospitals.*[15]

College of American Pathologists

CAP is a professional organization that provides peer-reviewed accreditation for hospital laboratories and independent laboratories, including blood banks. JCAHO recognizes accreditation by CAP as equivalent to its standards. The inspection process includes inspection and observation of laboratory safety compliance. CAP and JCAHO have adopted the National Fire Protection Association (NFPA) safeguards for fire safety.[16] CAP uses a comprehensive checklist for inspection of the blood bank for safety compliance.

American Association of Blood Banks

AABB's *Standards for Blood Banks and Transfusion Services* provides the basis for the inspection and accreditation of blood banks by a private, professional organization. Blood banks voluntarily comply with the AABB's inspection and accreditation, and accreditation is a high recognition of standards. AABB publications have served as principal guidelines for blood banks and transfusion services since 1958. These include the *Standards*, the *Accreditation Requirements Manual*, and the *Technical Manual*. Safety is a large component of the inspection process of the AABB.

Accreditation and Regulatory Equivalency Process

To provide for a comprehensive inspection for the regulatory and accreditation process, federal agencies may recognize an accreditation body as equivalent in standards and grant deemed status to this organization. AABB, JCAHO, and CAP accreditation standards are recognized, which may reduce the number of times a blood bank is inspected. The FDA, however, follows an unannounced inspection process and does not recognize accrediting agencies or accept HCFA inspections for donor and manufacturing facilities. The organization may inspect registered transfusion services if deemed necessary.

BLOOD BANK SAFETY PROGRAM

The blood bank safety program must be a comprehensive program, which includes policies and procedures of all regulatory bodies and any voluntary compliance accrediting agencies. In addition, any state and local laws must be taken into consideration. Most important, the safety program must be one that employees and employers endorse. Adherence to the safety program reduces any occupational hazards of the workplace and maintains a safe environment. The program should incorporate the OSHA regulations as outlined in Box 16-2.[17]

An individual or individuals responsible for the program must be appointed by the director or administrator of the blood bank. A written safety program that itemizes the requirements must be available to all blood bank personnel. The document should enumerate current safety policies, which need to be cross-referenced in each preanalytical, analytical, and postanalytical procedure in the laboratory. Safety program administrators need to consider not only the technical staff but potential risk for donors, ancillary personnel, volunteers, and visitors.

Physical Space, Safety Equipment, Protective Devices, and Warning Signs

Physical Space

The physical design of the blood bank and organization of tasks can reduce many potential hazards. Ready access to eye washes, showers, and hand washing is essential.

Areas of blood contamination should be separated from noncontaminated areas, including food service areas. The PHS has set criteria, according to risk, into biosafety levels (BSLs) for laboratory areas with potential exposure to infectious agents by risk (Box 16-3).[18] Most laboratory work with blood requires BSL 2 precautions, which should be applied in the blood bank as outlined in Box 16-4.

Laboratory Attire

Most tasks in the blood bank can be safely performed while wearing laboratory attire that protects the worker from common infectious hazards. A fluid-resistant laboratory coat, gown, or apron, whether disposable or made of cotton material, is recommended. Laboratory coats should be large enough to completely close in front, or aprons may be worn over long-sleeved uniforms. These personal barrier protection garments should be changed immediately if they are contaminated with blood or toxic substances. All outerwear worn during the performance of blood-banking tasks should be considered contaminated. Therefore such garments should not be worn outside of the laboratory into public

BOX 16-2 ***Occupational Safety and Health Administration Regulations for Protection from Bloodborne Pathogens Requirements***

Employers must:

- Provide a hazard-free workplace
- Educate and train staff
- Evaluate all procedures for potential exposure risks
- Evaluate each employment position for potential exposure risks
- Implement labeling procedures and post signs
- Apply universal precautions for handling all body substances
- Provide personal protective equipment, such as gloves or other barriers, without cost to the employee
- Make hepatitis B vaccine prophylaxis available to all staff who have occupational exposure, unless previously vaccinated or immune, and provide hepatitis B immune globulin treatment for percutaneous injury at no cost to the employee

BOX 16-3 ***Public Health Service Laboratory Biosafety Levels of Potential Exposure***

LEVEL 1

Work that involves agents of no known or of minimal potential hazard to laboratory personnel and the environment. Work is usually conducted on open surfaces, and no containment equipment is needed.

LEVEL 2

Work that involves agents of moderate potential hazard to personnel and the environment. Personnel wear laboratory coats and gloves as indicated, access to work areas is limited, and containment equipment should be used for procedures likely to create aerosols.

LEVEL 3

Work that involves indigenous or exotic agents that may cause serious or potentially lethal disease as a result of exposure by inhalation. Requires protective clothing, decontamination of wastes, and containment equipment for all procedures.

BOX 16-4 ***Biosafety Level 2 Precautions as Applied in the Blood Bank Setting***

Precautions include the following:

1. Bench tops consist of nonabsorbent material and are decontaminated daily with EPA-approved hospital disinfectant.
2. Laboratory rooms have closable doors. An air system with no recirculation is preferred but not required. Sinks and waste decontamination facilities are available within the area. Procedures that may create aerosols (e.g., opening evacuated tubes, centrifuging, mixing, or sonicating) are performed within a biologic safety cabinet or equivalent, or workers wear masks, goggles, gloves, and gowns during such procedures. (Note that open tubes of blood should not be centrifuged. If whole units of blood or plasma are centrifuged, overwrapping is recommended to contain leaks.)
3. Laboratory coats, gowns, and gloves are used routinely. Persons with open skin lesions on their hands and arms need to have all open areas securely bandaged. All staff members must wash their hands every time gloves are removed and after completing activities. Protective clothing must be removed before leaving the work area.
4. Mouth pipetting is not permitted.
5. All blood specimens are placed in well-constructed containers with secure lids to prevent leaking during transport. Blood is packaged appropriately for shipment in accordance with CDC requirements for etiologic agents or clinical specimens.
6. Infectious waste is not compacted and is decontaminated before disposal in leak-proof containers. Proper packaging includes double, seamless, tear-resistant, orange or red bags enclosed in protective cartons. Both the carton and the bag inside display the biohazard symbol. Throughout delivery to an incinerator or autoclave, infectious waste is handled only by suitably trained persons. If a waste management contractor is used, the agreement should clearly define respective responsibilities of the staff and the contractor.
7. No eating, drinking, smoking, application of cosmetics, or manipulation of contact lenses occurs in the work area. All food and drink are stored outside the restricted area, and laboratory glassware is never used for food or drink. Personnel are instructed to avoid touching faces, ears, mouth, eyes, or noses with hands or other objects, such as pencils and telephones.

BOX 16-4 Biosafety Level 2 Precautions as Applied in the Blood Bank Setting—cont'd

8. High-risk activities are appropriately segregated from low-risk activities, and the boundaries are clearly defined.
9. Needles and syringes are used and disposed of in a safe manner. Needles are never bent, broken, sheared, replaced in sheath, or detached from syringe before being placed in puncture-proof, leak-proof containers for controlled disposal. Procedures are designed to minimize exposure to sharp objects.
10. Any accidental exposure to suspected or actual hazardous material is reported to the laboratory director or responsible person immediately.

EPA, Environmental Protection Agency; *CDC*, Centers for Disease Control and Prevention.

areas. If nondisposable protective garments are used, they must be removed and stored in a suitable container and laundered in a manner that ensures decontamination. To contain the risk of infectious materials outside of a BSL 2 area, home laundering is prohibited, since unpredictable methods of transportation and handling can spread contamination, and laundering techniques may not be effective.[17]

SAFETY FACT: RULES OF THUMB

Hair should be secured away from the face and off the shoulders.

Jewelry should be kept to a minimum, and rings that could perforate gloves should not be worn.

Open-toed shoes are not permitted in areas where blood exposure exists.

Cosmetics should not be applied in the laboratory.

Personal Protective Equipment, Eyewashes, and Showers

Safety glasses, face shields or masks, splash barriers, and goggles are devices categorized as personal protective equipment (Fig. 16-1). Safety glasses or goggles should be worn when splashes are likely to occur during a task. Masks are better, since they protect the mouth, nose, and eyes. Face shields are made of shatterproof plastic and wrap around the face, thus offering greater protection. Permanently mounted splash barriers over the bench area are preferred when task performance risks splashing or aerosol contamination. Opening tubes of blood and using corrosive liquids warrant this protection for the employee. The shields should be cleansed and decontaminated on a regular basis.

If a splash does occur, the blood bank should have the availability of a shower and an eyewash device. An eyewash device should be capable of providing a gentle stream or spray of aerated water for an extended period time. Safety showers are for treating immediate first-aid needs of personnel contaminated with hazardous materials and for extinguishing clothing fires. Procedures and indications for use must be posted, and routine maintenance checks must be performed.

Biologic Safety Cabinets

Biologic safety cabinets (BSCs) are containment devices that facilitate safe handling of infectious materials and reduce the risk to personnel and the laboratory environment. Procedures that expose opened tubes of blood or units known to be positive for hepatitis B surface antigen or human immunodeficiency virus (HIV) are examples of blood bank procedures in which a BSC may be useful.

Employees need training in the operation of the BSC for maximum protection. The effectiveness of the BSC is a function of directional airflow inward and downward through a high-efficiency filter. Disruption of the airflow prevents maximum efficiency and usefulness of the cabinet.

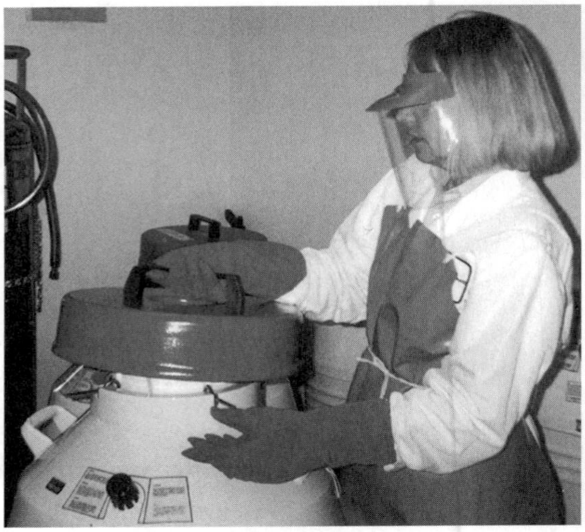

Fig. 16-1 Personal protective equipment. Gloves, gown, and face shield used while working with liquid nitrogen frozen red blood cell samples.

Courtesy of Micro Typing Systems, Inc., Pompano Beach, Fla.

SAFETY FACT: RULE OF THUMB
Blood bank personnel should wear gloves as a protective barrier when handling any blood or blood products.

Gloves and Hand Washing

Blood bank personnel should wear gloves as a protective barrier when handling any blood or blood products. OSHA does not require the routine use of gloves by phlebotomists working with healthy, prescreened donors or, if gloves are worn, the changing of unsoiled gloves between donors.[17] However, all employees likely to be exposed to blood should follow good practice by wearing gloves as another measure of precaution, since even prescreened "healthy" donors may have had contact with an infectious agent and may be unaware of the contact. A prudent part of the safety procedure of the blood bank includes the policy that all employees must wear gloves when tasks are likely to involve exposure to blood. Gloves used in a contaminated area should not be worn to a "clean" area or when using or touching telephones, doorknobs, or computer terminals.

Even when gloves are worn, hand washing remains the most effective defense in infection control and safety. Bloodborne pathogens generally do not penetrate intact skin, and thus, hand washing prevents their transfer to mucous membranes, such as nasal passages or broken skin areas. Hand washing also reduces the transmission of infectious agents to others. Hands should be washed after the removal of gloves in the following situations: following task completion; before leaving a work area; before, between, and after seeing patients; and immediately after contact with blood.

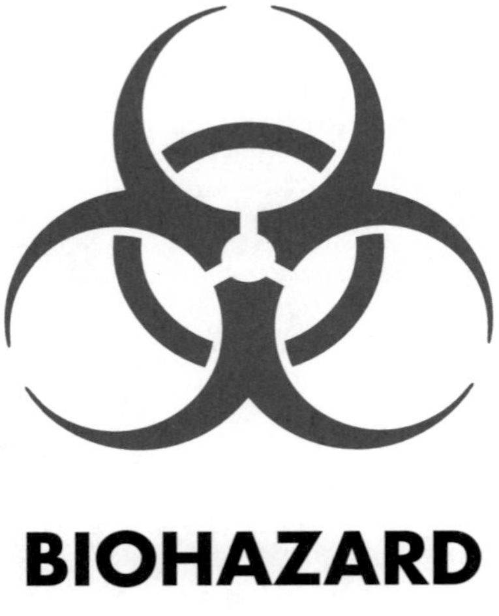

BIOHAZARD

Fig. 16-2 Biohazard symbol.

Warning Signs

Many regulatory agencies have designed warning signs and posted them in the laboratory for identification of hazardous materials or areas. OSHA emphasizes the importance of alerting personnel to potential danger with labels and signs. Biohazard warning labels, signs, and containers are fluorescent orange or red with lettering or symbols in a contrasting color (Fig. 16-2). Signs are intended to alert workers and others to take necessary precautions. NFPA has developed a sign identification system for hazardous materials with flammability risk.

SAFETY FACT: RULE OF THUMB
All laboratory surfaces and reusable equipment should routinely be cleaned and decontaminated daily and as needed while performing tasks and as spills occur.

Decontamination

All laboratory surfaces and reusable equipment should routinely be cleaned and decontaminated daily and as needed while performing tasks and as spills occur.

A list of EPA-approved disinfectant solutions can be obtained in the EPA publication *Registered Hospital Disinfectants and Sterilants*.[19] An economic and effective disinfectant is a fresh solution of 1:10 dilution of sodium hypochlorite (bleach), which can be used for general disinfection or for spills following the steps listed in Box 16-5.[20]

Chemical Storage and Hazards

The blood bank houses chemicals that may be of significant hazard (Table 16-1).[21] Chemical hazards are most often classified by their corrosiveness, ignitability, reactivity, and toxicity. Containment of chemicals is based on the nature of these hazards. Corrosiveness refers to any substance that can cause visible destruction or irreversible alteration in human tissues at the site of contact. Corrosives are stored near the floor (below eye level). Workers must wear protective equipment when handling corrosives. Pouring and pipetting of corrosives should occur under a chemical fume hood.

Ignitability has been classified by NFPA based on hazard potential of combustible or flammable liquids. Specifically designed flammable solvent containers are available and should be used in place of glass containers. Safety cans are required for more than one pint of Class A flammables, such as ether, and more than one quart of Class B flammables, such as acetone or ethanol. A flammable storage cabinet contains its contents during an ignition for approximately 10 minutes to allow personnel to vacate the area. These cabinets are required if the laboratory is storing more than 10 gallons of flammable liquids.

Toxicity is used to identify substances that, if inhaled, ingested, or contacted in small amounts, can cause serious biologic effects. Toxicity may be short term or long term. Short-term toxins are irritants and cause a local inflammatory effect on tissues at the site of contact and include sensitizers that cause an allergic reaction. Long-term toxins include substances that can cause change in genetic material and include tumorigens, carcinogens, and neoplasminogens.

OSHA published the Occupational Exposure to Hazardous Chemicals in Laboratories in 1990.[22] The regulations necessitate standards in the workplace to

BOX 16-5 ***Steps Taken in Case of Blood Spill***

If a blood spill should occur, the following steps should be taken in the order listed:

1. Leave the area for 30 minutes if an aerosol has been created, and post warnings to keep the area clear. Remove any contaminated clothing. If the spill occurs in the centrifuge, immediately turn off the power and leave the cover closed for 30 minutes. The use of overwraps helps prevent aerosols and widespread leakage.
2. Wear appropriate protective clothing and gloves. If sharp objects are involved, gloves must be puncture resistant, and a broom or other instrument should be used during cleanup to avoid injury.
3. Completely cover the spill with absorbent material. Remove the absorbent layer and any broken glass with a brush and pan.
4. Clean the area with detergent.
5. Flood the area with disinfectant, such as a freshly prepared 1:10 dilution of sodium hypochlorite (bleach) solution, and let it stand for 15 to 20 minutes.
6. Wipe up the disinfectant.
7. Safely dispose of all materials in accordance with biohazard guidelines. All blood-contaminated items must be autoclaved or incinerated.

Table 16-1 Sample List of Hazardous Chemicals in the Blood Bank

CHEMICAL	HAZARD
Ammonium chloride	Irritant
Bromelain	Irritant, sensitizer
Calcium chloride	Irritant
Carbon dioxide	Corrosive
Carbonyl iron powder	Oxidizer
Chloroform	Toxic, suspected carcinogen
Chloroquine	Irritant, corrosive
Chromium (III) chloride hexahydrate	Toxic, irritant, sensitizer
Citric acid	Irritant
Copper sulfate (cupric sulfate)	Toxic, irritant
Dichloromethane	Toxic, irritant
Digitonin	Toxic
Dry ice (carbon dioxide, frozen)	Corrosive
Ethidium bromide	Carcinogen, irritant
Ethylenediaminetetraacetic acid	Irritant
Ethyl ether	Highly flammable, explosive, toxic, irritant
Ficin (powder)	Irritant, sensitizer
34.9% Formaldehyde solution	Suspected carcinogen, combustible, toxic
Glycerol	Irritant
Hydrochloric acid	Highly toxic, corrosive
Imidazole	Irritant
Isopropyl (rubbing) alcohol	Flammable, irritant
Liquid nitrogen	Corrosive
Lyphogel	Corrosive
2-Mercaptoethanol	Toxic, stench
Mineral oil	Irritant, carcinogen, combustible
Papain	Irritant, sensitizer
Polybrene	Toxic
Potassium hydroxide	Corrosive, toxic
Saponin	Irritant
Sodium azide	Toxic, irritant, explosive when heated
Sodium ethylmercurithiosalicylate (thimerosal)	Highly toxic, irritant
Sodium hydrosulfite	Toxic, irritant
Sodium hydroxide	Corrosive, toxic
Sodium hypochlorite (bleach)	Corrosive
Sodium phosphate	Irritant, hygroscopic
Sulfosalicylic acid	Toxic, corrosive
Trichloroacetic acid	Corrosive, toxic
Trypsin	Irritant, sensitizer
Xylene	Highly flammable, toxic, irritant

minimize employee exposure to hazardous chemicals by the formation of a chemical hygiene plan (CHP). The CHP requires procedures for the following:

- The use of hazardous chemicals
- Personal protective equipment availability, use, and maintenance
- Employee education and training
- Medical consultation when exposure exceeds defined limits of safety
- The responsible person for the chemical hygiene plan

The CHP is to be a part of the blood bank safety program.

The Hazard Communications Standard (29 CFR 1910.1200) created a "right to know" procedure for the worker who handles or is exposed to hazardous chemicals. Material safety data sheets (MSDSs) are supplied by manufacturers, importers, or distributors of all toxic substances. MSDSs are required by OSHA and contain information including the chemical names, hazards, and personal protective equipment to be used and the spill cleanup details. The MSDS must be made readily available in the workplace to all employees.

Radiation Safety

Very few laboratory tests incorporate radionuclides. The blood bank, however, uses gamma irradiators for the irradiation of blood components. Employee safety needs to be emphasized with proper training in the use of the equipment, personal protective equipment, and exposure monitoring.

Blood irradiators vary in the amount of radiation scatter and leakage. The Nuclear Regulatory Commission requires training for all personnel using irradiators and records indicating exposure. Though monitors may not be required for some equipment, leak detection is necessary.

Fire Prevention and Control

Many combustible materials exist in a laboratory, including ignitable liquids and flammable gases. These materials should be clearly labeled following NFPA standards.[16] Portable fire extinguishers should be readily available for workers to extinguish small fires. Most fire extinguishers are of the multipurpose classification (ABC), which are recommended for all types of fires. An update in the use of fire extinguishers should be included in the annual safety training for all clinical laboratory employees. Fire blankets should be available for employees in the event that clothing or the person is on fire. A fire alarm system and sprinkler system should be installed in the laboratory as safety measures.

Biohazardous Wastes

Blood bank safety programs must include policies for handling all waste materials from areas where waste is contaminated with blood or body fluids. All laboratory personnel should be trained in a waste management program that protects staff and meets federal, state, and local regulatory requirements. Untrained personnel should not come in contact with or be responsible for biohazardous waste materials. The EPA identifies infectious wastes in 10 categories (Box 16-6).[23]

Until a national policy for the handling of medical waste is developed, each institution must adhere to state and local regulations and develop an infectious waste disposal program following those restrictions. The plan should identify potentially infectious material, indicate proper handling, transportation, and storage of such material, and prescribe the appropriate disposal of the material.

Correct identification of material is important to segregate potentially infectious waste from mainstream waste and to control cost and volume of infectious waste. Proper handling ensures that medical waste marked as biohazardous materials is placed in designated containers. Containers should be leak proof. Incineration and decontamination by autoclaving are currently recommended for disposing of blood samples and blood products. The EPA estimates that about 70% of hospital waste is incinerated on site, and incineration and decontamination are the methods of choice.[12] An alternative to these methods is decontamination by autoclaving before removal to a landfill. Some local laws require that

BOX 16-6

Environmental Protection Agency Infectious Waste Categories

- Isolation wastes
- Cultures and stocks of etiologic agents
- Blood and blood products
- Pathologic wastes
- Other wastes from surgery and autopsy
- Contaminated laboratory wastes
- Sharps
- Dialysis unit wastes
- Discarded biologics
- Contaminated equipment

infectious waste be not only decontaminated but also rendered unrecognizable as medical waste. For those laboratories that do not have the facilities for incineration or autoclaving large volumes, contracts with private carriers can be instituted. These contracts should include the responsibilities of the institution and those assumed by the carrier for transportation and disposal of the infectious materials.

SAFETY FACT: RULE OF THUMB
Food or drink should not be allowed in the blood storage or testing areas.

Storage and Transportation of Blood and Blood Components

Storage

Storage of blood and blood components for transfusion should be separate from reagents, specimens, and any other unrelated materials. Ideally a separate refrigerator should be used; however, if one is not available, areas within the refrigerator must be segregated to reduce spills or accidents. Refrigerators should be large enough to hold the anticipated blood storage need.

Transportation

Blood and blood components transferred within an institution for transfusion purposes do not require packaging and labeling as for shipping. Specimens should be transported in a plastic bag to prevent spills or leakage. To avoid contamination, paperwork should not be placed in the bag.

Any shipping of diagnostic materials or etiologic agents to or from the laboratory must follow the regulations of the DOT and USPS.[24,25] Regulations define a diagnostic specimen as "any human or animal material including, but not limited to, excreta, secreta, blood and its components, tissue, and tissue fluids shipped for the purposes of diagnosis."[24] If the specimen contains an "etiologic agent" (defined as a viable microorganism or its toxin that may cause human disease), packages must be sent in a triple-packaged, securely closed, watertight, primary container enclosed in a second durable watertight container; the container must be able to withstand shock, pressure changes, and other conditions found in ordinary handling during transportation.

Blood banks should contact the carrier for correct packaging and label identification requirements.

SAFETY FACT: RULE OF THUMB
An accident report should be initiated in **ALL** accidents and injuries involving employees or other persons.

Personal Injury and Reporting

In the event that an employee or other person is injured or possible injury or infection exists, an accident report should be initiated. These reports are required by worker's compensation, OSHA, and other regulatory and accrediting bodies. Most medical reports must be kept for a period of 30 years,[26] and OSHA requires incident reports to be kept 5 years beyond the calendar year of occurrence of the accident.[27]

Routine investigation of a minor incident and follow-up to correct the risk may thwart a major accident later. Personnel should be encouraged to report all incidents no matter how insignificant they may seem, since accident reporting is an essential part of maintaining a safe working environment. Each incident should be treated with a thorough investigation in a nonthreatening manner to the employee.

Employee Education

Employee education makes good sense, but it is also a mandate of OSHA and other regulatory and accrediting agencies.[17] The blood bank safety program should be reviewed with new employees during their orientation and training be-

BOX 16-7 ***Occupational Safety and Health Administration (OSHA) Requirements for Healthcare Employees***

OSHA requires employers to provide all employees' fundamental knowledge. Employees should:

- Have access to a copy of pertinent regulatory texts and an explanation of the contents
- Understand the employer's exposure control plan and know how to obtain a copy of the written plan
- Understand how hepatitis and HIV viruses are transmitted and how often; know the symptoms and consequences of HBV and HIV infection; be offered vaccination against HBV
- Recognize tasks that pose infectious risk and distinguish them from other duties
- Know what protective clothing and equipment is appropriate for the procedures he or she is performing
- Know and understand the limitations of protective clothing and equipment (e.g., ordinary gloves do not protect against needlestick injuries); employers and staff who use protective equipment should be forewarned against a false sense of security
- Know where protective clothing and equipment are kept and know how to use them properly to remove, handle, decontaminate, and dispose of contaminated material
- Be familiar with and understand all requirements for work practices and protective equipment specified in SOPs for the task they perform, including the meaning of signs and labels
- Know what appropriate actions to take and which persons to contact if exposure to blood or other potentially infectious materials occurs
- Know the corrective actions to take in the event of spills or personal exposure to fluids, tissues, and contaminated sharps, and know the appropriate reporting procedures and medical monitoring recommended when parenteral exposure may have occurred
- Know the right of access to medical records

HIV, Human immunodeficiency virus; *HBV*, hepatitis B virus; *SOPs*, standard operating procedures.

fore independent work is permitted. All employees whose tasks carry risk of infectious exposure should annually review the safety program as a condition of OSHA. The supervisor or responsible safety officer should document all employee participation in this education, and performance evaluations should include the employee's adherence to the blood bank's safety policies and procedures.

Education for employees must be designed for the specific tasks in which each employee or employee group is engaged. In accordance with OSHA all employees must have fundamental knowledge of all safety standards and practices listed in Box 16-7.

CHAPTER SUMMARY

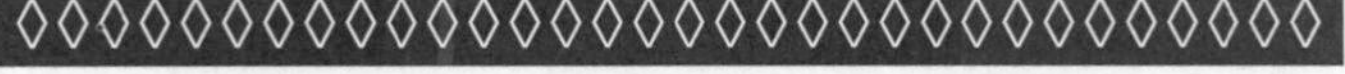

No blood bank is so safe that it cannot be made safer. Laws and regulations set forth by OSHA, CDC, HCFA, FDA, EPA, DOT, USPS, and state and local authorities, as well as the voluntary accreditation standards of AABB, CAP, and JCAHO, outline the requirements for blood banks and other laboratories.

A blood bank must have a written safety program that includes elements from the laws, regulations, and standards. Most important, this safety program must have policies and procedures that include:

- A CHP
- When and how to use personal protective equipment, including gloves and outer wear, BSCs, and accident safety devices such as eyewashes and showers

- Evaluation of all procedures and employee positions for risks
- The posting of signs and correct labeling
- Universal precautions
- Decontamination of required areas
- Infectious/biohazardous waste containment and disposal
- Reporting of accidents and injuries including an exposure control plan
- A fire safety plan
- Radiation safety

The most important element of a blood bank safety program is employee education. All employees must participate in safety education as a part of new employee orientation and yearly thereafter as a condition of OSHA. Employees and employers must embrace and adhere to the blood bank safety program. Safety is not only a matter of regulations and standards; it is common sense.

CRITICAL THINKING EXERCISES

EXERCISE 16-1

Prepare a blood bank safety program.

EXERCISE 16-2

Evaluate a blood bank or laboratory safety program that is currently in place in a blood bank or laboratory to which you have access.

EXERCISE 16-3

Compare laws and regulations to accreditation standards for safety in the blood bank.

EXERCISE 16-4

Contact local county authorities, research what laws apply to the disposal of biohazardous waste, and compare these to the laws of an adjoining county.

STUDY QUESTIONS

1. Ultimately the responsibility for safety in the laboratory belongs to:
   a. CDC
   b. the employer or laboratory director
   c. OSHA
   d. the employee

2. Using U.S. mail for sending diagnostic specimens requires meeting specifications of the:
   a. USPS for all specimens
   b. DOT for all specimens
   c. USPS for HIV- and HBV-positive specimens only
   d. DOT for HIV- and HBV-positive specimens only

3. Classes of medical waste as stipulated by EPA include:
   a. microbiology and pathology laboratory waste; blood specimens and blood products; and laboratory gowns and coats
   b. all blood specimens and blood products; soiled laboratory gowns and coats; and tissues
   c. microbiology and pathology laboratory waste; blood specimens and blood products; and all sharps
   d. blood and blood products; sharps; and laboratory gowns and coats

4. The *Technical Manual* often used for principal guidelines in the blood bank is a publication of:
   a. CAP
   b. JCAHO
   c. AABB
   d. OSHA

5. All blood banks as mandated by law must have a:
   a. water fountain
   b. written laboratory safety program
   c. BSC
   d. foot-operated hand wash

6. Goggles, face shields, and splash barriers are:
   a. personal protection equipment
   b. not necessary unless working with HIV- or HBV-positive specimens
   c. mandated at all times when working with blood specimens and blood products
   d. provided by the employee if needed

7. Laboratory work in a BSL I, as defined by the PHS, includes:
   a. the preparation of a 0.9% sodium chloride solution
   b. aliquoting patient plasma or serum
   c. antibody testing by immediate spin
   d. anti-D rapid tube tests

8. The policy of treating all body substances as potentially harmful, regardless of the patient diagnosis, is known as the:
   a. OSHA Exposure Program
   b. isolation guidelines
   c. AABB safety policy
   d. universal precautions

9. The most effective defense for infection control and safety is wearing gloves and:
   a. goggles
   b. laboratory coats
   c. posting warning signs
   d. hand washing

10. One of the most economical and easy disinfectants to use is a:
    a. 1:10 fresh solution of sodium hypochlorite (bleach)
    b. 1:5 solution of household Lysol
    c. 1:15 solution of sodium hydroxide
    d. detergent and water mixture

11. A substance that can cause visible destruction or irreversible alteration in human tissues at the site of contact is:
    a. corrosive
    b. ignitable
    c. toxic
    d. reactive

12. The reporting of an accident or injury should occur when any:
    a. injury may result in a fatality
    b. injury involves possible infection with HIV or HBV
    c. accident involves nonemployees or jeopardizes a patient
    d. accident or injury occurs

13. One of the best ways to protect employees and keep a safe laboratory environment is to provide employees with:
    a. health insurance
    b. safety education
    c. rest breaks
    d. fluid-repellent laboratory coats

14. All employees whose tasks carry risk of infectious exposure are required to participate in the blood bank safety program yearly as a condition of the:
    a. AABB
    b. OSHA
    c. CAP
    d. FDA

15. OSHA requires employers to provide all employees the following fundamental knowledge, EXCEPT:
    a. an exposure control plan for HIV or HBV exposure
    b. right of access to medical records when HIV or HBV is indicated
    c. exercising the "right to know" act on employees' medical records
    d. what personal protective equipment to use in all procedures

REFERENCES

1. The Coroner's Verdict in the St. Louis Tetanus Cases, 1901 New York Medical Journal 74, *JAMA* 37:1255, 1902.
2. Public Health Service Act of 1944, Public Law, 42 USC 262, 1944.
3. Food, Drug and Cosmetic Act of 1938, Public Law, 21 USC 321 (amended through November 17, 1998).
4. Occupational Safety and Health Act of 1970, Public Law, 29 USC 651, 1970.
5. US Department of Labor, Occupational Safety and Health Administration: *Approved state plans for enforcement of state statutes,* 29 CFR 1952, Washington, DC, 1998, US Government Printing Office.
6. Centers for Disease Control and Prevention: Recommendations for preventing HIV transmission in health care settings, *Morbidity and Mortality Weekly Report* 36(2S):1, 1987.
7. Centers for Disease Control and Prevention: *Guidelines for isolation precautions in hospitals,* (CDC) 59(214):55552, Washington, DC, 1995, US Government Printing Office.
8. Centers for Disease Control and Prevention/National Institutes of Health: *Biosafety in microbiological and biomedical laboratories,* ed 3, HHS Publication Number (CDC) 93-8395, Washington, DC, 1993, US Government Printing Office.
9. US Department of Health and Human Services, Health Care Financing Administration, Public Health Service: *Clinical laboratory regulations improvement amendments of 1988, final rule,* 42 CFR 493, Washington, DC, 1992, US Government Printing Office.
10. Public Health Service Act: *Clinical laboratory improvement amendments of 1988,* 42 USC 263a, section 353, Washington, DC, 1988, US Government Printing Office.
11. US Environmental Protection Agency: *Medical waste tracking act,* 40 USC 6992, Washington, DC, 1988, US Government Printing Office.
12. Tilton RC, Balows A, Hohnadel DC, Reiss RF: *Clinical laboratory medicine,* St Louis, 1992, Mosby.
13. Centers for Disease Control and Prevention: *Shipping standards,* 55:42, Washington DC, 1990, US Government Printing Office.
14. Joint Commission on Accreditation of Healthcare Organizations: *Accreditation manual for pathology and clinical laboratory services,* Oakbrook, Ill, 1992, Joint Commission on Accreditation of Healthcare Organizations.
15. Joint Commission on Accreditation of Healthcare Organizations: *Comprehensive accreditation manual for hospitals,* Oakbrook, Ill, 1992, Joint Commission on Accreditation of Healthcare Organizations.
16. National Fire Protection Association: *Safety standards for laboratories in health related institutions,* NFPA Publication No. 56C, Quincy, Mass, 1987, National Fire Protection Association.

17. US Department of Labor, Occupational Safety and Health Administration: *Occupational exposure to blood-borne pathogens, final rule,* 29 CFR 1910.1030, Washington, DC, 1992, US Government Printing Office.
18. US Environmental Protection Agency: *Good laboratory practice standards,* 40 CFR 792, Washington, DC, 1998, US Government Printing Office.
19. Environmental Protection Agency: *Registered hospital disinfectants and sterilants* (TS767C), Washington, DC, 1992, Antimicrobial Program Branch.
20. National Committee for Clinical Laboratory Standards: *Protection of laboratory workers from infectious disease transmitted by blood, body fluids and tissue,* ed 2, NCCLS document M29-T2, Villanova, Penn, 1991, National Committee for Clinical Laboratory Science.
21. Vengelen-Tyler V, editor: *Technical manual,* ed 12 , Bethesda, Md, 1996, American Association of Blood Banks.
22. US Department of Labor, Occupational Safety and Health Administration: *Occupational exposure to hazardous chemicals in laboratories,* 29 CFR 1910.1450, Washington, DC, 1990, US Government Printing Office.
23. Environmental Protection Agency: Standards for the tracking and management of medical waste, *Federal Register* 54(56):12326, 1989.
24. US Department of Transportation: *Research and special programs administration,* 49 CFR 100-199, Washington, DC, 1998, US Government Printing Office.
25. US Postal Service: *Mailability of etiologic agents,* 39 CFR 111, Washington, DC, 1998, US Government Printing Office.
26. US Department of Labor, Occupational Safety and Health Administration: *Occupational safety and health standards,* 29 CFR 1910, Washington, DC, 1998, US Government Printing Office.
27. US Department of Labor, Occupational Safety and Health Administration: *Recording and reporting occupational injuries and illnesses,* 29 CFR 1904.6, Washington, DC, 1998, US Government Printing Office.

SUGGESTED READING

Snyder JR, Wilkinson DS: *Management in laboratory medicine,* ed 3, Philadelphia, 1998, Lippincott.

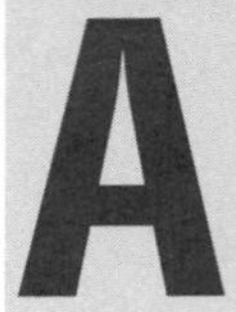

APPENDIX
Answers to Study Questions

Chapter 1

1. **d**
2. **a**
3. **b**
4. **c**
5. **a**
6. **a**
7. **b**
8. **a**
9. **c**
10. **a**
11. **a**
12. **b**
13. **d**
14. **b**
15. **a**
16. **c**
17. **a**
18. **d**
19. **d and e**
20. **e**
21. **a**
22. **d**
23. **d**
24. **e**
25. **e**

Chapter 2

1. **c**
2. **b**
3. **a**
4. **c**
5. **d**
6. **c**
7. **b**
8. **c**
9. **a**
10. **b**
11. **d**
12. **a**
13. **b**
14. **a**
15. **c**

Chapter 3

1. **d**
2. **b**
3. **d**
4. **b**
5. **a**
6. **b**
7. **a**
8. **c**
9. **d**
10. **c**
11. **b**
12. **b**
13. **a**
14. **a**
15. **c**

Chapter 4

1. **c**
2. **d**
3. **a**
4. **d**
5. **a**
6. **d**
7. **c**
8. **b**
9. **c**
10. **b**
11. **c**
12. **d**
13. **a**
14. **d**
15. **c**
16. **a**
17. **b**
18. **d**
19. **c**
20. **b**

Chapter 5

1. **d**
2. **a**
3. **d**
4. **a**
5. **a**
6. **b**
7. **b**
8. **d**
9. **d**
10. **a**
11. **a**
12. **b**
13. **a**
14. **c**
15. **a**

Chapter 6

1. **c**
2. **c**
3. **a**
4. **a**
5. **d, e, and g**
6. **d**
7. **d**
8. **c**
9. **d**
10. **c**
11. **a**
12. **d**
13. **a**
14. **c**
15. **d**
16. **a**
17. **c**
18. **c**
19. **b**
20. **d**

Chapter 7

1. **a**
2. **c**
3. **d**
4. **d**
5. **a**
6. **c**
7. **c**
8. **c**
9. **b**
10. **d**
11. **a**
12. **c**
13. **c**
14. **d**
15. **c**

Chapter 8

1. **b**
2. **c**
3. **c**
4. **d**
5. **a**
6. **b**
7. **c**
8. **c**
9. **b**
10. **d**
11. **f**
12. **f**
13. **f**
14. **f**
15. **t**
16. **f**
17. **t**
18. **f**
19. **f**
20. **t**

Chapter 9

1. **TD**
2. **A**
3. **TD**
4. **TD**
5. **PD**
6. **TD**
7. **A**
8. **TD**
9. **PD**
10. **PD**
11. **d**

12. **b**
13. **d**
14. **t**
15. **f**

Chapter 10

1. **d**
2. **a**
3. **e**
4. **b**
5. **a**
6. **c**
7. **d**
8. **b**
9. **a**
10. **a**

Chapter 11

1. **b**
2. **b**
3. **e**
4. **f**
5. **g**
6. **g**
7. **c**
8. **a**
9. **c**
10. **e**
11. **d**
12. **b**
13. **a**
14. **d**
15. **f**
16. **d**
17. **g**
18. **b**
19. **d**
20. **c**
21. **d**
22. **c**
23. **b**

Chapter 12

1. **a**
2. **c**
3. **d**
4. **b**
5. **d**
6. **c**
7. **d**
8. **a**
9. **c**
10. **c**
11. **a**
12. **b**
13. **d**
14. **a**
15. **b**

Chapter 13

1. **c**
2. **b**
3. **c**
4. **c**
5. **d**
6. **c**
7. **a**
8. **a**
9. **a**
10. **c**
11. **c**
12. **a**
13. **b**
14. **d**

Chapter 14

1. **a**
2. **a**
3. **a**
4. **c**
5. **d**
6. **d**
7. **c**
8. **a**
9. **d**
10. **c**

Chapter 15

1. **c**
2. **d**
3. **b**
4. **a**
5. **c**
6. **e**
7. **c**
8. **a**
9. **c**
10. **b**
11. **a**

Chapter 16

1. **b**
2. **a**
3. **c**
4. **c**
5. **b**
6. **a**
7. **a**
8. **d**
9. **d**
10. **a**
11. **a**
12. **d**
13. **b**
14. **b**
15. **c**

APPENDIX B
Glossary

ABO antibodies: anti-A, anti-B, and anti-A,B. Patients will possess the ABO antibody to the ABO antigen lacking on their red blood cells (e.g., group A individuals possess anti-B).

ABO discrepancy: occurs when ABO phenotyping of red blood cells does not agree with expected serum testing results for the particular ABO phenotype.

Acanthocytosis: presence of abnormal red blood cells with spurlike projections in the circulating blood.

Accuracy: degree to which a measurement represents the true value of the attribute being measured.

Acquired agammaglobulinemia: the absence of gamma globulin and antibodies associated with malignant diseases such as leukemia, myeloma, or lymphoma.

Acquired B phenotype: group A_1 individual with diseases of the lower gastrointestinal tract, cancers of the colon and rectum, intestinal obstruction, or gram-negative septicemia who acquires reactivity with anti-B reagents in ABO red blood cell testing and appears as group AB.

Acquired immunity: host defenses mediated by lymphocytes following exposure to an antigen that exhibits specificity, memory and self/nonself recognition.

Acute hemolytic transfusion reaction: complication of transfusion associated with intravascular hemolysis characterized by rapid onset with symptoms of fever, chills, hemoglobinemia, and hypotension; major complications include irreversible shock, renal failure, and disseminated intravascular coagulation.

Adsorption: attachment of antibody to red blood cell antigens and the subsequent removal from the serum.

Agglutination: visible clumping of particulate antigens.

Agglutinogen: group of antigens or factors.

Alleged father: man accused of being the biologic father; the putative father.

Alleles: alternate forms of a gene at a given locus.

Alloantibodies: antibodies with specificities other than self; stimulated by transfusion or pregnancy.

Allogeneic donation: donation for use by the general patient population.

Allogeneic: blood or tissue from the same species that is not genetically identical.

Alternative pathway: activation of complement that is initiated by foreign cell–surface constituents.

American Association of Blood Banks: professional organization that accredits and provides educational and technical guidance to blood banks and transfusion services.

Amniocentesis: process of withdrawal of amniotic fluid by aspiration for the purpose of analysis.

Amorphic: describes a gene that does not express a detectable product.

Amplicon: amplified target sequence of DNA produced by the PCR.

Anamnestic response: secondary immune response.

Anaphylatoxins: complement split products, C3a, C4a, and C5a, that mediate degranulation of mast cells and basophils, which results in smooth muscle contraction and increased vascular permeability.

Antibody: protein (immunoglobulin) that recognizes a particular epitope on an antigen and facilitates clearance of that antigen.

Antibody identification: procedure that determines the identity of a red blood cell antibody detected in the antibody screen by reacting serum with commercial panel cells.

Antibody potentiators: reagents or methods that enhance or speed up the antibody-antigen reaction.

Antibody screen test: test to determine presence of alloantibodies.

Antigen: substance (usually foreign) that binds specifically to an antibody or a T cell receptor.

Antigenic determinants: site on an antigen that is recognized and bound by a particular antibody or T cell receptor (also called the *epitope*).

Antigen-presenting cells: cells that process and present antigenic peptides in association with class II MHC molecules and activates T cells.

Antigram: profile of antigen typings of each donor used in the manufacturing of commercially supplied screening and panel cells.

Antithetical: opposite allele.

Apheresis donation: donation of a specific component of the blood; parts of the whole blood that are not retained are returned to the donor.

Audit trail: record-keeping system that recreates every step in the manufacturing process.

Audits: systematic investigations to determine whether policies and procedures are being performed and supported properly.

Autoadsorption: attachment of the patient's antibodies to the patient's own red blood cells and subsequent removal from the serum.

Autoantibodies: antibodies to self-antigens.

Autocontrol: testing a person's serum with his or her own red blood cells to determine if an autoantibody is present.

Autoimmune hemolytic anemia: immune destruction of autologous or self red blood cells.

Autologous: pertaining to self.

Autologous donation: donation by a donor reserved for the donor's later use.

Autosomes: chromosomes other than the sex chromosomes.

Avidity: sum total of the strength of binding of two molecules (e.g., antigen and antibody).

B cell clone: B cells producing antibodies with the same specificity.

B lymphocytes: lymphocytes that mature in the bone marrow, differentiate into plasma cells, and produce antibodies.

B(A) phenotype: group B individual who acquires reactivity with anti-A reagents in ABO red blood cell testing; in these individuals the B gene transfers trace amounts of the immunodominant sugar for the A antigen and the immunodominant sugar for the B antigen.

Biphasic hemolysin: an antibody, such as the Donath-Landsteiner antibody, that requires a period of cold and warm incubations to bind complement with resulting hemolysis.

Blood group systems: groups of antigens on the red blood cell membrane that share related serologic properties and genetic patterns of inheritance.

Blood warmer: medical device that prewarms donor blood to 37° C before transfusion.

Bombay phenotype: rare phenotype of an individual who genetically has inherited *h* allele in homozygous manner; individual's red blood cells lack H and ABO antigens.

Bone marrow transplant: procedure that transplants bone marrow from healthy donors to stimulate the production of blood cells.

Bradykinin: potent vasodilator of the kinin family.

Calibration: process of standardizing an instrument against a known value.

Carbohydrates: simple sugars, such as monosaccharides and starches (polysaccharides).

Cell separation: technique used to separate transfused cells from autologous or patient cells.

Cellular immunity: adaptive immunity in which T lymphocytes recognize and react with the antigen through direct cell-to-cell interaction.

Change control: system to plan and implement changes in procedures, equipment, policies, and methodologies to increase effectiveness and prevent problems.

Chemical mediators: factors secreted by certain cells that when activated promote or inhibit a response from another cell or tissue.

Chemokines: group of cytokines involved in the activation of white blood cells during migration across the endothelium.

Chemotactic: movement of cells in the direction of the antigenic stimulus.

Chromosomes: structures within the nucleus that contain DNA.

Chronic granulomatous disease: inherited disorder where the phagocytic white blood cells are able to engulf but not kill certain microorganisms.

***cis*:** two or more genes on the same chromosome of a homologous pair.

***cis*-Product antigens:** compound antigens produced when two genes are inherited on the same chromosome.

Classical pathway: activation of complement that is initiated by antigen-antibody complexes.

Clinical Laboratory Improvement Act: enacted to ensure that laboratory tests are consistently reliable and of high quality.

Clinical significance: antibodies that are capable of causing a decreased survival of transfused cells as in a transfusion reaction.

Clinically insignificant: antibody that does not cause red blood cell destruction or clearance

Clone: family of cells or organisms having genetically identical constitution.

Closed system: collection of blood in an airtight, sterile system.

Cluster of differentiation: cell membrane molecule used to differentiate human leukocyte subpopulations; determined by specific monoclonal antibodies.

***Code of Federal Regulations*:** FDA publication outlining the legal requirements of blood banking facilities.

Codominant: equal expression of two different inherited alleles.

Cold alloantibodies: red blood cell antibodies specific for other human red blood cell antigens that typically react at or below room temperature.

Cold autoantibodies: red blood cell antibodies specific for autologous antigens that typically react at or below room temperature.

Cold hemagglutinin disease: autoimmune hemolytic anemia produced by an autoantibody that reacts best in colder temperatures (less than 37° C)

Compatibility testing: all steps in the identification and testing of a potential transfusion recipient and donor blood before transfusion in an attempt to provide a blood product that survives in vivo and provides its therapeutic effect in the recipient.

Competency assessment: evaluation of the employee's ability and knowledge to perform a procedure or skill.

Competitive EIA: enzyme-linked immunosorbent assay technique used to determine the presence or quantity of an antigen or antibody. In this test a lower absorbance indicates detection of the marker.

Complement system: group of serum proteins that participate in an enzymatic cascade, ultimately generating the membrane attack complex that causes lysis of cellular elements.

Components: parts of whole blood that can be separated by centrifugation; consists of red blood cells, plasma, cryoprecipitated antihemophilic factor, and platelets.

Compound antigens: distinct antigens produced when two other antigens are encoded by the same gene.

Confidential Unit Exclusion: method that allows donors to exclude their unit from the general inventory following donation in a confidential manner.

Congenital agammaglobulinemia: genetic disease characterized by the absence of gamma globulin and antibody in the blood.

Congenital hypogammaglobulinemia: genetic disease characterized by reduced levels of gamma globulin in the blood.

Constant region: nonvariable portion of the heavy and light chains of an immunoglobulin and T cell receptor.

Continuous quality improvement/total quality management: plans that provide the framework for establishing quality assurance in an organization.

Cord blood cells: whole blood obtained from the umbilical vein or artery of the fetus.

Corrected count increment: relative increase in platelet count adjusted for the number of platelets transfused and the size of the patient.

Crossing over: exchange of genetic material during meiosis between paired chromosomes.

Crossmatch: procedure that combines donor's red blood cells and patient's serum to determine the serologic compatibility between donor and patient.

Cryoprecipitate: blood component recovered from a controlled thaw of fresh frozen plasma; the cold-insoluble precipitate is rich in coagulation Factor VIII, von Willebrand factor, Factor XIII, and fibrinogen.

Cryoprotective: solution added to protect against cell damage that occurs at or below freezing temperatures.

Cytokines: secreted proteins that regulate the intensity and duration of the immune response by mediating interactions between cells.

Deacetylating: removal of the acetyl group (CH_3CO-).

Diastolic pressure: filling of the heart chamber; the second sound heard while taking a blood pressure.

Differential adsorption: adsorption or attachment of antibodies in the serum to specific known antigens, usually to different aliquots of red blood cells.

Differential DAT: Immunohematologic test that uses monospecific anti-IgG and monospecific anti-C3 reagents to determine the cause of a positive DAT with polyspecific antiglobulin reagents.

Direct antiglobulin test: test used to detect antibody bound to red blood cells in vivo

Direct exclusion: exclusion of paternity when a child has a trait that neither parent demonstrates.

Directed donation: donation reserved for use by a specific patient.

Divalent: combining power of two.

Document control: plan for the management of all documents in an organization that addresses the design, responsibility, storage, removal, and revision of all records, forms, and procedures.

Dolichos biflorus: plant lectin with specificity for the A_1 antigen.

Dominant: gene product expressed over another gene.

Dosage effect: stronger agglutination when a red blood cell antigen is expressed from homozygous genes.

Edema: tissue swelling caused by an increase in fluid from the vasculature.

Eluate: antibody recovered in a solution for further testing by an antibody identification technique.

Elution: process that dissociates antigen-antibody complexes on red blood cells; freed IgG antibody is tested for specificity.

Enhancement media: reagents that enhance or speed up the antibody-antigen reaction.

Epitope: single antigenic determinant; functionally, it is the part of the antigen that combines with the antibody.

Erythroblastosis fetalis: hemolytic disease of the newborn.

Extravascular hemolysis: removal of red blood cells from circulation by the phagocytic cells of the reticuloendothelial system (liver and spleen).

False negative result: test result that incorrectly indicates a negative reaction (the lack of agglutination); an antigen-antibody reaction has occurred but is not demonstrated.

False positive result: test result that incorrectly indicates a positive reaction (the presence of agglutination or hemolysis); no antigen-antibody reaction occurred.

Fetomaternal hemorrhage: escape of fetal cells into the maternal circulation, usually occurring at the time of delivery.

Food and Drug Administration: agency responsible for the regulation of the blood banking industry and other manufacturers of products consumed by humans.

Frozen plasma: blood component prepared from whole blood that contains only the plasma portion of whole blood and is frozen after separation.

Gene: basic unit of inheritance on a chromosome.

Genetic loci: sites of a gene on a chromosome.

Genotype: actual genetic makeup; determined by family studies.

Glycolipids: compounds containing carbohydrate and lipid molecules.

Glycophorin: glycoprotein that projects through the red blood cell membrane and carries many blood group antigens.

Glycoproteins: compounds containing carbohydrate and protein molecules.

Glycosyltransferase: enzyme that catalyzes the transfer of glycosyl groups (simple carbohydrate units) in biochemical reactions.

Good manufacturing practices: methods used in, and the facilities or controls used for, the manufacture, processing, packing, or holding of a drug (including a blood product) to ensure that it meets safety, purity, and potency standards.

Granulocyte concentrates: blood component collected by cytapheresis; contains a minimum of 1.0×10^{10} granulocytes.

Half-life: time required for the concentration of a substance to decrease by half.

Haplotype: linked set of genes inherited together because of their close proximity on a chromosome.

Haptoglobin: plasma protein with sole function of binding free hemoglobin and carrying the molecule to the hepatocytes for further catabolism.

Heavy chains: larger polypeptide of an antibody molecule composed of a variable and constant region; five major classes of heavy chains determine the isotype of an antibody.

Hemapheresis: whole blood is removed from a donor or patient and separated into components; one or more of the components are retained, and the remainder is returned.

Hemolysis: lysis or rupture of erythrocytes.

Hemolytic disease of the newborn: disease caused by destruction of fetal or neonatal red blood cells by maternal antibodies.

Hemorrhage: bleeding through ruptured or unruptured blood vessel walls.

Hemotherapy: treatment of a disease or condition by the use of blood or blood derivatives.

Heterozygous: two alleles for a given trait are different.

Hinge region: portion of the immunoglobulin heavy chains between the Fc and Fab region; provides flexibility to the molecule to allow two antigen-binding sites to function independently.

Histamine: compound that causes constriction of bronchial smooth muscle, dilation of capillaries, and decrease in blood pressure.

Homozygous: two alleles for a given trait are identical.

Humoral immunity: adaptive immunity in which B lymphocytes and plasma cells produce specific antibodies that recognize and react with an antigen.

Hybridoma: hybrid cell formed by the fusion of a myeloma cell and an antibody-producing cell; used in the production of monoclonal antibodies.

Hydatid cyst fluid: fluid obtained from a cyst of the dog tapeworm.

Hypogammaglobulinemia: less than normal levels of gamma globulin in the blood associated with malignant diseases (chronic leukemias and myeloma) and immunosuppression therapy.

Iatrogenic blood loss: blood loss caused by treatment (e.g., collection of samples for testing).

Icterus: pertaining to or resembling jaundice.

Idiotypes: sets of antigenic determinants characterizing each unique antibody or T cell receptor.

Immediate spin phases: source antigen and source antibody used in immunohematologic testing are combined, immediately centrifuged, and observed for agglutination.

Immediate spin: interpretation of agglutination reactions immediately following centrifugation and without incubation.

Immunodominant sugar: sugar molecule responsible for specificity.

Immunogen: antigen in its role of eliciting an immune response, whether humoral, cellular, or both.

Immunogenicity: ability to stimulate an immune response.

Immunoglobulins: antibodies; proteins secreted by plasma cells that bind to specific epitopes on antigenic substances.

Immunohematology: study of blood group antigens and antibodies.

In vitro: reaction in an artificial environment, such as in a test tube.

In vivo: referring to a reaction within the body.

Incompatible crossmatches: occur when agglutination or hemolysis is observed in the crossmatch of donor red blood cells and patient serum, indicating a serologic incompatibility. The donor unit would not be transfused.

Independent assortment: random behavior of genes on separate chromosomes during meiosis that results in a mixture of genetic material in the offspring.

Independent segregation: passing of one gene from each parent to the offspring.

Indirect antiglobulin test: test used to detect antibody bound to red blood cells in vitro.

Indirect EIA: enzyme-linked immunosorbent assay technique used to determine the presence or quantity of an antibody.

Indirect exclusion: failure to find an expected marker in a child when the alleged father is apparently homozygous for the gene.

Innate immunity: nonspecific host defense that exists before exposure to an antigen; involves the anatomic and inflammatory response.

Intravascular hemolysis: destruction of red blood cells and release of hemoglobin within the vascular compartment through immune or nonimmune mechanisms; antibodies of the ABO system can cause this type of hemolysis.

ISBT-128: International Society of Blood Transfusion recommendations regarding the uniform labeling of blood products for international bar code recognition by computers.

Ischemia: decreased supply of oxygenated blood to an organ or body part.

ISO 9000: quality philosophy that establishes standards for manufacturing, trade, and communication.

Kappa chains: one of the two types of light chains that make up an immunoglobulin.

Kinins: group of proteins associated with contraction of smooth muscle, vascular permeability, and vasodilation.

Lambda chains: one of the two types of light chains that make up an immunoglobulin.

Landsteiner's rule: rule stating that normal, healthy individuals possess ABO antibodies to the ABO antigens lacking on their red blood cells.

Lattice formation: combination of antibody and a multivalent antigen to form crosslinks and result in visible agglutination.

Lecithin/sphingomyelin ratio: ratio of lecithin to sphingomyelin that indicates lung maturity.

Lectins: plant extracts useful as blood banking reagents; they bind to carbohydrate portions of certain red blood cell antigens and agglutinate the red blood cells.

Light chains: smaller polypeptide of an antibody molecule, composed of a variable and constant region; two major types of light chains exist in humans (kappa and lambda).

Liley graph: graph used to predict severity of HDN during pregnancy by evaluation of the amniotic fluid.

Linkage disequilibrium: occurrence of a set of genes inherited together more often than would be expected by chance.

Linked: when two genes are inherited together by being very close on a chromosome.

Lipids: fatty acids and glycerol compounds.

Look-back: identification of persons who have received seronegative or untested blood from a donor subsequently found to be positive for HIV or HCV.

Lot: unit of blood from one donor and all of its parts or components.

Lymphocytes: mononuclear leukocyte that mediates humoral or cell-mediated immunity.

Major histocompatibility complex: group of genes located on chromosome 6 that determine the expression of the human leukocyte antigen and complement proteins.

Medical directors: designated physicians responsible for the medical and technical policies of the blood bank.

Meiosis: cell division in gametes that results in half the number of chromosomes present in somatic cells.

Membrane attack complex: C5 to C9 proteins of the complement system that mediate cell lysis in the target cell.

Memory B cells: antigen-specific lymphocytes formed after a humoral response; capable of responding to the antigen more quickly and with greater affinity.

Mitosis: cell division in somatic cells that results in the same number of

Mixed field: agglutination pattern where a population of the red blood cells has agglutinated and the remainder of the red blood cells is unagglutinated.

Monoclonal antisera: single clones of B cells that secrete one antibody.

Mononuclear phagocytes: leukocytes that circulate (monocytes) or are fixed (macrophages) that are involved in phagocytosis and antigen presenting.

Multiparous: having multiple pregnancies.

Multiple myeloma: malignant neoplasm of the bone marrow characterized by abnormal proteins in the plasma and urine.

Neutralization: blocking antibody sites and thus causing a negative reaction.

Neutrophil: circulating granulocyte involved in the early immune response.

Non–red blood cell stimulated: immunologic stimulus for antibody production is unrelated to a red blood cell antigen.

Nonsecretor: individual who inherits the genotype *sese* and does not express soluble forms of H antigen in secretions.

Norepinephrine: hormone that increases blood pressure by vasoconstriction.

Nucleotide: phosphate, sugar, and base that constitute the basic monomer of the nucleic acids DNA and RNA.

Null phenotypes: absences of a particular blood group system from the red blood cell membrane.

Obligatory gene: gene that should be inherited from the father to prove paternity.

Occupational Safety and Health Administration: agency responsible for ensuring safe and healthful working conditions.

Oligosaccharide chain: compound formed by a small number of simple carbohydrate molecules.

One-stage enzyme technique: antibody identification technique that requires the addition of the enzyme to the cell and serum mixture.

Open system: collection or exposure to air that would shorten the expiration because of potential bacterial contamination.

Opsonins: substance (antibody or complement protein) that binds to an antigen and enhances its phagocytosis.

Parenterally: by routes other than the digestive tract, including needle-stick and transfusion.

Paroxysmal cold hemoglobinuria: rare autoimmune disorder characterized by hemolysis and hematuria associated with exposure to cold.

Partial D: D antigen that is missing part of its typical antigenic structure.

Passively transfused: when an antibody is transferred to the recipient from the plasma portion of a blood product during transfusion.

Paternity index: chance that the alleged father is the biologic father compared to the chance that an untested man is the father.

Pedigree chart: diagrammatic method of illustrating the inheritance patterns of traits in a family study.

Perinatally: exposure before, during, or after the time of birth.

Phagocytic cells: cells that engulf microorganisms, other cells, and foreign particles; include neutrophils, macrophages, and monocytes.

Phenotype: observable expression of inherited traits.

Phototherapy: treatment of elevated bilirubin or other conditions with light rays.

Plasma cell: antibody-producing B cell that has reached the end of its differentiating pathway.

Platelet concentrates: platelets obtained from a whole blood donation; contains a minimum of 5.5×10^{10} platelets.

Platelets pheresis: platelet-rich product obtained by cytapheresis; contains 3.0×10^{11} platelets.

Polyagglutination: agglutination of red blood cells by most human sera regardless of blood type.

Polyclonal antisera: several different clones of B cells that secrete antibodies.

Polymerase chain reaction: technique for the amplification of a specific targeted DNA sequence.

Polymorphic: genetic system that expresses more than two phenotypes.

Polymorphonuclear neutrophils: another name for neutrophils.

Potency: strength of an antigen-antibody reaction.

Potentiators: reagents added to the serum-cell mixture to enhance antibody uptake during the incubation phase of the IAT.

Preventive maintenance: maintenance that maximizes the duration of the equipment or facility, decreases "downtime," and avoids unnecessary costly repairs.

Prewarming techniques: techniques in which patient serum and test cells are prewarmed separately before combining to prevent reactions of cold antibodies binding at room temperature and activating complement.

Primary immune response: immune response induced by initial exposure to the antigen.

Proficiency testing: surveys performed to ensure that a laboratory's test methods and equipment are working as expected.

Proteolytic enzymes: enzymes that denature certain proteins.

Prozone: excess antibody causing a false negative reaction.

Punnett square: square used to calculate the frequencies of different genotypes and phenotypes among the offspring of a cross.

(*p*) value: probability value; value that provides a confidence limit for a particular event.

Quality assurance: activities providing confidence that all systems influencing the quality of a product are working as expected.

Quality control: testing to determine the accuracy and precision of the equipment, reagents, and procedures.

Rabbit stroma: red blood cell membranes from rabbits used for adsorption of I antigen.

Random man: untested man whose phenotype is unknown; the gene frequency is the same as that of the general population of the same race.

Reaction phase: observation of agglutination at certain temperatures, following incubation, or after the addition of antihuman globulin.

Recalls: manufacturers' removal of products from the market that may compromise the safety of the recipient.

Receptors: molecule on the cell surface that has a high affinity for a particular ligand.

Recessive: gene product expressed only when inherited by both parents.

Recipient: patient receiving the transfusion.

Red blood cell stroma: red blood cell membrane that remains following hemolysis.

Refractoriness: unresponsiveness to platelet transfusions due to HLA- or platelet-specific antibodies or platelet destruction from fever or sepsis.

Refractory: unresponsive to platelet transfusions.

Regulator gene: gene inherited at another locus or chromosome that affects the expression of another gene.

Respiratory distress syndrome: inability to maintain stable pulmonary alveolar structures, caused by low levels of surfactant, lecithin, and other pulmonary lipids in premature infants.

Restriction endonuclease: bacterial enzyme that recognizes and cleaves at specific DNA nucleotide sequences.

Restriction fragment length polymorphism: variation of size of the fragments within a gene, for a given population, produced by restriction enzymes.

Reticulocytosis: increase in the number of reticulocytes in the circulating blood.

Reticuloendothelial system: system of phagocytic cells, associated with the liver, spleen, and lymph nodes, that clear inert particles.

Rh immune globulin: immune serum globulin consisting of anti-D that is given to prevent the formation of anti-D by Rh-negative individuals.

Root-cause analysis: investigation and subsequent identification of the factors that contributed to an error.

Rouleaux: aggregation of red blood cells that may result from the presence of abnormal proteins in the patient; red blood cells appear as stacked coins.

Rule of three: confirming the presence of an antibody by demonstrating three cells that are positive and three that are negative.

Rule out: to eliminate the possibility that an antibody exists in the serum based on its nonreactivity with a particular antigen.

Saline replacement technique: test to distinguish rouleaux and true agglutination.

Sandwich EIA: enzyme-linked immunosorbent assay technique used to determine the presence or quantity of an antigen.

Secondary immune response: immune response induced following a second exposure to the antigen, which activates the memory lymphocytes for a quicker response.

Secretor: individual who inherits *Se* allele and expresses soluble forms of H antigens in secretions.

Segment: sealed piece of integral tubing from the donor unit bag that contains a small aliquot of donor blood; used in the preparation of red blood cell suspensions for crossmatching.

Selected cells: cells chosen from another panel to confirm or eliminate the possibility of an antibody.

Sensitization: binding of antibody or complement components to a red blood cell.

Serotonin: potent vasoconstrictor liberated by platelets.

Serum to cell ratio: ratio of antigen on the red blood cell to antibody in the serum.

Sialic acid: constituents of the sugars attached to proteins on red blood cells that lend a negative charge to the red blood cell membrane.

Specificity: ability of an antibody to distinguish between two antigens.

Standard operating procedures: written procedures to help ensure the complete understanding of a process and achieve consistency in performance from one individual to another.

***Standards for Blood Banks and Transfusion Services*:** publication of the American Association of Blood Banks that outlines the minimal standards of practice in areas relating to transfusion medicine.

Stem cell: cell from which differentiated cells divide.

Stem cell transplant: procedure that uses peripheral blood stem cells in lieu of bone marrow to stimulate the production of blood cells.

Sulfhydryl reagents: reagents that disrupt the disulfide bonds between cysteine amino acid residues in proteins; dithiothreitol, 2-mercaptoethanol, and 2-aminoethylisothiouronium bromide function as sulfhydryl reagents.

Supernatant: fluid above cells or particles following centrifugation.

Suppressor genes: genes that suppress the expression of another gene.

Surrogate markers: disease markers such as antibodies or elevations in enzymes that may be used as indicators for other potential infectious diseases; often used when direct testing is not available.

Syntenic: genetic term referring to genes closely situated on the same chromosome without being linked.

Systolic pressure: contraction of the heart; the first sound heard while taking a blood pressure.

T cytotoxic cells: lymphocytes responsible for the destruction of host cells that have become infected by virus or other intracellular pathogen.

T helper cells: lymphocytes that interact with mononuclear phagocytes to destroy intracellular pathogens and with B cells to signal cell division and antibody production.

T lymphocytes: lymphocytes that mature in the thymus and express specific receptors; involved in cellular immunity.

***Technical Manual*:** publication of the American Association of Blood Banks that provides a reference to current acceptable practices in blood banking.

Thalassemia: inherited disorder causing anemia because of a defective production rate of either alpha- or beta-hemoglobin polypeptide.

Therapeutic apheresis: removal of blood from a patient and retainment of the portion that may be contributing to a pathologic condition; remainder is returned along with a replacement fluid such as colloid or fresh frozen plasma.

Titers: extent to which an antibody may be diluted before it loses its ability to agglutinate with antigen.

Tn-polyagglutinable red blood cells: type of polyagglutination that results from a mutation in the hematopoietic tissue, characterized by mixed field reactions in agglutination testing.

***Trans*:** genes inherited on opposite chromosomes of a homologous pair.

Transferase: class of enzymes that catalyzes the transfer of a chemical group from one molecule to another.

Transfusion reaction: any unfavorable response by a patient to the infusion of blood or blood products.

Two-stage enzyme technique: treatment of the red blood cells with an enzyme before the addition of the serum.

***Ulex europaeus*:** plant lectin with specificity for the H antigen.

Universal donors: group O donors for red blood cell transfusions; these red blood cells may be transfused to any ABO phenotype because the cells lack both A and B antigens.

Universal precautions: policies of treating all body substances as potentially infectious and applying safety measures to reduce possible exposure.

Universal recipients: blood cells from any ABO phenotype; this recipient lacks circulating ABO antibodies in plasma.

Valency: number of epitopes per molecule of immunogen.

Validation: establishing that a specific process consistently produces a product that meets predetermined specifications.

Variable region: amino-terminal portion of immunoglobulins and T cell receptor chains that are highly variable and responsible for the antigenic specificity of these molecules.

Vasoactive amines: products such as histamines released by basophils, mast cells, and platelets that act on the endothelium and smooth muscle of the local vasculature.

Vasodilatation: increase in the diameter of blood vessels.

Waldenström's macroglobulinemia: overproduction of IgM by the clones of a plasma B cell in response to an antigenic signal; increased viscosity of blood is observed.

Weak D: weak form of the D antigen that requires the IAT for its detection.

Wharton's jelly: gelatinous tissue contaminant in cord blood samples that may interfere in immunohematologic tests.

Whole blood: blood collected from a donor before separation into its components.

Zeta potential: electrostatic potential measured between the red blood cell membrane and the slipping plane of the same cell.

Zone of equivalence: maximum agglutination or precipitation; equilibrium between antigen and antibody binding.

INDEX

H

U

V

W

X

Z